Social Determinants of Health

Edited by Pranee Liamputtong

Social Determinants of Health

Edited by Pranee Liamputtong

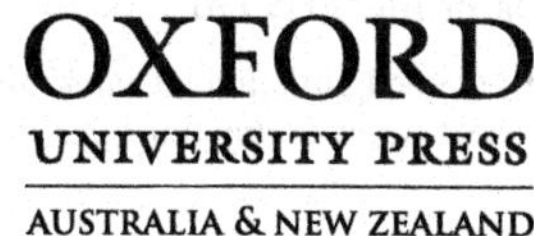
AUSTRALIA & NEW ZEALAND

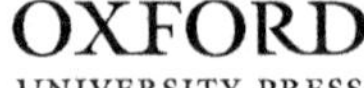

Oxford University Press is a department of the University of Oxford.
It furthers the University's objective of excellence in research,
scholarship, and education by publishing worldwide. Oxford is a registered
trademark of Oxford University Press in the UK and in certain other countries.

Published in Australia by
Oxford University Press
Level 8, 737 Bourke Street, Docklands, Victoria 3008, Australia.

First published 2019
Reprinted 2022(D)

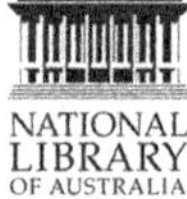

A catalogue record for this
book is available from the
National Library of Australia

ISBN 9780190313524

Edited by Adrienne de Kretser
Cover image credit Shutterstock
Typeset by Newgen KnowledgeWorks Pvt. Ltd., Chennai, India
Proofread by Carol Goudie
Indexed by Mary Russell
Printed and bound in Australia by Ligare Book Printers Pty Ltd

DEDICATION

To my late father Saeng Liamputtong, and my mother Yindee Liamputtong
To my daughters Zoe Sanipreeya Rice and Emma Inturatana Rice

CONTENTS

List of Figures and Tables

Figures

Tables

List of Case Examples

Preface

Not all illnesses are caused by biological and environmental agents. Situated within the new public health perspective, the health, illness and well-being of individual persons, groups and communities are determined by a diverse range of complex individual, social, cultural, environmental and economic factors and healthcare systems. This is known as determinants of health. The health and well-being of individuals is also influenced by a number of social determinants. There are a number of factors, including social, cultural, economic and political, which can impact health. According to the World Health Organization, social determinants of health can be described as 'the circumstances in which people grow, live, work, and age, and the systems put in place to deal with illness. The conditions in which people live or die are, in turn, shaped by political, social and economic forces'. They are also the root cause of health inequities, the unjust and preventable discrepancies in health status that we have witnessed within and between nations. The social determinants approach was chosen because it allows readers to better understand the many factors which impact on the health of people and to appreciate the relationships between these factors.

Social Determinants of Health provides an introduction to some of the important ideas which underlie the field of public health today. Chapters included in the book focus on social, cultural, economic and environmental determinants of health. They portray the ways in which the experience of health is determined by the characteristics of the society in which we live. The conceptual framework is international but the examples and case studies are often (but not exclusively) Australian. This book is intended for students who want to understand the forces which combine to shape the health of individuals, communities and populations. As such, it provides the basis for a career in any of the health sciences where insight into the meaning of health will allow for the development of effective practice and greater sensitivity to the needs of the individuals and the communities.

This book is intended to support the first year of tertiary study of public health. It will be beneficial as a starting point for those students who intend to concentrate on public health as a career and who need a strong foundation of knowledge on which to build. It will be equally useful as an introduction to the field for students who intend to enter other branches of the health sciences, with no further, detailed study of public health. It will also serve as a reference for any interested reader who requires a brief but in-depth introduction to any of the included topics and wishes to understand the nature of health and well-being in modern society.

In an edited volume like this, diversity in conceptualisation and expression style is inevitable but all chapters are linked by a common thread—the social determinants of health. An issue that was identified during the review process was the book's use of 'older' references in the chapters. These 'older' references have been retained as they are seminal works or theoretical pieces that continue to impact how we see and experience the world. We only refer to these pieces when we discuss some original ideas or theoretical perspectives.

Pranee Liamputtong
Sydney
February 2019

About the Editor

Pranee Liamputtong is a medical anthropologist and Professor of Public Health at the School of Science and Health, Western Sydney University. Previously, Pranee held a Personal Chair in Public Health at the School of Psychology and Public Health, College of Science, Health and Engineering, La Trobe University, Melbourne until January 2016. She also previously taught in the School of Sociology and Anthropology and worked as a public health research fellow at the Centre for the Study of Mothers' and Children's Health (now the Judith Lumley Centre), La Trobe University. Pranee has a particular interest in issues related to cultural and social influences on childbearing, childrearing, and women's reproductive and sexual health. She works mainly with refugee and migrant women in Sydney and Melbourne and with women in Asia (mostly in Thailand, Malaysia and Vietnam). She has published several books and a large number of papers in these areas.

Some of her books in the health and social sciences include: *The Journey of Becoming a Mother Amongst Women in Northern Thailand* (Lexington Books, 2007); *Community, Health and Population* (with Sansnee Jirojwong, Oxford University Press, 2009); *Infant Feeding Practices: A Cross-Cultural Perspective* (Springer, 2011); *Motherhood and Postnatal Depression: Narratives of Women and Their Partners* (with Carolyn Westall, Springer, 2011); *Health, Illness and Well-Being: Perspectives and Social Determinants* (with Rebecca Fanany and Glenda Verrinder, Oxford University Press, 2012); *Women, Motherhood and HIV/AIDS: A Cross-Cultural Perspective* (Springer, 2013); *Stigma, Discrimination and HIV/AIDS: A Cross-Cultural Perspective* (Springer, 2013); *Contemporary Socio-Cultural and Political Perspectives in Thailand* (Springer, 2014); *Children, Young People and Living with HIV/AIDS: A Cross-Cultural Perspective* (Springer, 2016); and *Public Health: Local and Global Perspective*s (Cambridge University Press, 2016, 2nd edn 2019).

Pranee is a qualitative researcher and has also published several method books. Her most recent method books include: *Researching the Vulnerable: A Guide to Sensitive Research Methods* (Sage, 2007); *Performing Qualitative Cross-Cultural Research* (Cambridge University Press, 2010); *Focus Group Methodology: Principles and Practice* (Sage 2011, 2016); *Qualitative Research Methods*, 4th edn (Oxford University Press, 2013); *Using Participatory Qualitative Research Methodologies in Health* (with Gina Higginbottom, Sage, 2015); *Research Methods in Health: Foundations for Evidence-Based Practice*, 3rd edn (Oxford University Press, 2017); and *Handbook of Research Methods in Health Social Sciences* (Springer, 2019).

About the Contributors

David Brain is a Health Economist at the Queensland University of Technology. He is committed to finding ways to make improvements to the health of the wider community by critically appraising the way services are delivered within the Australian healthcare system. He has published economic evaluations across a range of clinical disciplines and is actively involved in teaching at the undergraduate level. He has an aversion to waste and the politicisation of healthcare.

Susan Chong is a Lecturer in Public Health at La Trobe University, Melbourne. Susan has a PhD in public health and teaches students undertaking a Bachelor degree in Health Sciences. Her current research interests are in community systems strengthening, HIV and AIDS policy and advocacy, HIV treatment cascade and treatment-seeking behaviour of people living with HIV.

Tinashe Dune is a Clinical Psychologist and Health Sociologist with significant expertise in sexuality, and sexual and reproductive health. Her work focuses on the experiences of marginalised and hidden populations, using mixed methods and participatory action research frameworks. She is well-known for her work on improving diversity and inclusivity in health and education.

Sally Fitzpatrick is a Research Fellow at the Translational Health Research Institute, Western Sydney University, and a team investigator in the Aboriginal Health and Wellbeing Stream of Maridulu Budyari Gumal – The Sydney Partnership for Health, Education, Research and Enterprise (SPHERE). Sally is fifth-generation Australian-born. Her research is focused on the student experience of Aboriginal health and well-being coursework and its impact on practice.

Christopher Fox is a Senior Lecturer in Sexual Health (Sexology) in the Faculty of Medicine and Health at the University of Sydney. He has extensive teaching experience in public health, sociology and psychology. He has consulted on a number of research projects on gender, health and sexuality, and liaised with community organisations on development and evaluation, management, policy and public health/health promotion.

Deborah Gleeson is a Senior Lecturer in Public Health at La Trobe University, Melbourne. She has a Master of Public Health and a PhD in health policy. Deborah teaches subjects in the Bachelor of Health Sciences, Master of Public Health and Master of Health Administration disciplines. Her research focuses on national and international health, and public health policy issues, particularly the impact of international trade agreements on public health and access to medicines.

Emma George is a Lecturer in Health and Physical Education at Western Sydney University. Emma teaches across a range of Health Science subjects, with a focus on physical activity, nutrition, health promotion and evidence-based research methodology. Emma's research expertise includes men's health, intervention design, implementation and evaluation, mixed methods research, and community engagement.

Liz Hanna holds an honorary position as Senior Research Fellow at the Australian National University, Canberra, where she supervises PhD candidates researching climate change and human health. She has a background in Intensive Care nursing, and has a Master of Public Health and a PhD in which she examined exposures, risk avoidance behaviours and health sector preparedness to respond. Liz chairs the Environmental Health Working Group of the World Federation of Public Health Associations.

Peter Higgs has a background in community development and has worked with marginalised populations for over 25 years in Melbourne, Sydney, Vietnam, Indonesia and China. His field-based social research has been focused on working with people who inject drugs. His current research interests involve working with cohorts of people who inject drugs including older people, ethnic Vietnamese and people living with hepatitis C.

Somsri Kitisriworapan was an Associate Professor at Kasetsart University Demonstration School, Thailand. Somsri taught social science, history and Thai language at both primary and secondary levels at the Demonstration School as well as in the Faculty of Education of Kasetsart University. Her main interest is in the health and psychology of children and her research has involved children's understanding of social and health issues. She retired in 2018 but continues to be involved in some academic works.

Elizabeth Martin is a maternity services researcher with expertise in economic evaluation and an extensive professional background in the Australian healthcare system. She has experience in health promotion and communicable disease program and policy development, implementation and evaluation. She has worked with rural and urban Aboriginal and Torres Strait Islander communities. Elizabeth currently teaches undergraduate and post-graduate students in health policy, healthcare systems and cost-effectiveness analysis at the Queensland University of Technology.

Freya MacMillan is a Lecturer in Health Science at Western Sydney University, where she teaches in Health Promotion and Interprofessional Health Science. Her research focuses on the development and evaluation of life-style interventions for the prevention and management of diabetes in those most at risk. Particularly relevant to this chapter, she has expertise in working with community to develop appropriate and appealing community-based interventions.

Kate McBride is a Lecturer in Population Health in the School of Medicine, Western Sydney University. Kate teaches population health, basic and intermediate epidemiology and evidence-based medicine to undergraduate and postgraduate students. Kate's research expertise is in epidemiology, public health and the use of mixed methods to improve health at a population level through the prevention and reduction of chronic and non-communicable disease prevalence.

Debra Miles is an Associate Professor in Social Work at James Cook University, Townsville, Australia. Her teaching foci include human rights and social work practice, feminist social work and women's studies. Her research areas of interest include working with women and children, Aboriginal and Torres Strait Islander issues and international social work education.

Yvonne Parry is a Senior Lecturer at Flinders University, Adelaide. She uses mixed methods to research the area of health access and the influence of the broader determinants of health on health supply and access. She actively promotes the inclusion of consumer experiences in the development and assessment of health access and service provision. She is acknowledged internationally for the translation of her research findings into evidence-based knowledge for student learning and expanded student placement experiences.

Linda Portsmouth is a Senior Lecturer in Health Promotion in the School of Public Health at Curtin University, Perth. Her lecturing and research interests include the social determinants of health, behaviour change communication, health communication media development, social marketing, and health promotion with Aboriginal and Torres Strait Islander peoples.

Lisa Jackson Pulver AM is an Aboriginal woman with family connections from her mother to northern New South Wales, and through her father to Wiradjuri people in south-western New South Wales and to the Jacksons and Campbells in southern South Australia and western Victoria. She is Deputy Vice-Chancellor, Indigenous Strategy and Service at the University of Sydney and is a Co-founder and inaugural Research Lead of *Maridulu Budyari Gumal*—The Sydney Partnership for Health, Education, Research and Enterprise's Aboriginal Health and Wellbeing Stream. She remains an active researcher, educator and advisor.

Genevieve Steiner is a multi-award winning NHMRC-ARC Dementia Research Development Fellow at NICM, Western Sydney University. Gen uses functional neuroimaging and physiological research methods to investigate the biological bases of learning and memory processes that will inform the prevention, diagnosis and treatment of cognitive decline in older age. She also conducts many clinical trials including herbal and life-style medicines that may reduce the risk of dementia.

Dusanee Suwankhong is a Lecturer in Public Health at Thaksin University, Thailand. She obtained her PhD from La Trobe University, Melbourne. She has conducted many research projects, in collaboration with Pranee Liamputtong, in Thailand. Her research interests include traditional medicines, breast cancer, HIV/AIDS, motherhood, school-age children, and Thai kick-boxing. She has published many papers in these areas.

Megan Williams is Head of the Indigenous Health Discipline at the Graduate School of Health, University of Technology Sydney, and a Wiradjuri descendant through her father's family. She has over 20 years' experience combining health service delivery, evaluation and research, particularly at the nexus of justice and health. She contributes to research on the health and well-being of Aboriginal young people, including in residential rehabilitation and through program evaluations using the Ngaa-bi-nya Aboriginal framework.

Eileen Willis is Emeritus Professor at the College of Nursing and Health Sciences, Flinders University, Adelaide. Her research interests are in Indigenous health and in the impact of health reform on the work of health professionals. She is a member of the European consortium on rationed nursing care and has published widely on the topic. Her most recent publication is *Understanding the Australian Healthcare System* (Elsevier, 2015, with Reynolds and Keleher).

Cassandra Wright has a background in health promotion and public health and has experience in conducting both qualitative and quantitative research, with a focus on program evaluation. Her PhD was focused on using new media and technology in health promotion. Her primary research interest is health promotion in both local and international contexts, with a specific interest in diverse and disadvantaged populations.

About the Book

This book comprises 14 chapters, separated into Part I, Social Determinants of Health and Conceptual Frameworks; and Part II, Social Determinants of Health and Applications. **Chapter 1** is an introduction to the issues, written by Pranee Liamputtong. It focuses on the concepts of health, illness, well-being and determinants of health. Discussions on how individuals understand health, illness and well-being are provided. Health determinants include biological, behavioural, environmental, social, cultural and economic factors. The author points out that these determinants do not operate in their own space but intersect to produce health and illness in individuals and populations.

Part I of the book comprises six chapters which discuss the conceptual frameworks relating to the social determinants of health. Health as a social construct is discussed in **Chapter 2** by Cassandra Wright and Peter Higgs. This chapter focuses on the social model of health. The authors suggest that western societies commonly focus on biological aspects of health and illness; this is known as the biomedical model. In response to growing evidence of the deficiencies of this model in explaining patterns of disease and inequitable susceptibility, alternative models of understanding health have emerged, which encompass a broader range of influences such as individual psychological factors, behaviour, family factors, social factors, environmental factors, economic factors and political factors. The chapter also examines the debate regarding agency and structure. The last section of the chapter discusses the sociological imagination, a term that means thinking about the social factors which shape an issue including historical, cultural, structural and critical factors.

Culture as a social determinant of health is discussed in **Chapter 3** by Pranee Liamputtong and Dusanee Suwankhong. The authors suggest that all human beings have to deal with good health, illness, disease, sickness and death. In all human groups, there exists a set of beliefs about the nature of health and illness, its cause and cures, and its relations to other aspects of life. They are conditions which shape an aspect of social experience and cultural knowledge. As such, concepts of health, illness and well-being are likely to reflect a marked cultural influence. What is seen as health or illness in one location, or by the members of one group, is not always perceived the same way in another. Culture not only influences how individual health consumers perceive health conditions and appropriate treatments, but also the healthcare providers' perspectives. Cultural differences between the healthcare providers and their patients can lead to cross-cultural misunderstandings and conflicts which ultimately impact on the quality of healthcare provision. This chapter brings readers through several important issues relevant to culture and health. In the first part, it discusses the concepts of culture, the relevance of culture and health, illness and well-being, the explanatory model of illness (EM), culture-bound and culture-reactive syndromes, and cultural idiom of distress. The chapter then looks at the folk healing system and religion, health and healing. The last part focuses on cultural competence and its relevance to healthcare.

Chapter 4 introduces deviance, discrimination and stigma as social determinants of health. Pranee Liamputtong and Somsri Kitisriworapan discuss health issues and behaviour that are seen as 'difference'. The main focus is on deviance, difference, stigma and discrimination. The chapter first introduces notions of deviance, difference and stigma, then discusses the impact of deviance and stigma on the health and well-being of those who are stigmatised. It also discusses stigma and HIV/ AIDS, and what has been done to combat HIV-related stigma as a case example. It suggests that stigma is associated with stereotyping and prejudice. It is employed by individuals to define certain attributes of others as unworthy; as such, these people are seen as 'tainted'. Stigma is socially constructed and is attributable to cultural, social, historical and situational factors. Stigmatised individuals are subject to feelings of shame and guilt. A major consequence of stigmatisation is discrimination, which occurs when an individual is treated unfairly and unjustly due to the perception that the individual is deviant from others. Many health issues such as HIV and AIDS are perceived as deviance. Individuals living with HIV/AIDS are socially constructed as the 'other'. The chapter also points out that health and illness conditions which tend to produce stigma are those that are connected with negative characteristics, have uncertain or unknown causes and limited treatment, and produce intense reactions such as fear and disgust. Individually, the effects of stigma and social exclusion can be destructive. They can result in isolation, low self-esteem, depression, self-harm, poor academic achievement and social relationships, and poor physical and mental health. The impact of stigma on the public health of the stigmatised individuals and groups is huge. In the area of HIV/AIDS, for example, it is now clear that the stigmatisation of certain groups such as sex workers, injecting drug users, and gay men would only make them more susceptible to HIV infection and push them out of reach of those who attempt to help them modify the behaviours that put them and others at risk.

Health and social justice are discussed by Debra Miles in **Chapter 5**. In 2005, the World Health Organization (WHO) established the Commission on Social Determinants of Health, which released its report in 2008. Charged with the responsibility of developing a pathway to global health equity, the Commission clearly and unequivocally pointed to social justice as an essential element that allows people to live healthy lives uninhibited by illness and premature death. This chapter explores the relevance and usefulness of human rights-based approaches in guiding action to address health inequities and to improve the underlying social determinants of health. A conceptual framework informed by human rights principles offers sustainable opportunities to create positive change and develop successful local and global initiatives that improve social determinants of health, well-being and equity. This chapter discusses the nature of social justice and human rights concepts as they are relevant to understanding and influencing social determinants of health. Later sections highlight direct links between human rights violations, social injustice and health disparities, and explore the possibilities offered by policy approaches informed by human rights.

Kate McBride, Freya MacMillan, Emma George and Genevieve Steiner introduce health promotion and social determinants of health in **Chapter 6**. Health promotion refers to 'the process of enabling people to increase control over, and to improve, their health, moving beyond a focus on individual behaviour towards a wide range of social and environmental interventions' (World Health Organization 2005). In this chapter, the authors discuss the basic principles of health promotion and theoretical models underpinning health promotion approaches, before examining the five Ottawa Charter for Health priority action areas. These five areas—developing personal skills, strengthening community action, creating supportive environments, re-orienting healthcare services towards prevention of illness and promotion of health, and building healthy public policy—are explored using obesity as a focus.

In **Chapter 7**, the economic determinants of health and disease are discussed by Elizabeth Martin and David Brain. The authors argue that as the focus of economics is on the welfare of society, there is an inextricable link between the social and economic determinants of health. They define economics and challenge the notion that economic growth is the solution to addressing the social determinants of health. They also examine how economists have contributed to identifying the economic determinants of health, and where changes need to be made in society to improve health outcomes. The chapter ends with a focus on the economic determinants of gender-based health inequality, and the close relationship between social and economic factors in forming the health outcomes of women.

Part II comprises seven chapters that focus more on the application of social determinants of health. In **Chapter 8**, social determinants of Australia's First Peoples' health are discussed by Lisa Jackson Pulver, Megan Williams and Sally Fitzpatrick. The authors contend that contemporary western understandings of social determinants of health need to be expanded and extended to more fully reflect the experiences of Aboriginal and Torres Strait Islander people, Australia's First Peoples. This chapter explores three different yet interrelated sets of factors implicated in the health and well-being of Australia's First Peoples: cultural, historical and structural determinants. It explores First Peoples' experience of determinants, and presents examples of strengths-based, community-led services, programs and research. It then extends our understanding of determinants using a socio-ecological model of health that incorporates multi-level empowerment, with a particular focus on social support and the centrality of the value of relatedness. This provides a scaffold for discussion about how all health and social care providers can develop confidence in engaging with and providing support to First Peoples' families and communities, and be a good partner within and through their practice.

Tinashe Dune and Pranee Liamputtong discuss gender, sexuality and social determinants of health in **Chapter 9**. This chapter brings readers through several important issues relevant to gender and sexuality. They suggest that every society attaches expectations to gender. This expectation is the result of a series of socio-cultural constructs assumed to be natural characteristics of masculinity or femininity. Constructions of gender are also linked to constructions of sexuality, with women being perceived as lesser and opposite to men, thus making them 'natural' sexual partners. But sexuality goes far beyond biological sex, intercourse or procreation processes, as exemplified by the diversity that exists across these, and many more, aspects of gender and sexuality. Importantly, societal constructions of gender and sexuality often restrict or penalise experiences and manifestations of gender or sexuality that diverge from what is expected. Clearly, gender and sexuality are key social determinants of health that determine the ways in which a society defines and therefore perceives and treats a person across their life-span. The chapter discusses gender and sexuality as well as acknowledging the range of diversity within these concepts and their impacts on health and well-being. It also discusses the role of gender and sexuality through a case example which explores social constructions related to health outcomes.

In **Chapter 10**, Christopher Fox introduces the concept of life-course determinants to health. He suggests that this is one of the social determinants that is often forgotten. Life-course determinants can account for some of the chronic disease experienced in later life. Often, people are placed in a position to take responsibility for the causes of chronic disease. With a life-course approach, we can see that the 'causes' are not always a result of the individual but a function of experiences earlier in life. Readers are introduced to ideas of how experiences in the womb and from birth can have a major impact much later in life. The chapter discusses key concepts and ideas that underpin life-course determinants and shows how to apply the ideas in practice. The chapter includes a life-mapping process to explore the impacts of the reader's life on their health in later adulthood.

Chapter 11, written by Liz Hanna, is about health and the living environment. This chapter provides an understanding of the deep relationship between humanity and the planet upon which we evolved, flourished and developed successful, complex human societies. It explores how the social determinants of health are intricately linked with environmental health determinants. In keeping with the UN Sustainable Development Goals, the chapter takes a global planetary view of the environment as this determines global health—wherever we live. It ends with strategies for the health sector to minimise health harm and boost resilience among the most vulnerable communities.

In **Chapter 12**, Linda Portsmouth suggests that mass media is a social determinant of health. It is one of the many features of a society that impacts on people's knowledge, attitudes and beliefs about health—and thus on their health behaviours. The mass media that people are exposed to, and interact with, has had a measurable impact on their health choices and outcomes. Many people gain much of their understanding of health from what they see and hear on television, the internet, radio, newspapers and magazines. Mass media is pervasive and persuasive, reaching population-wide with health information in a way that promotes and normalises the health concepts portrayed. Mass media plays a role in the socialisation of children and adolescents, influencing them as to what to expect and what is expected of them in their society. News and current affairs, entertainment, the internet—and the advertising that pays for most of it—often contain messages of significance to public health. Public health professionals seek to explore the impact of mass media—aiming to describe, quantify and counter any negative influence on population health. The chapter also studies the effective techniques utilised by media professionals and how to work in partnership with media professionals. This enables public health professionals to successfully communicate health messages via the mass media in a way that promotes population health. They seek to influence news and current affairs content to increase people's awareness of health issues, often advocating for a change in policy or legislation. They also seek to influence existing entertainment and develop entertainment-education media, and have successfully developed advertising (among other social marketing activities) to promote health. Working closely with members of population groups at risk allows health professionals to develop concepts, messages and media materials that will communicate most effectively with that particular group.

Chapter 13, written by Yvonne Parry and Eileen Willis, discusses social determinants and the healthcare system. It suggests that social factors are major determinants of health for individuals and populations. In order to demonstrate how a nation's healthcare system can be understood as a social determinant of health, the chapter draws on the World Health Organization's Commission on Social Determinants of Health (CSDH) framework. The first section of the chapter summarises the CSDH argument that the healthcare system is a determinant of health that impacts on availability and access to health services. Second, it describes the Australian healthcare system, specifically Medicare. It then identifies features of the Australian healthcare system that are positive social determinants of health, and those features that contribute to and maintain inequalities in health. The final section provides examples of public policy that might contribute to good health outcomes.

In the last chapter, **Chapter 14**, Deborah Gleeson and Susan Chong discuss social determinants of health from a global perspective. The chapter explores the global distribution of health and disease and the influence of social determinants of health on these patterns. It examines the global burden of both infectious and non-communicable diseases, focusing on differences between developing and developed countries. It also discusses the role of global economic, political and health system factors in shaping global health inequities, and concludes by examining current action to address the social determinants at the global level.

Acknowledgments

In bringing this book to life, I owe gratitude to many people. I thank Debra James, the Higher Education Publishing Manager for Oxford University Press, who believed in the value of this book, contracted me to edit it, and provided ongoing support throughout my journey. I am grateful to all contributors who worked hard to make this book possible. I also thank Dr Mofi Islam, who saw the value of this book for his undergraduate teaching and provided suggestions about the content that students will find valuable.

The idea for the book came from my previous text, *Health, Illness and Well-Being: Perspectives and Social Determinants*, which was co-edited by Rebecca Fanany and Glenda Verrinder and published by Oxford University Press in 2012. In *Social Determinants of Health*, the new text, Chapter 1 contains sections published from the previous book for which I was the main writer. It has been updated with new content and references to suit students and lecturers who are currently studying and researching in the fields of social determinants, sociology of health, primary health and public health. I would like to thank Rebecca Fanany and Glenda Verrinder for their work as co-editors of the previous text.

I dedicate the book to my parents, who brought their children up amid poverty in Thailand. They believed that only education would improve the lives of their children and hence worked hard to send us to school. I have made my career thus far because of their beliefs and the opportunity that they provided for me. I thank them profoundly. I also dedicate this book to my two daughters, who have been part of my life, and thank them for understanding the ongoing busy life of their mother.

Pranee Liamputtong
Sydney
February 2019

Chapter 1

Health, Illness and Well-being: An Introduction to Social Determinants of Health

Pranee Liamputtong

Topics covered

This chapter covers the following topics:

- an introduction to health, illness, well-being and disease
- determinants of health
- biological determinants
- environmental determinants
- social determinants of health
- gender, ethnicity and social class
- health inequality and social justice
- the social gradient

Key terms

behavioural determinants
biological determinants
determinants of health
disease
environmental determinants
ethnicity
gender
health
health inequality
illness
individual determinants
sex
sickness
social class
social determinants
social gradient in health
social justice
well-being

Introduction

Health
There is no definite meaning of health. Its meaning can be different depending on individuals, social groups and cultures, and can differ at different times. However, the World Health Organization (1978, p. 2) defines health as 'a state of complete physical, mental and social well-being and not merely the absence of disease or infirmity'.

The concept of **health** has different meanings to different people (Jirojwong & Liamputtong 2009; Wiley & Allen 2017). Each individual perceives and experiences health, illness and well-being differently from others (Jones & Creedy 2012; see also Chapter 2 in this volume). Some individuals see health as a general sense of well-being such as 'feeling good' (Winkelman 2009, p. 14). Health may mean being active and fit for some people. For others, health means having a balance in their lives, being productive or able to fulfil their responsibilities (Levin & Browner 2005; Taylor 2008; Jirojwong & Liamputtong 2009; Blaxter 2010; AIHW 2018). Additionally, members of different cultural groups may see health, illness and well-being differently (Winkelman 2009; see also Chapter 3).

In Australia, the notion that health is of primary importance is pervasive. This is reflected in the fact that health and illness are featured in all kinds of media. Often, there are reports or stories about health issues, health-related behaviours and experiences, the importance of fitness and health, new medical and scientific discoveries, healthcare services and government policies (Taylor 2008; Germov & Freij 2019; see also Chapter 13).

There are many things that can determine our health, illness and well-being. These range from societal influences to individual aspects such as genetic makeup as well as the healthcare to which we have access. These are referred to as the 'determinants of health' since they 'influence how likely we are to stay healthy or to become ill or injured' (AIHW 2016, p. 128; see section below on determinants of health and Chapters 2, 13 & 14). According to the Australian Institute of Health and Welfare (AIHW) (2016, p. 3), the health, illness and well-being of an individual comprise many aspects that 'result from complex interplay between biological, lifestyle, socio-economic, societal and environmental factors'.

I will take you through several important concepts. First, I introduce the meaning of health, illness, well-being and disease, followed by the determinants of health. Then I discuss relationships between health determinants, in particular the intersection of gender, ethnicity and social class. Last, I provide the social gradient in health and health inequalities.

Conceptualising health

According to Keleher and MacDougall (2016a), it is impossible to find a universal definition of health which can be applied to all individuals, locations and time. As health embraces many aspects, it is tricky to say exactly what health means. The meanings of health are 'dependent on the context in which the term is used and the people who use it' (Keleher & MacDougall 2016a, p. 4). The concept of health can change over time, and it differs between individuals, families, social groups and **cultures** (Jones & Creedy 2012). Hence, health is 'socially and culturally constructed' (Taylor 2008, p. 5; Turnock 2016; see Chapter 2). The Australian Institute of Health

Culture
A system of shared ideas, attitudes and practices that defines the social system of its members.

and Welfare (2010, p. 3) defines health as an essential component of well-being. It is about how we 'feel and function'. Health is not simply about the non-existence of injury or illness, but there are degrees of wellness and health. Health is situated within broad social and cultural contexts (Baum 2016). The state of health of individuals in a society contributes to the social and economic well-being of that particular society. The following quotes suggest that health is defined differently depending on the contexts within which the definition is located.

> Health is a social, economic and political issue and above all a fundamental human right. Inequality, poverty, exploitation, violence and injustice are at the root of ill-health and the deaths of poor and marginalised people (People's Health Movement 2011, p. 2).

> Health is not merely the absence of disease or distress; it is also a positive state of physical, emotional, mental, personal, and spiritual well-being and a balance with nature and the social world (Winkelman 2009, p. 18).

> Health is a personal and social state of balance and well-being in which a woman feels strong, active, creative, wise and worthwhile: where her body's vital power of functioning and healing is intact; where her diverse capacities and rhythms are valued; where she may decide and choose, express herself and move about freely (CHETNA 2011).

Keleher and MacDougall (2016a, pp. 5–6) outline different perspectives which can be used to conceptualise health. Several perspectives are relevant to this textbook (see Chapter 2). The lay or cultural perspective suggests that health is understood and interpreted differently by individuals depending on their experiences, life situations and cultural backgrounds. The biological perspective examines the role of genes and risk factors as well as their interactions with other health determinants (discussed later in this chapter). Closely related to the biological approach is the biomedical perspective. Within this approach, health and illness are perceived in terms of a person's medically defined pathology.

The behavioural perspective advocates that superior quality of life results from having good health, which is founded on risk factors and life-style behaviours. Health education is often the response to improving these determinants. The health promotion approach includes all of these perspectives and, in addition, pays attention to the powerful impact of a 'place' or location in determining health. Hence, we see projects such as 'Healthy Schools', 'Healthy Workplace' and 'Healthy Cities' (Baum 2016, p. 13; see Chapter 6). Research suggests that disadvantaged individuals such as poor people may have poorer health because they reside in places which are health-damaging (Baum 2016; Ratcliff 2017; AIHW 2018). The influence of location on health can be clearly seen in remote Indigenous communities in Australia and other parts of the world where important health facilities such as healthy food supply, clean water, good sewerage system, suitable accommodation and access to healthcare are insufficient or absent (Baum 2016; AIHW 2018). This also applies to poor people living in slums in many parts of the globe (Corburn & Riley 2016).

The Ottawa Charter for Health Promotion (WHO 1986) is considered the formal beginning of the new public health, which focuses on the social causes of illness and disease, health equity and social justice (Baum 2016; see Chapter 6). It suggests that social inequalities and health are situated within complex connections between social, economic, political and environmental determinants. As such, health is perceived as a 'complex outcome' which is influenced by factors including genetic, environmental, economic, social and political circumstances (Baum 2016, p. 17; Turnock 2016).

Disease, illness, health and well-being

Disease
A condition adversely affecting health that has measurable (clinical) symptoms.

Illness
A condition adversely affecting health as perceived by the individual in question.

Sickness
The term is often used interchangeably with disease and illness; sometimes it refers to both. Sickness embodies a sociological meaning and is related to the concept of the 'sick role' theorised by Talcott Parsons.

Three main terms tend to be used to describe an individual's experiences of ill symptoms—'disease', 'illness' and 'sickness'. The term **disease** refers to 'medically defined pathology' (Blaxter 2004, p. 20). It is a malfunctioning of biological mechanisms (Jirojwong & Liamputtong 2009; Brown & Closser 2016; Wiley & Allen 2017). The term disease incorporates 'a set of signs and symptoms and medically diagnosed pathological abnormalities' (Baum 2016, p. 4). On the other hand, **illness** involves the subjective experience of ill health (symptoms and suffering) of an individual (Taylor 2008; Blaxter 2010; Baum 2016; Brown & Closser 2016; Wiley & Allen 2017). Individuals feel that 'something is not right with their health' (Jones & Creedy 2012, p. 4). Primarily, it is about how a person lives through the disease. Often, it involves personal, social and cultural reactions to a disease (Baum 2016; Brown & Closser 2016). Illnesses can disrupt people's lives, which may lead individuals to seek medical care and encourage behavioural changes so that the discomfort can be alleviated (Wiley & Allen 2017). An ailing person may have to rely on others for their basic needs in daily living (Spector 2017). Additionally, the subjective experience of illness is influenced by cultural contexts: 'There are culturally specific and culturally appropriate ways of being ill and expressing that experience' (Wiley & Allen 2017, p. 16; see also Chapter 3).

Sickness is often used interchangeably with disease and illness and sometimes it refers to both. It, however, embodies a sociological meaning (Wiley & Allen 2017). Sickness is related to the concept of the 'sick role' theorised by Talcott Parsons (1951, 1979). According to Parsons, a sick person must fulfil 'a socially recognised set of expectations'. To be able to embrace the sick role, an individual must have a disease which is perceived as credible by the social group. The individual must also seek help in order to restore their health. The individual will be exempted from normal responsibilities including work, household chores or other duties which are expected of well persons (Wiley & Allen 2017).

Health, when situated within a biomedical framework of biological determinants, can be seen as 'the absence of disease or pathology' in a person (Taylor 2008, p. 10). It suggests that if the person does not have a disease, they are healthy. Taylor (2008, p. 10) contends that this view implies two main assumptions. First, there are two opposite states of being—an individual is either healthy or ill. Within this view, health and illness are seen as uniform and permanent concepts. Second, it implies that having good health is the norm and being ill is deviant. Thus, illness connotes 'abnormality, deficiency or impairment' (Scambler 2003; Blaxter 2010). As Blaxter (2004, p. 7) contends, 'the objective observation of a lack of "normality" meets a very ancient and universal tendency to see the sick person as in some way morally tainted or bewitched. Possibly, they are responsible for their own condition' (see also Chapter 4).

The concept of health as the absence of disease has been perceived as being 'too narrow' (Taylor 2008, p. 11). Health should be seen as a more credible and holistic condition (Levin & Browner 2005; Taylor 2008; Blaxter 2010; Wiley & Allen 2017). This is reflected in the definition of health proposed by the WHO (1948, p. 2), which advocates that health is a 'a state of complete physical, mental and social well-being and not merely the absence of disease or infirmity'. This definition suggests that it is not only the biological functioning of individuals that determines the state of their health, but also their social and psychological conditions. These components do not function separately but interact with each other in complicated processes (Taylor 2008; Wiley & Allen 2017; discussed further in next section).

This view of health is reflected in the mental health area. There has been an attempt to define mental health in a way that moves beyond the focus on biological factors (Baum 2016). The Victorian Health Promotion Foundation's initial mental health promotion plan included the following positive definition: 'Mental health is the embodiment of social, emotional and spiritual well-being. Mental health provides individuals with the vitality necessary for active living, to achieve goals and to interact with one another in ways that are respectful and just' (VicHealth 1999, p. 4; see also VicHealth 2015).

The WHO definition of health incorporates the concept of **well-being**. This concept is seen as more expansive than that of health because it signifies an individual's sense of general contentment with life (Taylor 2008; Heil 2014; Wiley & Allen 2017). Well-being, Heil (2014, p. 41) suggests, refers to 'satisfactory states of being' that focus on 'positive connotations'. It underscores the 'subjective and experiential state of being in the world'. Well-being is used in a subjective sense in that there is nothing wrong, and can be completely separated from the objectively measured health or disease status of an individual (Heil 2014). People may possess a sense of personal well-being even when they are in very deprived situations; for example, during stressful life events or when confronted with acute or chronic disease (Wiley & Allen 2017). In a way, it could be said that well-being symbolises the opposite of illness (Jones & Creedy 2012). A sense of well-being in one society may be seen differently in another. For example, possessing a considerable expanse of body fat might be perceived as 'overweight' and requiring medical treatment in one society, but seen as a sign of excellent health in another (Wiley & Allen 2017, p. 15).

Well-being
A positive conceptualisation of health: feeling healthy, happy or doing well in life. It can be completely separated from the objectively measured health or disease status of an individual.

Case Example 1.1

Sophie

Sophie is a 78-year-old woman who has experienced a range of symptoms in the last few years. She suffers from severe tinnitus (ringing sounds) in both ears, and hearing loss in one ear. She has high blood pressure, which is being controlled by prescribed medication. Although she is slower with everyday activities and often has body aches and pains, she still eats and sleeps well. She is poor but she has good support from her children. She thinks what she has been experiencing is part of growing old. She does not think she is ill.

- What do you think about Sophie's idea of her health?
- In your view, should Sophie's conditions be categorised as illness? Discuss.

Stop and Think

- What does health mean to you?
- What does illness mean to you?
- What does well-being mean to you?
- How do you know if someone is healthy or not?

Determinants of health

Situated within the new public health perspective, the health, illness and well-being of individual persons, groups and communities are determined by a diverse range of complex individual, social, cultural, environmental and economic factors and healthcare systems (AIHW 2016; Germov 2019; Hallet et al. 2019; Liamputtong 2019). This is referred to as determinants of health (Wilkinson & Marmot 2003; Marmot & Wilkinson 2006; Keleher & MacDougall 2016b; Oldroyd 2019). Conceptually, the focus of this perspective is on factors which could influence and determine the health of people, instead of on the state and outcomes of their health. It also underscores the prevention of ill health, rather than the measurement of illness (Taylor 2008; Keleher & MacDougall 2016b; Oldroyd 2019).

Determinants of health
A range of individual, social, economic, environmental and cultural conditions that have the potential to contribute to or detract from the health of individuals, communities or whole populations.

The **determinants of health** are characteristics or factors which can bring about a change in the health and illness of individuals and populations, for the better or worse (Keleher & MacDougall 2016b; AIHW 2018; Oldroyd 2019). Determinants of health include biological and genetic factors; health behaviours (such as risky life-styles, abuse of alcohol and cigarette smoking); socio-cultural and socio-economic factors (such as gender, ethnicity, education, income and occupation); and environment factors (including housing, social support, social connection, geographical position and climate) (see Chapters 2, 7, 9, 10, 11, 13 & 14). Resources and systems also have effects on the health and well-being of individuals and populations. These include access to health services, healthcare policy and the healthcare system (AIHW 2016; Sendall 2019; see Chapter 13).

Essentially, these determinants are connected with conditions, which can either improve or hinder individuals' possibilities of having and sustaining good health. Some conditions have a direct impact on the health and illness of individuals; for example, direct contact with heat or asbestos in their environment, cigarette smoking or lack of physical activities. Other conditions have an indirect impact on individuals. They can increase or reduce the influences of other factors, for example, when individuals are poor and cannot access suitable healthcare (Oldroyd 2019). These conditions can interact and function in complex ways. For instance, when people do not have good health, they may not be able to participate in employment or physical activities. This in turn will have further impact on their health (Oldroyd 2019).

According to the Australian Institute of Health and Welfare (AIHW) (2010, p. 64), health determinants can be perceived as a 'web of causes'. They can also be described as part of broad causal 'pathways' which can influence health. Figure 1.1 presents a conceptual framework which shows the complex relationships of health determinants. The determinants are divided into four main categories. The direction of influence moves from left to right; that is, from the 'upstream' factors (such as culture, resources and affluence) to more 'downstream' or direct influences (such as body weight and blood pressure). The figure illustrates how one broad category (the broad features of society and environmental factors) can determine the nature of another main group (individuals' socio-economic characteristics, such as their level of education and employment). Both these broad categories in turn have impact on individuals' health behaviours, their psychological state and safety. These can then affect biomedical components, such as body weight and blood pressure, which have further health effects through different pathways. Along the different paths and states, these various factors interact with the genetic composition of the individuals. It should be noted that the direction of these influences can occur in reverse. For instance, an individual's health can have an impact on their levels of physical activity, employment status and wealth.

Health-promoting conditions can be divided into four main categories from the upstream factors such as ecosystem viability, equitable public policies and convivial communities, through to health-promoting mediating structures, for example caring relationships and service to others, through to health life-styles such as town planning to promote physical fitness and on to community-managed health services. It is argued that equitable public policies, for example, do much to promote healthy life-style choices (see Chapter 6).

Figure 1.1 Determinants of health

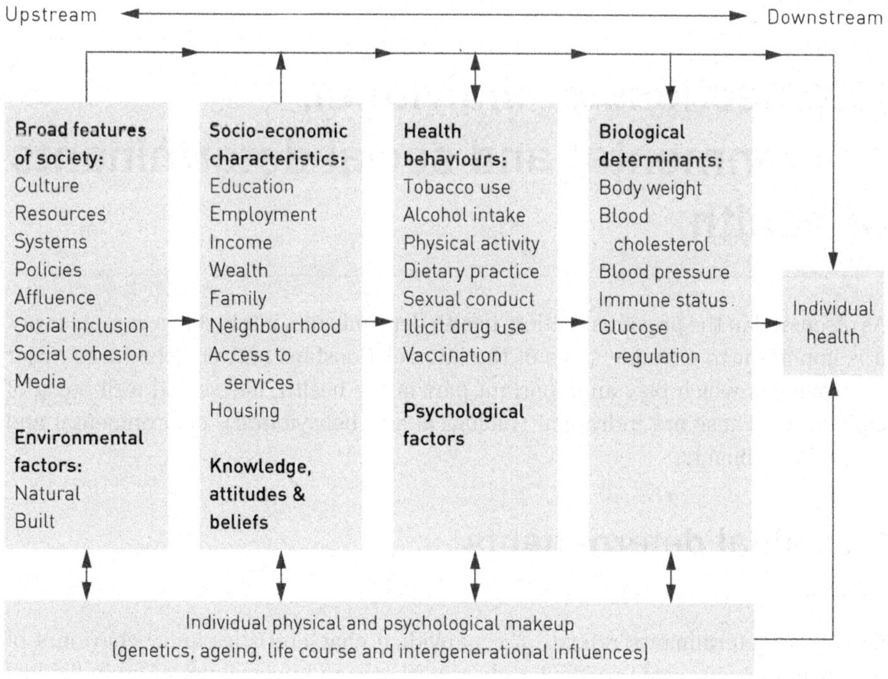

Upstream ⟷ Downstream

Broad features of society:
Culture
Resources
Systems
Policies
Affluence
Social inclusion
Social cohesion
Media

Environmental factors:
Natural
Built

Socio-economic characteristics:
Education
Employment
Income
Wealth
Family
Neighbourhood
Access to services
Housing

Knowledge, attitudes & beliefs

Health behaviours:
Tobacco use
Alcohol intake
Physical activity
Dietary practice
Sexual conduct
Illicit drug use
Vaccination

Psychological factors

Biological determinants:
Body weight
Blood cholesterol
Blood pressure
Immune status
Glucose regulation

Individual health

Individual physical and psychological makeup
(genetics, ageing, life course and intergenerational influences)

Adapted from AIHW (2010, p. 64); see also AIHW (2018, p. 6)

Case Example 1.2

Samantha

Samantha, a three-year-old child, was born into a poor family and lived in a remote part of the country. One day, while running in the street with her older brother, she was pierced by a sharp bamboo stick that was discarded on the ground. Her mother bandaged the wound. Several days later, the wound became infected. Samantha began to feel pain in her groin and had fever. Her mother tried to manage Samantha's pain and fever with whatever she had at hand. However, Samantha became very unwell so her mother took her to a hospital, which was many kilometres away. Tragically, Samantha died a few days after being admitted to hospital (adapted from Werner 1997).

Stop and Think

- What do you think contributed to Samantha's tragic death?
- Could her death have been prevented? How?
- Who or what should be blamed for her death?
- Was death equally likely to occur if Samantha had been born into a more affluent family and lived in an urban area like Melbourne or Perth?

Intersections of individual, environmental and social determinants of health

As discussed in the previous section, health determinants interact in a complex way. It is important to examine some of the interrelationships between the three major determinants which play an important part in the health, illness and well-being of individuals. These are individual (biological and behavioural), environmental and social determinants.

Individual determinants
The individual characteristics and behaviours of a person. Individual determinant examines how particular characteristics and behaviours of an in individual influence their health outcomes.

Individual determinants

Individual determinants refer to the individual characteristics and behaviours of a person, including how particular characteristics and behaviours of an individual influence their health outcomes. There are two basic types of health determinants that link to an individual determinant: biological and behavioural determinants.

Biological determinants

The **biological determinants** of health and disease include a diverse range of 'heterogeneous, intra-individual factors' which push, intervene or mitigate the passages towards health or disease of an individual (Swinburn & Cameron-Smith 2009, p. 248). Genes play a crucial role in underlying biological differences between individuals, but they also interact with other social and environmental components which influence the health and disease of persons (see examples below) (Swinburn & Cameron-Smith 2009; Fleming & Tenkate 2015; Bartley 2016). According to Swinburn and Cameron-Smith (2009, p. 248), 'the genetic and physiological systems within the body are dynamic, complex, and highly interconnected, with whole systems balancing and competing against each other' to achieve homeostasis. This is very similar to the complex processes of the social and environmental system outside the physical body of the individual.

Biological determinants
The inner physiological aspect of health and disease. Genes play a crucial role in underlying biological differences between individuals.

This can be seen in the case of HIV. HIV is dispersed in three ways: through sexual intercourse, blood transfusions (including through the use of needles and syringes), and from mother to child (Vaughan 2009; AIDSInfo 2017). While everyone can be infected with HIV, there are biological factors which increase an individual's susceptibility to infection. For instance, if an individual has another sexually transmitted infection (STI), such as chlamydia or gonorrhoea, the risk of becoming infected with HIV during sex is likely to be higher. If an individual has a blood disorder (and needs regular blood transfusions), they are at higher risk of contracting HIV. If a woman who is infected with HIV has health problems during pregnancy and breastfeeds her baby, there is a greater chance that the infection will be transmitted to the baby. The risk of HIV infection is also connected with the behaviours of individuals; for instance, having multiple sexual partners and having sex without a condom. Sharing equipment used for injecting drugs is a high-risk behaviour. Hence, although the biological factors are important, a focus on only biological risk factors will not stop the spread of HIV in populations (Vaughan 2009; see also Chapter 2).

Three biological determinants that play a role in the health and illness of individuals are race, sex and age. However, these are intertwined with social and environment determinants. Sometimes, it can be difficult to differentiate between the biological and other social and environmental conditions that determine people's health and illness.

Age is a clear biological determinant of the health of human beings (Miller 2009; West & Bergman 2009). Genes may have some impact on the causation of disease (Keleher & Joss 2009; Passarino et al. 2016). However, for many diseases the causes are environmental. For example, cognitive functioning decline among older people is not only the result of being old. It may also be affected by lack of practice, illness (such as depression), behaviours (such as the use of medications), psychological components (such as lack of confidence, motivation and low expectations), and social aspects (such as isolation and loneliness) (Cyarto & Batchelor 2019). (Race and gender will be discussed in a following section, under the social determinants of health.)

Biological determinants are fixed individual attributes that the person cannot control; for example, a family history of disease and heritable conditions, such as sickle cell disease. Some of these factors have an impact on the health of certain groups more than others. For example, sickle cell disease is especially common among people whose ancestors came from sub-Saharan Africa.

Behavioural determinants

Behavioural determinants
Personal attributes or behaviours that influence an individual's risk of experiencing poor health.

Individual behaviours play an important role in the health outcomes of a person. **Behavioural determinants** of health include personal characteristics (beliefs and values) and behavioural dispositions which can escalate or reduce good health, or the risk of poor health outcomes. These include protective or risk behaviours such as hygiene, exercise, diet, sexual practices and alcohol and other drug use (licit and illicit), as well as responses to health issues such as help-seeking and compliance with healthcare and medical treatment (Bidewell 2019; Hallet et al. 2019). According to McGinnis and colleagues (2002), the behavioural choices of an individual are a major determinant of health. They contend:

> The daily choices we make with respect to diet, physical activity, and sex; the substance abuse and addictions to which we fall prey; our approach to safety; and our coping strategies in confronting stress are all important determinants of health (p. 82).

Behavioural factors can increase our risk of both chronic diseases and infectious diseases. For example, cigarette smoking increases the risk of chronic diseases such as heart disease and lung cancer, while unprotected sex increases the risk of sexually transmitted infections such as HIV. Unlike the biological determinants of health, behavioural determinants are modifiable characteristics, and an individual has some control over their health and well-being.

Some characteristics of an individual, such as knowledge, attitudes and skills, have a great impact on their health behaviours. These determinants can assist an individual to preserve healthy behaviour and obtain the best possible health outcomes. Health promoters are particularly interested in influencing the knowledge, attitudes and skills of individuals in order to achieve long-term improvements in the person's health behaviour (see Chapter 6).

Environmental determinants

Environmental determinants
Physical environmental factors, such as climate and location, which can affect the health of individuals.

The important connection between the **environment** in which individuals live and their health and well-being has long been observed (McMichael 1993, 2000, 2001; McMichael et al. 2003; Nicholson & Stephenson 2009; Griffith et al. 2010; Fleming & Tenkate 2015; Ratcliff 2017; Hallet et al. 2019). Historically, environmental dangers to people's health tended to be related to issues of underdevelopment such as poor water quality, poor housing and the absence of sanitation. Although these 'traditional' threats have been managed successfully in more affluent areas within developed countries, there are still problems among socially disadvantaged and vulnerable groups of developed nations, and in the poorer countries of the globe

(Nicholson & Stephenson 2009; WHO 2017a; Hallet et al. 2019). This can be seen clearly in the environmental threats faced by some Indigenous people in Australia and elsewhere (Bertolatti et al. 2015; WHO 2017a). 'Modern' threats have emerged because of overconsumption and overdevelopment in developed nations (WHO 1997; Ratcliff 2017). These modern threats, including climate change, have become global hazards (McMichael 1993, 2000, 2001; McMichael et al. 2003; Eisenberg et al. 2007; Nicholson & Stephenson 2009; Fleming & Tenkate 2015; Baum 2016). Australia is a developed nation which is highly susceptible to the impacts of climate changes (Kennedy et al. 2010; Baum 2016; Talbot & Verrinder 2017; see Chapter 11).

Global climate changes can impact on many aspects of human life and health (Watts et al. 2015; Ratcliff 2017). Thermal extremes, such as heatwaves, can cause difficulty for many people, in particular the very young, very old, very poor and very sick (Goldsworthy et al. 2009; Nicholson & Stephenson 2009; Baum 2016; Talbot & Verrinder 2017). In 1959, a four-fold increase from the normal mortality rate resulted from a prolonged heatwave in Melbourne (McMichael 1993). Climate change and global warming are directly connected with the dispersion of infectious disease vectors and pests as well as with reduced food production (Talbot & Verrinder 2017). And this of course will affect people from poor areas and nations more than those from wealthier areas and locations with better resources (Hancock 1994; Baum 2016; Ratcliff 2017). Poor people who live in poor nations are disproportionately burdened by environmental problems and the related health impacts (Hancock 1994; Baum 2016; Ratcliff 2017). The WHO (1997, p. 198) puts it clearly: 'Impoverished populations ... are at greater risk from degraded environmental conditions. The cumulative effects of inadequate and hazardous shelter, overcrowding, lack of water supply and sanitation, unsafe food, air and water pollution and high accident rates impact heavily on the health of these vulnerable groups'.

Increasingly and globally, we have witnessed more environmental hazards and the health impacts of climate change resulting from human behaviours (Hallet et al. 2019). Severe drought, flooding, storms and extreme temperatures have become very common in recent years. This is what we have experienced in Australia—the Black Saturday bush fires in Victoria in January 2009, the widespread floods in Queensland, New South Wales and Victoria in January 2011, Cyclone Yasi in north Queensland and Cyclone Carlos in Darwin in February 2011, and extreme changes of weather in many Australian cities in 2017 and 2018 (see Chapter 11).

Social determinants of health

Not all illnesses are caused by biological and environmental agents. The health and well-being of individuals is also influenced by a number of **social determinants**. There are a number of factors, including social, cultural, economic and political, which can impact health (WHO 2015; AIHW 2018). This position goes beyond the restricted view of biological and genetic aspects of health (Wilkinson & Marmot 2003; Marmot & Wilkinson 2006; Marmot 2010; Keleher & MacDougall 2016b). Social determinants of health are described by the WHO (CSDH 2008, p. 1) as 'the

Social determinants
A number of factors, including social, cultural, economic and political, which can impact on the health of individuals.

circumstances in which people grow, live, work, and age, and the systems put in place to deal with illness. The conditions in which people live or die are, in turn, shaped by political, social and economic forces' (see also AIHW 2018, p. 179; WHO 2017b). Social determinants of health are created by 'the multilevel distribution of money, power, and resources' (Compton & Shim 2014, p. 4). This social condition is the most influential foundation of good health or illness (Cockerham 2013). Thus, social determinants can be perceived as 'causes of the causes—that is, as the foundational determinants which influence other health determinants' (AIHW 2016, p. 129; Marmot & Bell 2016). They are also the root cause of health inequities, the unjust and preventable discrepancies in health status that we have witnessed within and between nations (WHO 2017b; see also Chapter 14).

Social determinants of health are 'attributable to the structure and functioning of society' (Reidpath 2004, p. 22). For example, transportation can be seen as a social determinant of health since it can impact on individuals' physical activities, and this in turn can influence their nutritional intake and cardiovascular condition. Social expectations regarding sexual behaviours are also social determinants of health as they can influence individuals' approaches to risky sexual conduct. This can lead to marginalisation, stigma and discrimination (Reidpath 2004; see also Chapter 14).

Stop and Think

Have you ever looked at the homeless men who sleep on the local park bench with a blanket to cover their bodies, while their possessions are kept in some plastic bags next to them? When they wake, they tend to talk to themselves and do not seem to care about others around them. Have you ever thought about how they came to be like this? Have you been curious about what type of journey they have been through in their lives and what it would have been like for them before this misfortune, such as when they were somebody's son, father, husband or colleague? To develop an understanding of the life of these men necessitates some understanding of the social determinants of health (adapted from Lawn 2008, p. 36).

Important social determinants of health are related to positions of social life including gender, ethnicity and social class (Reidpath 2004; Cockerham 2013; Hill 2015; Schofield 2015). **Gender** is understood as a social construct, referring to the distinguishing characteristics of being a woman or a man (Schofield 2015; Stuber 2016; VicHealth 2017; Broom et al. 2019). Gender can be seen as the full range of personality traits, attitudes, feelings, values, behaviours and activities which are ascribed to women and men by the society in which they live (Stuber 2016; see also Chapter 9). It is different from **sex**, which is a 'biological construct premised upon biological characteristics enabling sexual reproduction' (Krieger 2003, p. 653; Stuber 2016). **Ethnicity** refers to a shared cultural background; it is a characteristic of a group within a society (Stuber 2016; Julian 2019). Ethnicity includes dimensions other than biological determinants (referred to as race). These include social, cultural and economic factors. Ethnicity is now accepted as a more appropriate

Gender
Socially and culturally constructed categories reflecting what it means to be 'masculine' and 'feminine', and associated expectations of roles and behaviours of men and women.

Sex
A biological construct based on biological characteristics that enable sexual reproduction.

Ethnicity
A shared cultural background which is a characteristic of a group within a society.

determinant of health than race (Jones & Creedy 2012; Schofield 2015). Gender and ethnic inequalities in health have been observed in many societies, including Australia (Hill 2015; Bartley 2016; Casado et al. 2016). **Social class** refers to the position of a person in a 'system of structured inequality' which is grounded in the unequal distribution of income, wealth, status and power (Stuber 2016; Germov 2019). Income, poverty and wealth are closely connected with health; people who live in poverty are likely to have worse health status than those who are better-off (Wilkinson & Marmot 2003; Marmot 2010; Cockerham 2013; Mackenbach 2015; Schofield 2015; Baum 2016; Marmot & Bell 2016; Germov 2019). The Australian Institute of Health and Welfare (AIHW 2018, p. 256) states that 'people from poorer social or economic circumstances are at greater risk of poor health, have higher rates of illness, disability and death, and live shorter lives than those who are more advantaged' (see also Mackenbach 2015; Ratcliff 2017; Chapter 7).

Social class
The position of a person in a system of structured inequality; it is grounded in unequal distribution of income, wealth, status and power.

None of these social determinants exist in isolation (Reidpath 2004). They intersect in a way that can create inequalities in health among people (Hill 2015; Schofield 2015). For example, women from a low socio-economic background are likely to be in poorer health than those from a higher social class (Baum 2016; Germov 2019). Men from ethnic minority groups and lower social classes are likely to be disadvantaged in terms of health and well-being in comparison to white Anglo-Celtic men with higher incomes (Jones & Creedy 2012; Julian 2019). We have witnessed ample examples of these interrelationships. The most influential indicator of health inequalities is life expectancy at birth. Between 2010 and 2012 in Australia, life expectancy was 69.1 years for Indigenous males and 73.7 years for Indigenous females—10.6 and 9.5 years less than for their non-Indigenous counterparts (AIHW 2018). Indigenous Australians also fare worse in health issues. The health inequalities of Indigenous Australians are the consequences of 'poorer socio-economic status, long-standing marginalisation from mainstream society and healthcare and, in many instances, geographical location and isolation' (Taylor 2008, p. 18; see also Genat & Cripps 2009; MacDonald 2010; Saggers et al. 2011; Chirgwin & D'Antoine 2019; Gray et al. 2019; Chapter 8).

Social gradient in health and health inequalities

As we have witnessed, a number of circumstances and conditions have created basic inequalities that not only contribute to the ill health of people, but establish a recurrence of adverse physical and mental health consequences for many individuals and groups within the current socio-cultural, economic and political contexts around the globe including in Australia (Bartley 2016; WHO 2017b). As such, there exists health inequality among populations. This section discusses two issues that are relevant to inequalities in health among individuals, communities and nations.

Social gradient in health

The health status of people coincides with a social gradient. Those who are situated lower on the ladder of the social hierarchy have a shorter life expectancy and greater risk of ill health than those who are higher up the social ladder (Marmot & Bell 2016). Individuals with a higher position in society will enjoy better health outcomes, both physical and mental, than those with a lower position (Fisher & Baum 2010; Compton & Shim 2014; AIHW 2018; Oldroyd 2019). The nature and magnitude of this social gradient differs between nations but it usually includes wealth, income, education, occupation, gender and ethnicity as well as area of residence (Marmot & Bell 2016).

Social gradient in health
Differences in social status that lead to different health outcomes. Individuals who are lower in the social hierarchy tend to have worse health outcomes than those located at higher social levels.

The **social gradient in health** impacts on the lives of people in both rich and poor countries. Within Australia and other western countries, the social gradient not only affects people from lower socio-economic backgrounds but also those in marginalised groups, including Indigenous people and people from culturally and linguistically diverse backgrounds including migrants and refugees (Shepherd et al. 2012; Castañeda et al. 2015; Moore et al. 2015; Khan et al. 2017; AIHW 2018). The social gradient in health has a significant impact on those in poorer areas of the globe. The greater the social disadvantages, the worse health will be the result (Oldroyd 2019). This means that 'not only the poorest but the majority have worse health and shorter lives than the best off in society' (Marmot & Bell 2016, p. 238).

Health inequality, health inequity and social justice

Health inequality
'Health differences' which are closely connected with social disadvantage and advantage.

Health inequalities refer to 'health differences' which are closely connected with social disadvantage and advantage (Braveman 2016, p. 38). This inequality disproportionately influences the health of the most disadvantaged members of society. Due to their low levels of wealth, prestige, influence or acceptance in society, people who are socially disadvantaged are adversely affected by health inequalities. These people include individuals from low-income backgrounds, members of ethnic minority and sexual minority groups, people with disabilities, women and many community groups who have historically been marginalised, discriminated against or excluded from others. Often, health inequalities are the consequences of social inequalities. Generally, those from more advantaged groups will have better health than those from disadvantaged groups (Keleher & MacDougall 2016a; AIHW 2018). Health inequality unfairly impinges on the health of people in poorer countries (Turnock 2016). This inequality has contributed to the psychosocial burden of many people (Kawachi & Kennedy 2006; Cushing et al. 2015).

Intrinsically, health inequalities are interwoven with health inequities (Braveman 2016). Health inequities refer to inequalities in health which are presumed to be unfair or arising from some kinds of injustice (Keleher & MacDougall 2016a). For example, people with disabilities and those from culturally and linguistically diverse backgrounds experience health inequities because of inadequate or lack of access to healthcare; people living in rural areas confront health inequities due to the unfair distribution of health services. In order to reduce or eliminate health inequalities, we must move toward health equity.

As inequalities are the consequence of inequitable societies, they are addressed through the concept of **social justice** (Braveman 2016; Taket 2019). It has been suggested that social justice approaches to health are crucial for public health and any healthcare system, so that individuals will have the right to good health outcomes (Wilkinson 2005; Wilkinson & Pickett 2009; CSDH 2014; Keleher & MacDougall 2016; see also Chapter 5). Justice means an equitable distribution of burdens and benefits among populations. Injustices occur when a burden unwarrantedly impacts on only some individuals and groups, and they lack access to benefits to which they are entitled (Turnock 2016).

Social justice
Systemic and structural social arrangements that improve equality. They include the fair distribution of resources, equal access to opportunities and rights, and protection of the marginalised and vulnerable.

Stop and Think

Consider the following examples. What do these tell you about our society and our own values?

- Rachel is an old woman who has been widowed for more than 10 years. She has little education and has always been poor. She does not own her own house, and has been renting a house in a suburb in Sydney. Recently, her lease was terminated because the owner wishes to renovate the house and increase the rent. Rachel does not have another place to move into and it has been very difficult to find rental accommodation in Sydney.
- Due to some difficulties in his life, Jack has become an alcoholic. He has been drinking heavily recently and, as a result, has been asked to leave his job. He is separated from his wife and two young children, and has been living on his own in a small flat. Because of his drinking problem and the difficulty he has caused his family, his colleagues and social network do not wish to have anything to do with him. He has virtually lost all of his social support.

Case Example 1.3

Barriers to breast cancer screening program among Thai migrant women

Early breast cancer detection is recognised as a common way to prevent breast cancer. However, the general trend in terms of numbers for screening for breast cancer among Asian women (e.g. from Malaysia, Iran, Jordan and China) is relatively low. It has been shown that less than 20 per cent of these women use the programs for early detection. The main reason for the low participation rate is the cultural attitude towards screening practices, especially shame from exposing breasts to strangers. However, there may be other factors that prevent migrant women seeking care to prevent breast cancer.

In a study with Thai migrant women in Melbourne, Suwankhong and Liamputtong (2018) showed that there were many barriers that prevent Thai migrant women from attending early breast cancer detection programs involving mammography, although the program was seen by the women as important. The women in this study had little familiarity with the health service systems in Australia. They expected to receive medical services at a single health location or facility, as this was the system they were familiar with in Thailand. Also, screening services were often located too far away from their areas of residence. Due to their low incomes, many women did not have a car, and it was difficult for them to travel to different healthcare facilities. Because of these difficulties, the women lacked interest in the program or were unwilling to find out further about the screening facilities that might be available.

The authors also found that language problems prevented many women from attending breast cancer screening programs. Most women had limited proficiency in English and were unable to communicate effectively with healthcare providers. They were unable to understand medical terms that would help them understand symptoms and illnesses in the necessary detail. Interpreters were not always available. When an interpreter was provided, the women were not satisfied with the interpreter nor with the interpretations. The interpreters were said to provide unclear explanations. They were said to deliver only very superficial health information. The women had no confidence that the interpreters explained what the doctor had actually told them. Often, the interpreters were not Thai. A Lao interpreter might be used, who did not possess a good understanding of the Thai language and culture. The women believed that this could create poor understanding of the issues and might also give them wrong recommendations for health practices. The women in the study sought to remedy this by consulting friends, co-workers and family members. This study suggested that language barriers are an important factor concerning the use of screening programs for breast cancer among Thai migrant women.

This study revealed that although breast cancer screening is seen as the best way to reduce deaths from breast cancer among women worldwide, there are many barriers to Thai migrant women using these programs. It is important for healthcare providers to understand their perceptions, experiences and living situations. This will lead to the provision of appropriate health prevention programs that will increase accessibility and better meet the circumstances of migrant women.

Reflection Exercise

> Of all forms of inequality, injustice in healthcare in the most inhumane.
>
> (Martin Luther King, cited in WHO 2015, p. 1).

Below is an example of how social determinants of health can significantly impact healthcare costs in the US. Homeless people who are un- or under-insured tend to forgo preventive care and rely on the emergency room to deal with major health issues. Once their acute conditions are addressed, recovery is hampered by a paucity of stable housing and constrained access to follow-up care. Furthermore, these conditions might interfere with mental health issues and substance abuse. The consequence is an immense rate of complications that require costly re-hospitalisations, and little or no improvement in overall health or quality of life in the end.

Witnessing the meanness and inefficiency of this cycle, ShelterCare, a non-profit human services organisation in Eugene, Oregon, looked for change. The ShelterCare Medical Recuperation program, a medical respite care program which determinedly enhances well-being while reducing costs by integrating SDOH into the care of homeless people was developed in collaboration with Community Health Centers of Lane County (federally qualified health centers), Trillium Community Health Plan, the local coordinated care organization, and PeaceHealth Sacred Heart Medical Center, the local hospital. This 30-day program provides residents a safe, stable housing environment to assist them to recover. At the same time, a community health worker provides medical care coordination and an on-site case manager helps residents connect to community resources to help them regain long-term stability.

Phil, a homeless man, went to the hospital emergency department with an infected wound. After receiving critical medical treatment, the hospital referred him to the ShelterCare program, where he was provided with a small flat and three meals a day. The medical caregiver on site provided medications, changed dressings and organised follow-up appointments and transportation. She helped Phil establish care with a primary care provider. He had an untreated mental health issue and a substance abuse problem, and was referred to both counselling and an addiction treatment program.

At the same time, a case manager advocated for Phil with other social service and government agencies, assisting him through the process of applying for food stamps, Social Security, Medicaid, rental assistance, unemployment benefits and other services for which he might qualify. Phil was given a bus pass and ShelterCare staff took him shopping for toiletries and clothing. He participated in on-site training workshops that helped him create a resume, apply for jobs and gain knowledge about basic budgeting skills.

Although at the end of his month-long stay, Phil still had much work to do to regain full stability, he was one of the 80 per cent of program participants who left the program to move into permanent housing. By addressing the social determinants of health rather than continuing the cycle of emergency department visits, Phil's coordinated care costed 34 per cent less while helping him (and the greater community by extension) make progress toward a better quality of life.

Although the ShelterCare program is focused specifically on those experiencing a predetermined set of conditions (homelessness and the need for acute recovery assistance), it shows both the value and feasibility of an outcome-based, SDOH-integrated network approach to healthcare for all (Rohwer 2018).

- What does this case study tell you about the social determinants of health?
- Would this case be applicable in other social contexts, like in Australia? How?
- What other social issues might we be able to adapt this framework to, to reduce health inequalities and social justice in our society?
- Considering the determinants of health model given in Figure 1.2, how can we address health inequalities in population groups in our society?

Figure 1.2 Determinants of health

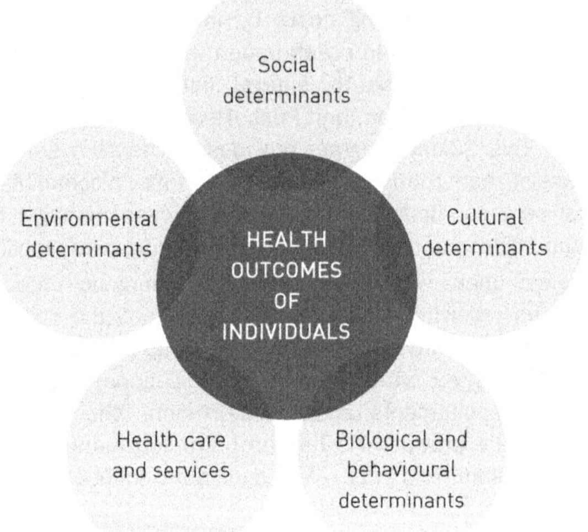

Summary

Health, illness and well-being are inevitable aspects of our lives and have always played a part in the life of all human beings. However, the concepts of health, illness and well-being are socially and culturally constructed because individuals and cultures see health, illness and well-being differently. Diverse factors can have an impact on the health, illness and well-being of individuals, groups and populations. These determinants of health include biological, environmental, social, cultural and economic factors. These determinants can affect how healthy or sick an individual can be. Within the social determinants of health, there are three crucial social structures which can affect people's health and well-being. These are gender, ethnicity and social class. These three factors do not operate in isolation but, rather, interrelate to the extent that they create inequality in health.

Tutorial exercises

1. Form a group of five with your peers in the class. Each of you writes down as many definitions of health as you can. Then compare your answers. Are there similarities in your definitions? Are they different? Discuss the similarities and differences that you have noted in the group, and how they have come about.
2. After finishing this chapter, walk around the university campus and note any determinant that can make you healthy or ill. What have you noticed?
3. It has been suggested that women live longer and men die sooner. What is your view about this suggestion? Is it true? What would be the determinants of this difference?
4. As a group, watch the documentary *The Shape of Water* (2006) (available online: http://www.theshapeofwatermovie.com). Discuss the possible determinants that can create inequalities and social justice in different groups of people.

Further reading

AIHW (Australian Institute of Health and Welfare) (2018). *Australia's Health 2018*. Canberra: Australian Institute of Health and Welfare. Accessed 20 June 2018 from http://www.aihw.gov.au/getmedia/7c42913d-295f-4bc9-9c24-4e44eff4a04a/aihw-aus-221.pdf.aspx?inline=true

Baum, F. (2016). *The New Public Health: An Australian Perspective*, 4th edn. Melbourne: Oxford University Press.

Bergholt, K. (2008). *Wellbeing: A Cultural History of Healthy Living* (translated by Jane Dewhurst). Cambridge: Polity Press.

Blaxter, M. (2010). *Health*, 2nd edn. Cambridge: Polity Press.

Cockerham, W.C. (2013). *Social Causes of Health and Disease*, 2nd edn. Cambridge: Polity Press.

Fisher, M., Baum, F.E., MacDougall, C., Newman, L., McDermott, D., & Phillips, C. (2017). Intersectoral action on SDH and equity in Australian health policy. *Health Promotion International*, 32, 953–963.

Germov, J. (Ed.) (2019). *Second Opinion: An Introduction to Health Sociology*, 6th edn. Melbourne: Oxford University Press.

Jones, K., & Creedy, D. (2012). *Health and Human Behaviours*, 3rd edn. Melbourne: Oxford University Press.

Keleher, H., & MacDougall, C. (Eds) (2016). *Understanding Health: A Determinants Approach*, 4th edn. Melbourne: Oxford University Press.

Liamputtong, P. (Ed.) (2019). *Public Health: Local and Global Perspectives*, 2nd edn. Melbourne: Cambridge University Press.

MacDonald, J.J. (2010). Health equity and the social determinants of health in Australia. *Social Alternatives*, 29(2), 34–40.

Marmot, M. (2016). *Boyer Lectures on Inequality and Health*. Retrieved from http://www.abc.net.au/radionational/programs/boyerlectures/series/2016-boyer-lectures/7802472

Marmot, M., & Wilkinson, R.G. (Eds) (2006). *Social Determinants of Health*, 2nd edn. Oxford: Oxford University Press.

Robertson, S. (2007). *Understanding Men and Health: Masculinities, Identity and Well-being*. Berkshire: Open University Press/McGraw Hill.

Solar, O., & Irwin, A. (2010). *A Conceptual Framework for Action on the Social Determinants of Health. Social Determinants of Health Discussion Paper 2 (Policy and Practice)*. Geneva: World Health Organization.

Stuber, J. (2016). *Exploring Inequality: A Sociological Approach*. New York: Oxford University Press.

Websites

www.unep.org/

This is the website of the UN Environment Program (UNEP). It provides a number of resources regarding environmental issues; for example, urban issues, waste, water quality, sanitation, air quality, climate change and ozone depletion.

www.who.int/social_determinants/en/

This is the website of the WHO's Commission on Social Determinants of Health. It is a good source of discussions on social determinants and provides crucial background papers and reports as well as examples of actions in relation to social determinants.

http://www.phmovement.org/

The website of the People's Health Movement provides discussions about health and inequalities in health. It contains information about health networks and activists who have concerns about the inequalities and inequities in health.

References

AIDSInfo (2017). *HIV/AIDS: The Basics*. Retrieved 17 June 2018 from http://aidsinfo.nih.gov/understanding-hiv-aids/fact-sheets/19/45/hiv-aids--the-basics

AIHW (Australian Institute of Health and Welfare) (2010). *Australia's Health 2010*. Australia's Health series No. 12. Cat No. AUS 122. Canberra: Australian Institute of Health and Welfare.

AIHW (Australian Institute of Health and Welfare) (2016). *Australia's Health 2016*. Canberra: Australian Institute of Health and Welfare. Accessed 15 November 2017 from http://www.aihw.gov.au

AIHW (Australian Institute of Health and Welfare) (2018). *Australia's Health 2018*. Canberra: Australian Institute of Health and Welfare. Accessed 20 June 2018 from http://www.aihw.gov.au/getmedia/7c42913d-295f-4bc9-9c24-4e44eff4a04a/aihw-aus-221.pdf.aspx?inline=true

Baer, H.A., Singer, M., & Susser, I. (2014). *Medical Anthropology and the World System: Critical Perspectives*, 2nd edn. Santa Barbara, CA: Praeger.

Baum, F. (2016). *The New Public Health: An Australian Perspective*, 4th edn. Melbourne: Oxford University Press.

Bartley, M. (2016). *Health Inequality: An Introduction to Concepts, Theories and Methods*. Cambridge: Polity Press.

Bertolatti, D., Hannelly, T., & Jansz, L. (2015). Environmental health and safety: social aspects. In J. Wright (Ed.), *International Encyclopedia of the Social and Behavioural Sciences*, 2nd edn (pp. 740–746). New York: Elsevier.

Bidewell, J. (2019). Individual decision-making in public health. In P. Liamputtong (Ed.), *Public Health: Local and Global Perspectives*, 2nd edn (Chapter 8). Melbourne: Cambridge University Press.

Blaxter, M. (2004). *Health*. Cambridge: Polity Press.

Blaxter, M. (2010). *Health*, 2nd edn. Cambridge: Polity Press.

Bleich, S.N., Jarlenski, M.P., Bell, C.N., & LaVeist, T.A. (2012). Health inequalities: trends, progress, and policy. *Annual Review of Public Health*, 33, 7–40.

Braveman, P. (2016). Health difference, disparity, inequality, or inequity: what difference does it make what we call it? In M. Buchbinder, M. Rivkin-Fish & R. Walker (Eds), *Understanding Health Inequalities and Justice: New Conversations Across the Disciplines* (pp. 33–63). North Carolina: University of North Carolina Press.

Broom, D., Freij, M., & Germov, J. (2019). Gendered health. In J. Germov (Ed.), *Second Opinion: An Introduction to Health Sociology*, 6th edn (pp. 133–160). Melbourne: Oxford University Press.

Brown, P.J., & Closser, S. (2016). Medical anthropology: an introduction. In P.J. Brown & S. Closser (Eds), *Understanding and Applying Medical*

Anthropology: Biosocial and Cultural Approaches, 3rd edn (pp. 13–24). Walnut Creek, CA: Left Coast Press.

Casado, D.L.P., Gonzalez, D.G., & Torre Esteve, M.D.L. (2016). The social class gradient in health in Spain and the health status of the Spanish Roma. *Ethnicity & Health*, 21(5), 468–479.

Castañeda, H., Holmes, S.M., Madrigal, D.S., DeTrinidad Young, M-E., Beyeler, N., & Quesada, J. (2015). Immigration as a social determinant of health. *Annual Review of Public Health*, 36, 375–392.

CHETNA (Centre for Health Education, Training and Nutrition Awareness) (2011). *Commitment to Women*. https://www.chetnaindia.org

Chirgwin, S., & D'Antoine, H. (2019). The health of indigenous people. In P. Liamputtong (Ed.), *Public Health: Local and Global Perspectives*, 2nd edn (Chapter 19). Melbourne: Cambridge University Press.

Cockerham, W.C. (2007). *Social Causes of Health and Disease*. Cambridge: Polity Press.

Cockerham, W.C. (2013). *Social Causes of Health and Disease*, 2nd edn. Cambridge: Polity Press.

Compton, M.T., & Shim, R.S. (2014). *The Social Determinants of Mental Health*. Washington, DC: American Psychiatric Publishing.

Corburn, J., & Riley, L. (2016). *Slum Health: From the Cell to the Street*. Berkeley, CA: University of California Press.

CSDH (Commission on Social Determinants of Health) (2008). *Closing the Gap in a Generation: Health Equity through Action on the Social Determinants of Health. Final Report of the Commission on Social Determinants of Health*. Geneva: World Health Organization.

CSDH (Commission on Social Determinants of Health) (2014). *Closing the Gap in a Generation: Health Equity through Action on the Social Determinants of Health. Final Report of the Commission on Social Determinants of Health*. Geneva: World Health Organization.

Cushing, L., Morello-Frosch, R., Wander, M., & Pasto, M. (2015). The haves, the have-nots, and the health of everyone: the relationship between social inequality and environmental quality. *Annual Review of Public Health*, 36, 193–209.

Cyarto, E., & Batchelor, F. (2019). Healthy ageing. In P. Liamputtong (Ed.), *Public Health: Local and Global Perspectives*, 2nd edn (Chapter 17). Melbourne: Cambridge University Press.

DHS (Department of Health and Human Services) (2018). *Healthy People 2020 Framework*. http://www.healthypeople.gov/2020/topics-objectives/topic/social-determinants-of-health

Eisenberg, J.N.S., Desai, M.A., Levy, K., Bates, S.J., Liang, S., & Naumoff, K. (2007). Environmental determinants of infectious diseases: a framework for tracking causal links and guiding public health research. *Environmental Health Perspectives*, 115(8), 1216–1223.

Fisher, M., & Baum, F. (2010). The social determinants of mental health: implications for research and health promotion. *Australian and New Zealand Journal of Public Health*, 44(12), 1057–1063.

Fleming, M.L. (2015a). Defining health and public health. In M.L. Fleming & E. Parker (Eds), *Introduction to Public Health* (2nd edn) (pp. 3–43). Sydney: Churchill Livingstone.

Fleming, M.L. (2015b). Social and emotional determinants of health. In M.L. Fleming & E. Parker (Eds), *Introduction to Public Health* (2nd edn) (pp. 140–159). Sydney: Churchill Livingstone.

Fleming, M.L., & Tenkate, T. (2015). Biological and environmental determinants. In M.L. Fleming & E. Parker (Eds), *Introduction to Public Health* (2nd edn) (pp. 117–139). Sydney: Churchill Livingstone.

Genat, B., & Cripps, K. (2009). Understanding the determinants of Aboriginal health. In H. Keleher & C. MacDougall (Eds), *Understanding Health: A Determinants Approach*, 2nd edn (pp. 87–100). Melbourne: Oxford University Press.

Germov, J. (2019). The class origins of health inequality. In J. Germov (Ed.), *Second Opinion: An Introduction to Health Sociology*, 6th edn (pp. 88–110). Melbourne: Oxford University Press.

Germov, J., & Freij, M. (2019). Media and health: moral panics, sinners, and saviours. In J. Germov (Ed.), *Second Opinion: An Introduction to Health Sociology*, 6th edn (pp. 422–445). Melbourne: Oxford University Press.

Goldsworthy, D., Jirojwong, S., & Liamputtong, P. (2009). Emerging population health issues and health promotion. In S. Jirojwong & P. Liamputtong (Eds), *Population Health, Communities and Health Promotion: Assessment, Planning, Implementation and Evaluation* (pp. 92–103). Melbourne: Oxford University Press.

Gray, D., Saggers, S., & Stearne, A. (2019). Indigenous health: the perpetuation of inequality. In J. Germov (Ed.), *Second Opinion: An Introduction to Health Sociology*, 6th edn (pp. 161–179). Melbourne: Oxford University Press.

Griffith, L., Raina, P., Wu, H., Zhu, B., & Stathokostas, L. (2010). Population attributable risk for functional disability associated with chronic conditions in Canadian older adults. *Age and Ageing*, 39(6), 738–745.

Hallet, J., Crawford, G., Pollard, C., & Hannelly, T. (2019). Behavioural, nutritional and environmental determinants of public health. In P. Liamputtong (Ed.), *Public Health: Local and Global Perspectives,* 2nd edn (Chapter 7). Melbourne: Cambridge University Press.

Hancock, T. (1994). Sustainability, equity, peace and the (green) politics of health. In C. Chu & R. Simpson (Eds), *Ecological Public Health: From Vision to Practice* (pp. 36–46). Griffith and Toronto: Institute of Applied Environmental Research and Centre for Health Promotion.

Heil, D. (2014). Well-being and wellness. In J. Germov (Ed.), *Second Opinion: An Introduction to Health Sociology*, 5th edn (pp. 43–64). Oxford University Press: Melbourne.

Helman, C.G. (2007). *Culture, Health and Illness*, 5th edn. London: Hodder Arnold.

Hill, S.E. (2015). Axes of health inequalities and intersectionality. In K.E. Smith, C. Bambra & S.E. Hill (Eds), *Health Inequalities: Critical Perspectives*. Oxford Scholarship Online. doi:10.1093/acprof:oso/9780198703358.001.0001

Jirojwong, S., & Liamputtong, P. (2009). An introduction: population health and health promotion. In S. Jirojwong & P. Liamputtong (Eds), *Population Health, Communities and Health Promotion: Assessment, Planning, Implementation and Evaluation* (pp. 3–25). Melbourne: Oxford University Press.

Jones, K., & Creedy, D. (2012). *Health and Human Behaviours*, 3rd edn. Melbourne: Oxford University Press.

Julian, R. (2019). Ethnicity, health, and multiculturalism. In J. Germov (Ed.), *Second Opinion: An Introduction to Health Sociology*, 6th edn (pp. 180–204). Melbourne: Oxford University Press.

Kawachi, I., & Kennedy, B.P. (2006). *The Health of Nations: Why Inequality is Harmful to your Health*. New York: New Press.

Keleher, H., & Joss, N. (2009). Determinants of healthy ageing. In H. Keleher & C. MacDougall (Eds), *Understanding Health: A Determinants Approach*, 2nd edn (pp. 367–378). Melbourne: Oxford University Press.

Keleher, H., & MacDougall, C. (2016a). Concepts of health. In H. Keleher & C. MacDougall (Eds), *Understanding Health*, 4th edn (pp. 3–18). Melbourne: Oxford University Press.

Keleher, H., & MacDougall, C. (2016b). Determinants of health. In H. Keleher & C. MacDougall (Eds), *Understanding Health*, 4th edn (pp. 19–34). Melbourne: Oxford University Press.

Kennedy, D., Stocker, L., & Burke, G. (2010). Australian local government action on climate change adaptation: some critical reflections to assist decision-making. *Local Environment*, 15(9–10), 805–816.

Khan, A.M., Urquia, M., Kornas, K., Henry, D., Cheng, S.Y., Bornbaum, C., & Rosella, L.C. (2017). Socioeconomic gradients in all-cause, premature and avoidable mortality among immigrants and long-term residents using linked death records in Ontario, Canada. *Journal of Epidemiology and Community Health*, 71, 625–632.

Krieger, N. (2003). Genders, sexes and health: what are the connections—and why does it matter? *International Journal of Epidemiology*, 32, 652–657.

Lawn, S. (2008). 'The needs of strangers': understanding social determinants of mental illness. *Social Alternatives*, 27(4), 36–41.

Levin, B.W., & Browner, C.H. (2005). The social construction of health: critical contributions from evolutionary, biological and cultural anthropology. *Social Science and Medicine*, 61(4), 745–750.

Liamputtong, P. (2019). Public health: an introduction to local and global contexts. In P. Liamputtong (Ed.), *Public Health: Local and Global Perspectives*, 2nd edn (Chapter 1). Melbourne: Cambridge University Press.

MacDonald, J.J. (2010). Health equity and the social determinants of health in Australia. *Social Alternatives*, 29(2), 34–40.

Mackenbach, J.P. (2015). Socioeconomic inequalities in health in high-income countries: the facts and the options. In R. Detels, M. Guillford, Q.A. Karim & C.C. Tan (Eds), *Oxford Textbook of Global Public Health*, 6th edn. Oxford: Oxford University Press.

Marmot, M. (2000). Social determinants of health: from observation to policy. *Medical Journal of Australia*, 172(8), 379–382.

Marmot, M. (2003). Understanding inequalities in health. *Perspectives in Biology and Medicine*, 46(3), S9–S23.

Marmot, M. (2004). *Status Syndrome: How your Social Standing Directly Affects your Health and Life Expectancy*. London: Bloomsbury Press.

Marmot, M. (2010). *Fair Society, Healthy Lives: The Marmot Review*. London: University College London.

Marmot, M., & Bell, R. (2016). Social inequalities in health: a proper concern of epidemiology. *Annals of Epidemiology*, 26, 238–240.

Marmot, M., & Wilkinson, R.G. (Eds) (2006). *Social Determinants of Health*, 2nd edn. Oxford: Oxford University Press.

McGinnis, J.M., Williams-Russo, P., & Knickman, J.R. (2002). The case for more active policy attention to health promotion. *Health Affairs,* 21(2), 78–93.

McMichael, A.J. (1993). *Planetary Overload*. Cambridge: Cambridge University Press.

McMichael, A.J. (2000). The urban environment and health in a world of increasing globalization: issues for developing countries. *Bulletin of the World Health Organization*, 78, 1117–1126.

McMichael, A.J. (2001). *Human Frontiers, Environments and Disease: Past Patterns, Uncertain Futures*. Cambridge: Cambridge University Press.

McMichael, A.J., Campbell-Lendrum, H., Corvalen, C., Ebi, K., Githeko, A.K., Schwraga, J.D., & Woodward, A. (Eds) (2003). *Climate Change and Human Health: Risks and Responses*. Geneva: World Health Organization.

Miller, C.A. (2009). *Nursing for Wellness in Older Adults*, 5th edn. Philadelphia: Wolters Kluwer/Lippincott Williams & Wilkins.

Moore, T.G., McDonald, M., Carlon, L., & O'Rourke, K. (2015). Early childhood development and the social determinants of health inequities. *Health Promotion International*, 30(S2), ii102–ii115. Doi:10.1093/heapro/dav031

Nicholson, R., & Stephenson, P. (2009). Natural environments as a determinant of health. In H. Keleher & C. MacDougall (Eds), *Understanding Health: A Determinants Approach*, 2nd edn (pp. 112–133). Melbourne: Oxford University Press.

Oldroyd, J. (2019). Social determinants of public health. In P. Liamputtong (Ed.), *Public Health: Local and Global Perspectives*, 2nd edn (Chapter 6). Melbourne: Cambridge University Press.

Parsons, T. (1951). *The Social Role*. Glencoe, IL: Free Press.

Parsons, T. (1979). Definitions of health and illness in the light of American values and social structure. In E.G. Jaco (Ed.), *Patients, Physicians and Illness* (pp. 97–117). New York: Free Press.

Passarino, G., De Rango, F., & Motesanto, A. (2016). Human longevity: genetics or lifestyle? It takes two to tango. *Immunity & Ageing*, 13(12). Doi:10.1186/s12979-016-0066-z

People's Health Movement (2011). *People's Charter for Health*. http://www.phmovement.org/files/phm-pch-english.pdf.

Powers, M., & Faden, R. (2008). *Social Justice: The Moral Foundations of Public Health and Health Policy*. New York: Oxford University Press.

Ratcliff, K.S. (2017). *The Social Determinants of Health: Looking Upstream*. Cambridge: Polity Press.

Reidpath, D.D. (2004). Social determinants of health. In H. Keleher & B. Murphy (Eds), *Understanding Health: A Determinants Approach* (pp. 9–22). Melbourne: Oxford University Press.

Rohwer, M.D. (2018). *Social Determinants of Health: A Case Study*. https://www.thelundreport.org/content/social-determinants-health-case-study

Rumbold, B., & Dickson-Swift, V. (2012). Social determinants of health: historical developments and global implications. In P. Liamputtong, R. Fanany & G. Verrinder (Eds), *Health, Illness and Well-being: Perspectives and Social Determinants* (pp. 177–196). Melbourne: Oxford University Press.

Saggers, S., Walter, M., & Gray, D. (2011). Culture, history and health. In R. Thackrah & K. Scott (Eds), *Indigenous Australian Health and Cultures: An Introduction for Health Professionals* (pp. 1–21). Sydney: Pearson.

Schofield, T. (2015). *A Sociological Approach to Health Determinants*. Melbourne: Cambridge University Press.

Scambler, G. (2003). Deviance, sick role and stigma. In G. Scambler (Ed.), *Sociology As Applied to Medicine* (pp. 192-202). Edinburgh: Saunders.

Sendall, M. (2019). Political determinants of public health. In P. Liamputtong (Ed.), *Public Health: Local and Global Perspectives,* 2nd edn (Chapter 9). Melbourne: Cambridge University Press.

Shepherd, C.C.J., Li, J., & Zubrick, S.R. (2012). Social gradients in the health of Indigenous Australians. *American Journal of Public Health*, 102(1), 107–117.

Smith, J., Griffiths, K., Judd, J., Crawford, G., D'Antoine, H., Fisher, M., Bainbridge, R., & Harris, P. (2018). Ten years on from the World Health Organization Commission of Social Determinants of Health: progress or procrastination? *Health Promotion Journal of Australia*, 29(1), 3–7.

Spector, R.E. (2017). *Cultural Diversity in Health and Illness,* 9th edn. New Jersey: Pearson Prentice Hall.

Stuber, J. (2016). *Exploring Inequality: A Sociological Approach*. New York: Oxford University Press.

Suwankhong, D., & Liamputtong, P. (2018). Barriers to seeking healthcare for breast cancer among Thai immigrant women in Melbourne. *Asian Pacific Journal of Cancer Prevention*, 19(3), 253–261.

Swinburn, B., & Cameron-Smith, D. (2009). Biological determinants of health. In H. Keleher & C. MacDougall (Eds), *Understanding Health: A Determinants Approach*, 2nd edn (pp. 248–269). Melbourne: Oxford University Press.

Syme, S.L. (2004). Social determinants of health: the community as an empowered partner. *Preventing Chronic Disease*, 1(1), 1–5.

Taket, A. (2019). Human rights, social justice and public health. In P. Liamputtong (Ed.), *Public Health: Local and Global Perspectives,* 2nd edn (Chapter 10). Melbourne: Cambridge University Press.

Talbot, L., & Verrinder, G. (2017). *Promoting Health: The Primary Care Approach*, 6th edn. Sydney: Elsevier Australia.

Taylor, S.D. (2008). The concept of health. In S. Taylor, M. Foster & J. Fleming (Eds), Healthcare Practice in Australia (pp. 3–21). Melbourne: Oxford University Press.

Turnock, B.J. (2016). *Public Health: What it is and How it Works,* 6th edn. Burlington, MA: Jones & Bartlett Learning.

Vaughan, C. (2009). Vulnerability and globalisation. In H. Keleher & C. MacDougall (Eds), *Understanding Health: A Determinants Approach*, 2nd edn (pp. 170–184). Melbourne: Oxford University Press.

VicHealth (1999). *Mental Health Promotion Plan. Foundation Document: 1990–2002*. Melbourne: VicHealth.

VicHealth (2015). *VicHealth Mental Health Strategy: 2015–2019*. Melbourne: VicHealth.

VicHealth (2017). *Gender Equality, Health and Wellbeing Strategy: 2017–19*. Melbourne: Victorian Health Promotion Foundation.

Watts, N., et al. (2015). Health and climate change: policy responses to protect public health. *The Lancet*, 386(10006), 1861–1914.

Werner, D. (1997). *Questioning the Solution: The Politics of Primary Healthcare and Child Survival with an In-depth Critique of Oral Rehydration Therapy*. Palo Alto, CA: Health Wrights.

West, G.B., & Bergman, A. (2009). Toward a systems biology framework for understanding aging and health span. *Journal of Gerontology Series A: Biological Sciences and Medical Sciences*, 64A(2), 205–208.

WHO (World Health Organization) (1948). *Constitution*. Geneva: World Health Organization.

WHO (World Health Organization) (1978). *Alma-Ata 1978: Primary Healthcare*. Geneva: World Health Organization.

WHO (World Health Organization) (1986). *Ottawa Charter for Health Promotion*. Geneva: World Health Organization.

WHO (World Health Organization) (1997). *Health and Environment in Sustainable Development, Five Years after the Earth Summit*. Geneva: World Health Organization.

WHO (World Health Organization) (2015). *Integrating Equity, Gender, Human Rights and Social Determinants into the Work of WHO: Roadmap for Action (2014–2019)*. Geneva: World Health Organization.

WHO (World Health Organization) (2017a). *Climate Change and Health, Update July 2017*. Retrieved from http://www.who.int/mediacentre/factsheets/fs266/en

WHO (World Health Organization) (2017b). *Social Determinants of Health*. Geneva: WHO. Retrieved from http://www.who.int/social_determinants/sdh_definition/en/

Wiley, A.S., & Allen, J.S. (2017). *Medical Anthropology: A Biocultural Approach*, 3rd edn. New York: Oxford University Press.

Winkelman, M. (2009). *Culture and Health: Applying Medical Anthropology*. San Francisco: Jossey-Bass.

Wilkinson, R.G. (2005). *The Impact of Inequality: How to Make Sick Societies Healthier*. New York: New Press.

Wilkinson, R.G., & Marmot, M. (Eds) (2003). *Social Determinants of Health: The Solid Facts*. Copenhagen: WHO Regional Office for Europe.

Wilkinson, R., & Pickett, K. (2009). *The Spirit Level: Why More Equal Societies Almost Always do Better*. London: Allen lane.

Part I

Social Determinants of Health and Conceptual Frameworks

Chapter 2

Health as a Social Construct

Cassandra Wright and Peter Higgs

Topics covered

This chapter covers the following topics:

- overview of how health is socially constructed
- different models of understanding health
- structure and agency debate
- how to apply a sociological imagination

Key terms

agency
biological model
biopsychosocial model
ecological model
HIV/AIDS
social model of health
socio-ecological model of health
structure–agency debate

Introduction: health as a social construct

We often think of health in terms of disease and medicine—being healthy means not having a disease, and being sick often means needing medicine. While both of these statements can be true, research from the public health field teaches us that health is much more complex than just biology. Similarly, when we are unwell, we often look for the biological pathogens that might have caused the illness (e.g. viruses, bacteria). But people's exposure, susceptibility and response to pathogens are shaped by social, cultural and environmental factors (see Chapter 1 in this volume). For example, if I catch a cold at work, I could think about not only the rhinovirus which is the biological pathogen, but also how my immune system is suppressed because I am rundown and stressed, the proximity of my colleagues in a small open-plan area, the weather being cold which means that people stay indoors, the pressure of workloads which leads to colleagues regularly coming into the workplace despite being sick, the way that this is managed by senior staff and so on. Just because a biological pathogen exists, this does not mean that it has to be passed on. In order to prevent it from being passed on, we have to look beyond individuals to see where the pathways to prevention lie.

Additionally, many things that create health and illness are not necessarily biologically caused although they may result in physical effects. Although there has been some investment in research to try to find genetic causes of obesity, there are far stronger bodies of evidence showing the relationships between obesity and not only diet and exercise behaviours, but also socio-economic status (Monteiro et al. 2004; McLaren 2007), occupation (Kirk & Rhodes 2011; Solovieva et al. 2013), density of takeaway outlets in the local area (Reidpath et al. 2002; Li et al. 2009), the walkability of the local area (Grasser et al. 2013; Rundle et al. 2009), pricing of fresh food (Powell et al. 2013), availability of fresh food (Walker et al. 2010), policies relating to taxation (Andreyeva et al. 2010) and advertising (Boyland et al. 2016). These days, health is often framed as being about behaviour, but this does not acknowledge the multitude of factors that influence the behaviour of not just one person, but whole populations (see Chapters 1 & 7).

These social factors and their influence on health and well-being are evident when we look at changes over time in patterns of disease, or when we compare groups in different circumstances or countries. For example, inequalities and inequities can be very visible if we compare an average Australian to someone in a low-income country, with no access to clean water, no sanitation and poor nutrition. The latter almost invariably involves lower life expectancy, higher rates of child mortality and higher rates of all kinds of communicable diseases. It is unjust but makes sense that a country with a lower income has less to spend on infrastructure such as clean water, sanitation and healthcare systems, which clearly affect the prevention and treatment of infectious diseases (see Chapter 14).

We do not have to look at extreme examples to see very stark differences in health. Extensive research has shown that there is a social gradient of health (Marmot 2005). This exists both within and between countries. If we go back to the example of looking at high- and low-income countries, and plot health outcomes of other countries which fall more in the middle in terms of income, the graph would show a clear relationship between increasing income and improved health outcomes. This social gradient has been demonstrated over and over again, even within one country, state or city. The famous Whitehall study undertaken by Sir Michael Marmot showed that among British government employees, there was a clear gradient whereby lower occupational and social grade was associated with higher mortality from a range of diseases including ischaemic heart disease (Reid et al. 1974; Marmot et al. 1978, 1984). Each step up the social ladder was associated with reduced risk of those diseases. Even 10 years later, those in the lowest grade had a mortality rate three times higher than those in the highest grade. The second Whitehall study investigated why this might be the case, and found that income was not the only thing that mattered (Marmot et al. 1991). While income was important for affording healthcare, other social factors also contributed to poor health in lower-ranking employees, such as stress, the work environment, social support and job demands (Bosma et al. 1997; Stansfeld et al. 1998, 1999). Since these seminal studies, a great deal of research has illustrated the powerful effect of social factors on health and well-being. Marmot went on to work with the World Health Organization to highlight the importance of 10 specific social determinants of health. These included the social gradient, stress, early life, social exclusion, work, unemployment, social support, addiction, food and transport (Wilkinson & Marmot 2003). Marmot and Wilkinson compiled evidence to show the relationships between each of these factors and a range of communicable and non-communicable illnesses including premature mortality, diabetes, coronary heart disease and poor mental health. More recent work by the WHO Commission on the Social Determinants of Health has also provided strong evidence for the relationship between health and gender equity, employment conditions, urbanisation and globalisation (Marmot et al. 2008). Each of these factors affects people's opportunities in life and what they are exposed to, which in turn affects their ability to lead healthy lives. Understanding how these factors influence health underpins the **social model of health**.

Social model of health
A model which focuses on the social forces which influence health and well-being.

HIV/AIDS
Human Immunodeficiency Virus (HIV) and Acquired Immunodeficiency Syndrome (AIDS) HIV is a blood-borne virus which emerged in the 1980s in North America and has since spread globally. It is a particularly prominent issue in sub-Saharan Africa. HIV causes the development of AIDS, which marks a certain point of depletion in the immune system and is fatal if left untreated.

Case Example 2.1

HIV: biological cause but social susceptibility

HIV/AIDS is one health issue with a clear biological pathogen—the Human Immunodeficiency Virus. We know that the virus is blood-borne, meaning that a person can contract the virus if they come in contact with the blood of an infected person. If two people came into contact with the blood of an infected person, we might think that they would be equally susceptible to contracting the virus. But if we look at patterns of infection and transmission in a population, it is clear that particular subgroups are more at risk than others. It is social factors which shape this risk. If we understand these social factors, we can deploy prevention efforts which protect against inherent increased risk. The HIV/AIDS epidemic exemplifies this when we compare the experiences of two different high-income countries—Australia and the US.

In both countries, there are two population groups with the highest risk of contracting HIV: men who have sex with men, and people who inject drugs (CDCP 2012; Kirby Institute 2017). These two groups are particularly vulnerable due to biological or behavioural factors. However, the overall rate of HIV infection within these two groups, and also outside those groups, is considerably different in Australia and the US. In both countries, men who have sex with other men make up the majority of HIV cases: 56 per cent of HIV notifications in the US (CDCP 2012) and about 68 per cent in Australia (Kirby Institute 2017). But in the US, among men who have sex with men, African-American men are far more likely to contract HIV than Caucasian men. One in 16 of all African-American men in the US will be diagnosed with HIV compared to one in 102 Caucasian men (CDCP 2012). There is no biological explanation for this; instead, a range of social factors has shown to be associated with increased HIV among African-American people. These include socio-economic issues associated with higher rates of poverty, which limits access to quality healthcare, housing and education, as well as social issues including stigma, discrimination and fear (Reif et al. 2006).

We also see vast differences between the US and Australia in the proportions of people who inject drugs (PWID) living with HIV (CDCP 2012; Kirby Institute 2017). In the US, about 20 per cent of people living with HIV have injecting drug use as their main risk factor for infection whereas in Australia the figure is less than 5 per cent. Explaining the factors for this mean we need to look beyond individual behaviours. This is where the impact of government policy can be seen to make a huge difference. In Australia, the introduction of programs that provide sterile injecting equipment free to PWID was begun very early in the epidemic (in the mid to late 1980s) (Plummer & Irwin 2006). This meant that although the proportion of PWID in both countries was roughly the same, those in Australia were far more likely to use sterile equipment than those in the US (Lurie & Drucker 1997).

Access to testing and treatment services are also very different in Australia and the USA. PWID in the US have trouble getting medical treatment for HIV because they are more likely to be homeless, incarcerated and uninsured (Cunningham et al. 2007; Stevens & Keigher 2009; Wolfe et al. 2010). The universal healthcare available in Australia means that while many PWID are also affected by homeless and histories of incarceration, they can still be provided with basic healthcare (AIHW 2016).

We see an entirely different epidemiological portrait if we look at HIV epidemiology in sub-Saharan Africa, which accounts for more than 70 per cent of the global burden of infection (UN 2014). While Australia and the US have a disproportionate burden of infection concentrated in men who have sex with men, in sub-Saharan Africa the young women are most at risk (Dellar et al. 2015; Kharsany & Karim 2016). In countries such as South Africa, the HIV prevalence is three times higher in females than males (Harrison et al. 2015). A range of social factors influence the susceptibility of young girls and women including poverty, power, gender norms, violence, occupations, age differences in relationships and educational opportunities (Harrison et al. 2015).

Alternative models of health

There are many different ways of conceptualising health, and various models have been proposed by experts from different disciplines over time. Here we present some of the most common models of health, and discuss their key foci in understanding health.

Biomedical model

Biological model
The traditional western mode of medicine, which understands disease and illness to be caused by external pathogens or disorders of organs and body systems.

The biomedical model is focused on the biological aspects of disease and ill health, and underpins the traditional approach to western medicine. Disease and illness is understood to be caused by external pathogens or disorders of organs and body systems. Therefore, when an individual experiences poor health, the key actions are to diagnose the condition and provide medical treatment, with the aim of curing the condition and thus returning the patient to a state of pre-disease health. Doctors, hospitals and medication are essential to creating health in this model, due to doctors' specialist knowledge and hospitals' specialist equipment. This model of health may be familiar, as it frames most modern healthcare in developed countries. In Australia, most health-related funding goes towards biomedically focused healthcare.

There are reasons why this model has been so popular in the past two centuries. The medical field has made impressive advancements in understanding the pathology of diseases down to cellular and genetic levels. Some infectious diseases and cancers which were previously incurable have either been eradicated or now require only simple and widely available interventions. However, there are also some limitations, which have been highlighted in the past 50 years especially (Germov 2019). First, the model tends to ignore the wider factors which can affect health (discussed above), and reduces health to being about disease. Second, it is reactive, rather than proactive. By this, we mean that the model waits for people to get sick, rather than promoting good health or preventing ill health. Third, interventions can be costly due to the emphasis on technology, medication and specialist healthcare workers.

Biopsychosocial model

Biopsychosocial model
A model which posits that ill health and disease are created through interactions between a person's biological, psychological and social factors.

The **biopsychosocial model** was proposed by Engel (1977), a doctor in the field of psychiatry, who was frustrated by the biomedical model's limitations. Drawing upon knowledge from the field of psychology, the biopsychosocial model posited that ill health and disease are created through interactions between a person's biological, psychological and social factors. Engel noted that biochemical alterations do not necessarily result in illness, and that illness results from the interplay of a range of factors at the molecular, individual and social levels. He noted the placebo effect as just one example of how psychological factors could influence a person's disease experience, and stated that psychosocial factors were 'more important determinants of susceptibility, severity and course of illness than had been previously appreciated' under the constraints of the biomedical model. The biopsychosocial model incorporated the relationship between doctor and patient as influential to health, and Engels championed a more compassionate, humanised approach to medicine. While this model is often touted as preferable, there are varying views on the extent to which it has been taken up in modern medicine (Borrell-Carrió et al. 2004).

While this model represents an advance towards a more holistic view of health, it is important to note that it still focuses on individual-level disease and treatment.

Ecological models

Ecological model
A model which understands health and well-being (not merely the absence of disease) to be shaped by human biology, personal behaviour, and psychosocial and physical environments. More recent updates (i.e. socio-ecological models) have added political and economic factors.

Similar to how the biopsychosocial model was developed in response to identified deficiencies in the biomedical model, ecological models were developed to further incorporate the emerging understanding of how social factors and environments shape and influence health. One of the earliest ecological models was Hancock's (1985) Mandala of Health, a 'bio-psycho-socio-environmental' model of heath. The Mandala of Health includes four elements which affect health:

- human biology
- personal behaviour
- psycho-social environment
- physical environment.

Hancock conceptualised personal behaviour as influenced by psycho-social environments, and emphasised a need to avoid victim-blaming in any efforts targeting life-style. He understood the psycho-social environment to include socio-economic status, peer influences, access to social support and exposure to advertising. The physical environment includes workplaces, neighbourhoods and housing. A further critical component of this model is its focus not only on the individual but also on the family, which is situated in the context of community and culture. The Mandala highlights the medical care system itself as influential on both biology and behaviour of individuals and families. Hancock's further iterations of the Mandala conceptualised the individual as comprising mind, body and spirit, and added the elements of the work context and economic environments (Hancock 1993). This model, although complex, has been widely used to explain and map the determinants of health.

Socio-ecological models

Socio-ecological model
A model conceptualising the influences on health in nested layers expanding out from the individual. These layers are seen to influence each other, and in turn shape an individual's health.

Socio-ecological models emerged from the field of development psychology, with Urie Bronfenbrenner pioneering the field through his ecological systems theory (Bronfenbrenner 1992). A key distinction of Bronfenbrenner's socio-ecological model is that it conceptualises influences on health in nested layers expanding out from the individual. These layers are seen to influence each other, and in turn shape an individual's health. Individual-level factors affecting health include gender, age and health status. Immediately surrounding the individual are the microsystem factors, such as family, peers, school, work and other organised structures and relationships. Next is the mesosystem, which includes interactions between two or more settings in the microsystem. The third layer, the exosystem, comprises social, political and economic factors such as industry, local politics and mass media. At the outer layer, the macrosystem, these social, political and economic factors interplay with attitudes and beliefs within society. Socio-ecological models are widely used in public health to tease out the determinants of health for issues, and commonly include the following five nested layers: individual (inner layer), interpersonal, organisational, community and public policy (outer layer) (McLeroy et al. 1988).

Stop and Think

- Which model of health do you think is most evident in your contacts with the healthcare system so far in your life?

Agency versus structure

Agency
The capacity and power of individuals to influence their own lives and shape their society.

Structure–agency debate
The debate on how much people's decisions are shaped by social institutions and culture compared to their individual will (agency).

While debates around why some people are not as healthy as others have been dominated by the professions that work to make individuals healthy, there are many other ways of thinking that can help to make sense of the amount of control we have over our own health. Sociologists, for example, study the relationship between society and individuals and have been at the forefront of discussions in health about human behaviour and ways in which behaviour change can be influenced (Germov 2019).

Clearly the social environments (also called structure) we live in play a crucial role in our health, but there are also important things that we as individuals and communities can do (also called **agency**) to impact on our health. This '**structure–agency debate**' has been heavily influenced by the work of US and European theorists for the past 100 years. This approach has framed much of the thinking about how much control we as individuals have over behaviour compared to the influences of our social environment. It highlights that the links between structure and agency are very tight and should not be looked at in isolation from each other. Both have an impact on health, especially on health inequality. The importance of structure and agency in discussions of health has recently expanded; the field of science and technology studies, especially the increasing influence of Actor Network Theory, has taken on many of the new ways of thinking about public health issues (Latour 2005).

The focus of this chapter is on the social model of health, which, as outlined earlier, has a history in social movements around community-building including the development of the Ottawa Charter (WHO 1986), an international agreement signed at the World Health Organization's first conference on health promotion, held in Ottawa, Canada in 1986 (see also Chapter 6). The Charter builds on the 'health for all' mantra promoted by WHO in the late 1970s and is a cornerstone in the view that health and social justice are inextricably linked (see Chapter 5).

There are a number of reasons why this sociologically framed view of health (informed by the field of medical sociology) is important for health workers to understand. These include understanding that where we live, our educational attainment, access to income, our gender and genetics, as well as our social relationships all affect health outcomes. An enormous amount of good research shows links between increased health status for people with more social and physical resources—the wider the gaps, the larger the difference in health. The most obvious example relates to increases in life expectancy as a measure of health: the more affluent a country is, the longer people's life expectancy is. But looking at health so crudely masks a range of other issues that impact on the health of citizens within countries where some communities are nowhere near as healthy as others. The work of Germov (2019, p. 3) is seminal in this area. He argues that the social model of health 'provides a second opinion to the conventional medical view of illness derived from biological and psychological explanations, by exploring the social origins of health and illness'.

One of the key principles of the WHO, enshrined in its Constitution, was that 'health is a state of complete physical, mental and social well-being and not merely the absence of disease' (WHO 1948). Indeed, access to health became enshrined as a human right in the 1948 Declaration of Human Rights. From the very earliest stages, bodies like the UN saw health as more than just an individual approach to illness.

The German political scientist Professor Ilona Kickbusch was very influential in the development of this charter. Her thinking and writing have shaped the development of ideas around the current social view of health. Much of her career has involved working within WHO and providing evidence on the important role of governments, social policy-makers and others in the development of healthier communities. Her promotion of the role of the WHO and the direction of the 'new public health' (Kickbusch 2003) have been crucial to the view that there is more to health than individual disease or illness. This understanding is vital if we are to build a foundation to better understand the impact of health, not just on individuals but on communities and neighbourhoods as well.

The view that 'everything about health is political' (Clark 2017) is an important one if we are to see the influence of society on our individual behaviours. The impact of growing up and living in one neighbourhood as compared to another has been clearly linked to individual health. Our task is to understand and confront how this has the potential to influence our health and well-being.

What control do we as individuals have over the behaviours and actions we take? Potential resources are sometimes referred to as 'social capital' (Eriksson 2011), a term which has seen a huge increase in the academic literature in the past 25 years. It is important to understand that as individuals we can all make choices about the way we live our lives and the things that we do to 'live healthy'. The concept of 'agency' is crucial—what capacity do we as individuals have to control our lives? We are clearly able to exercise agency, but are limited by the environments in which we live.

This does get confusing when we are using the social model of health, because it places so much emphasis on contributions which are outside the individual. Where are the parks and other recreational spaces in the community? What kinds of places can people use to shop locally? Where are the schools and other neighbourhood hubs?

Substantial work done by Jesuit Social Services in its 20 years of work on place-based disadvantage shows that there are ways in which we can measure the contributions to disadvantage in small local areas (postcodes) and see how these change over time (Vinson et al. 2015).

Case Example 2.2

Dropping Off the Edge

Dropping Off the Edge (DOTE) is a follow-up study from two previous reports investigating place-based disadvantage in Australia. The 2015 report shows that complex and entrenched disadvantage is experienced by a small but persistent number of locations (postcodes) in each Australian state and territory. It also highlights that there have been few signs of improvement over time. The report finds that the experience of disadvantage is unevenly distributed across the country.

When the report was launched in July 2015 there was an enormous amount of media interest and discussion about the kinds of things that impact on disadvantage, like educational opportunities, incarceration rates, unemployment and housing stress. These factors are clearly very important in people's health.

While the DOTE report analysed health indicators with a narrow focus on 'disability', it clearly understood that people's social and economic circumstances affect their health. Drawing on the social determinants of health as outlined by Marmot (2005), DOTE uses data from government sources to map disadvantage. It is a good example of why the Ottawa Charter has a settings approach to health. As noted by the WHO (1986, p. 3), 'health is created and lived by people within the settings of their everyday life; where they learn, work, play, and love'.

Changing individual patterns of behaviour has historically been a huge focus of governments and other organisations that are interested in people's health. For example, there have been campaigns to reduce the prevalence of smoking (Quit Victoria, https://www.quit.org.au/) or to encourage safe sex (https://playsafe.health.nsw.gov.au/), and more specific ones focused on gay and bisexual men (http://www.thedramadownunder.info/).

Much of the time these kinds of campaigns are focused entirely on individuals and on providing information so that they can make rational decisions to 'choose health'. But people still continue to make choices which do not appear rational. How can we explain this? One way is by having a broader view which incorporates many of the structures that impact on our lives. The perspective that there is much in our living environments that influences and impacts on these behaviours is crucial to understanding how to work as an agent of behaviour change.

Ultimately, understanding the opportunities that both structure and agency present to improve health and well-being in individuals as well as communities is important for everyone working in health. If all the emphasis is placed on individual choice, we neglect the other influencing factors. This leads to victim-blaming and ineffective responses, and does not allow for change.

Stop and Think

Individuals are often seen as the focus for behaviour change interventions. Think about conversations you have had around the dinner table or in the classroom about health and illness. How much emphasis do we place on the individual? For example, 'How do we get people who are overweight to lose weight? What can we do to stop people using illicit drugs?'

Some people are quick to blame an individual for their behaviours, but the goal of a health worker is to improve the health of people and the communities in which they live. There are complex reasons why people behave the way they do even if it seems to be irrational. We all know that smoking has many negative health consequences, yet there are people who continue to smoke.

- List other influencing structural factors which may influence individuals' 'agency' to improve their own health.
- What kinds of things hinder potential changes to individual behaviour?

Sociological imagination

The sociological imagination is a way of thinking. It means seeing the role that societal factors play in problems that seem at first to be personal issues. C. Wright Mills (1959) coined the term, but its core concept has been central to sociology throughout history. When we look at a health problem at an individual level, we only get superficial insight into what contributes to it. This can lead us to focus on only biology and behaviour, and ignore the many other factors in society which contribute to both individual and population health. Essentially, we are too 'zoomed in' to see the bigger picture. When we zoom out, it allows us to see patterns and trends in bigger populations. We can then apply our sociological imagination to unpack the broader influences on health, wellness and problems which affect many people rather than just one. This is useful not only because it enriches our understanding, but because it helps us to see where we can target population-level strategies to prevent a problem or reduce its impact. These solutions are more significant because they reach beyond an individual to affect many people at the same time.

In western cultures, using sociological imagination does not always come naturally; the tendency is to focus on health in a medical sense and lay the responsibility on individuals to make healthy choices. This has led to some issues being dismissed as personal problems, although we know that they can have social or cultural origins. For example, unemployment, drug use, gambling, depression and sexual harassment are just a few of the many social issues which are often dismissed as personal problems. In fact, each of these issues affects a great number of people in Australia, and disproportionately affects some subgroups of the population. Attempting to solve each at the individual level would not only be costly and time-consuming, but also would not address the society-level factors which shaped the problems.

What does applying a sociological imagination mean in practical terms? Famous British sociologist Anthony Giddens (1983) suggests looking at three components in a sociological analysis: historical, cultural and critical factors. Australian sociologist Evan Willis (2011) added a fourth dimension: structural factors. Unpacking these four components will help in understanding the societal influences shaping an issue. Figure 2.1 illustrates the questions relevant to each component, and shows that sometimes the components can overlap.

Figure 2.1 Four components of a sociological analysis

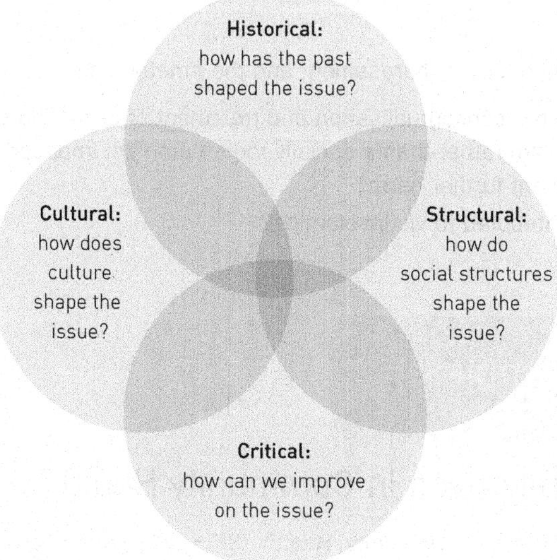

Adapted from Germov (2019).

We now unpack the issue of sexual harassment in Hollywood, using the four components to guide the investigation. One person reporting sexual harassment could be treated as a unique case—this could be classified as a personal problem. But if the reports are compiled (as encouraged by the #metoo campaign), it is clear that there are bigger problems than just one harasser and one person who has been harassed. In terms of historical factors, we might consider the long-standing gender inequalities in society. In the entertainment industry, there is a history of sexual objectification of women in film and media. Females have historically been less likely to be in positions of power in this industry, making up a small proportion of directors, producers, writers and executives. Next, the cultural factors might overlap with historical factors in the way that women are, and have been, valued in western society. We might consider our broader culture, and the specific culture of Hollywood and how men were raised to respect and treat women. We could investigate double standards for men and women in relation to sexual behaviour (i.e. men being socially rewarded for sexual 'conquests', and women being condemned for 'promiscuity'). Structural factors which might be relevant to this issue include policies for reporting harassment and the absence of protections for victims of harassment. Some sociologists might consider that factors such as race and class also constitute structural factors.

Finally, critical factors might involve improving gender equity in the entertainment industry, including improved cultural attitudes to and respect for women. We might consider the need for improved reporting systems and support for victims of harassment, as well as measures to deter it from occurring.

This activity involved applying sociological imagination by thinking about the society-wide issues which might influence an individual's behaviour or experience. The critical factors particularly help us to think about what we can do to improve a problem or prevent it from happening.

Stop and Think

Consider the issue of sexual harassment and the #metoo campaign.

- How has society's conceptualisation and treatment of sexual harassment as an individual problem rather than a socially rooted problem impeded our ability to effectively prevent further harm?
- How has it contributed to victim-blaming?

Case Example 2.3

Student Initiatives in Community Health

Student Initiatives in Community Health (SICH) (1975–1992) was a student-run organisation that promoted a social view of health by enabling students to meet people outside their main discipline of study. Importantly, it provided funding for hands-on experience for students in diverse, mostly community-based settings. SICH was established in the mid 1970s, around the same time as the 'Health for All' movement, with funding from the Commonwealth government. The impetus came from medical students who were concerned about deficiencies in their medical education. As noted by O'Sullivan (1979), there were two major concerns: the first was 'a lack of contact with students of other health and welfare disciplines during undergraduate years, allowing little chance for working as a member of an interdisciplinary team', and the second was a 'lack of exposure to people/patients/clients in their own home environment' (p. 98).

SICH quickly expanded to become a national organisation with groups on many campuses, involving students from a wide range of health and welfare courses in regular meetings. One of the major annual events was the national conference. The other major activity was the Vacation Employment Scheme, where students were offered opportunities to have paid placements in health-related organisations.

SICH provided many students with the opportunity to learn skills they were not being taught, such as submission-writing, talking to government policy-makers and learning how government structures operate. SICH was active in encouraging students to become involved and informed about the political background to health and welfare. It was a great example of community development principles in action, with the organisation being run by students for students.

SICH was a precursor to the many current examples of student-based organisations, for example, Students for Sensible Drug Policy has been active both globally (https://ssdp.org/) and across Australia (http://ssdp.org.au/) for 20 years.

Reflection Exercise

Even for health and social care workers who are clinically trained, it is important to understand that health is more than disease. By understanding the multitude of factors beyond the individual which contribute to health, workers can provide more evidenced, client-centred and empathetic practice. Although western medicine still tends towards the biomedical model of health, there are opportunities to integrate a broader understanding of health into your work. For example, a health worker such as a doctor, physiotherapist or dietitian is likely to encounter patients who struggle with obesity alongside other health conditions. Our society has trained us to attribute this to 'poor' behaviour choices, and recommend improved diet and physical activity. A practitioner who has a better understanding of a social model of health will recognise that there are likely to be other contributing factors which shape the patient's behaviours. Do they work long hours? Are there adequate, affordable and accessible facilities for physical activity? Are they a carer, and how does this affect their leisure time? Do they face stigma or even ridicule when entering spaces such as gyms? These broader factors may not be easily solved by one health worker, but recognising them can encourage more empathetic practice.

- Can you think of two ways that you might be able to creatively work with individual patients who are struggling to lose weight? Who else might you need to 'team up' with the do this?

Sometimes health workers need to be activists, too. For instance, associations for health workers (e.g. Australian Medical Association, Dietitians Association of Australia) can be extremely effective at advocating for environmental and policy changes, which can help entire populations to achieve health. It is impossible to do this if the focus is on only one individual, and their behaviour!

- At any one time, there are more than a dozen Australian parliamentary inquiries accepting public submissions. Can you find a Commonwealth government inquiry that is currently accepting public submissions, where your expertise can make a difference? Think broadly about the way public health can impact change.

Summary

Western societies commonly focus on biological aspects of health and illness; this is known as the biomedical model. In response to growing evidence of the model's deficiencies in explaining patterns of disease and inequitable susceptibility, alternative models of understanding health have emerged, which encompass a broader range of influences such as individual psychological factors, behaviour, family factors, social factors, environmental factors, economic factors and political factors. In public health, we try to understand health and well-being with a socio-ecological model of health, acknowledging the complex web of factors which influence individual, community and population well-being. However, there are debates about the capacity of individuals to exercise free will against strong social forces. This is known as the structure–agency debate. The sociological imagination is a term that means thinking about the social factors which shape an issue, including historical, cultural, structural and critical factors.

Tutorial exercises

1. Go to a news website, and pick an article that relates to health in some way. Try applying a sociological imagination analysis to better understand the issue and how it has been shaped by social forces. Unpack the historical, cultural, structural and critical factors involved in the issue.

2. Pick a health topic which is predominantly thought of as biologically caused (e.g. malaria, sexually transmitted infections, influenza). For most of these issues, a lot of money and effort are invested in medications, blood tests, vaccinations and clinical treatment when someone is already infected. What are the limitations of looking at this issue in terms of only biology? What social factors can be targeted to prevent the spread of such illnesses?
3. 'Obesity, gambling problems and drug use are caused by bad genes or poor choices'. Prepare a counter-argument for this statement, using the socio-ecological model of health.
4. How can clinical healthcare workers employ a social or socio-ecological model of health in the way that they work? Pick a specific discipline (e.g. doctor, dietitian) and brainstorm how its practitioners can encompass this holistic view of health into their practice, even if they continue to work in a predominantly clinical role.

Further reading

AIHW (Australian Institute of Health and Welfare) (2018). *Australia's Health 2018*. Canberra: AIHW.

Bambra, C., Gibson, M., Sowden, A., Wright, K., Whitehead, M., & Petticrew, M. (2010). Tackling the wider social determinants of health and inequalities: evidence from systematic reviews. *Journal of Epidemiology and Community Health*, 64(4), 284–291. doi:10.1136/jech.2008.082743

Baum, F. (2016). *The New Public Health: An Australian Perspective*, 4th edn. Melbourne: Oxford University Press.

Germov, J. (2019). Imagining health problems as social issues. In J. Germov (Ed.), *Second Opinion: An Introduction to Health Sociology*, 5th edn (pp. 2–23). Melbourne: Oxford University Press.

Marmot, M., & Wilkinson, R. (Eds) (2006). *Social Determinants of Health*. Oxford: Oxford University Press.

Moore, S., & Kawachi, I. (2017). Twenty years of social capital and health research: a glossary. *Journal of Epidemiology and Community Health*, 71(5), 513–517. doi:10.1136/jech-2016-208313

Rydin, Y., Bleahu, A., Davies, M., Dávila, J., Friel, S., De Grandis, G., Groce, N., Hallal, P., Hamilton, I., Howden-Chapman, P., Lai, K.M., Lim, C.H., Martins, J., Osrin, D., Ridley, I., Scott, I., Taylor, M., Wilkinson, P., & Wilson, J. (2012). Shaping cities for health: complexity and the planning of urban environments in the 21st century. *Lancet*, 379(9831), 2079–2108.

Willis, E. (2011). *The Sociological Quest: An Introduction to the Study of Social Life*, 5th edn. Sydney: Allen & Unwin.

Wright Mills, C. (2000). *The Sociological Imagination*. New York: Oxford University Press.

Walker, R.E., Keane, C.R., & Burke, J.G. (2010). Disparities and access to healthy food in the United States: a review of food deserts literature. *Health and Place*, 16(5), 876–884.

WHO (World Health Organization) (1948). *Constitution.* Geneva: World Health Organization.

WHO (World Health Organization) (1986). World Health Organization: Ottawa charter for health promotion. *Journal of Health Promotion*, 1, 1–4.

Wilkinson, R.G., & Marmot, M. (2003). *Social Determinants of Health: The Solid Facts.* Denmark: World Health Organization.

Willis, E. (2011). *The Sociological Quest: An Introduction to the Study of Life*, 5th edn. Sydney: Allen & Unwin.

Wolfe, D., Carrieri, M.P., & Shepard, D. (2010). Treatment and care for injecting drug users with HIV infection: a review of barriers and ways forward. *Lancet*, 376(9738), 355–366.

Wright Mills, C. (1959). *The Sociological Imagination*. New York: Penguin.

Chapter 3

Culture as a Social Determinant of Health

Pranee Liamputtong and Dusanee Suwankhong

Topics covered

This chapter covers the following topics:

- definitions of culture
- cultural influence on health, illness and well-being
- explanatory model of illness
- culture-bound syndrome
- cultural idiom of distress
- ethnomedicine and folk healing system
- religion, health and healing
- cultural competence

Key terms

cultural awareness
cultural competence
cultural idiom of distress
cultural relativism
cultural sensitivity
culture
culture-bound syndrome
emic
ethnocentrism
ethnomedicine
explanatory model of illness
folk healing
religion
symbolic healing

Introduction

All human beings have to deal with good health, illness, disease, sickness and death. In all human groups, no matter how small or large, whether technologically primitive or advanced, there exists a set of beliefs about the nature of health and illness, its cause and cures, and its relations to other aspects of life (Helman 2007; John 2017; Wiley & Allen 2017). They are conditions which shape an aspect of social experience and cultural knowledge. As such, concepts of health, illness and well-being are likely to reflect a marked cultural influence (Helman 2007; Winkelman 2009; Jones & Creedy 2012). What is seen as health or illness in one location, or by the members of one group, is not always perceived the same way in another (Jones & Creedy 2012; Fleming 2015; Spector 2017; Wiley & Allen 2017).

Culture, as theorised by Winkelman (2009, p. 2), is 'the foundation of everyone's health concerns and practices'. Culture has influence on how individuals and groups experience physical and emotional afflictions, how they deliberate them and, more importantly, from whom they seek help (Ventriglio et al. 2015; John 2017). According to Hunt (2007), culture can affect a person's experience and understanding of a health problem and therefore affect their expectations in relation to therapy. Thus, cultural factors are pivotal to understanding the health and social issues such as drug addiction, problems of the homeless, obesity, HIV/AIDS epidemic, infant mortality, mental illness and sexual violence that confront the world today (Winkelman 2009). Understanding how culture influences health can help health- and social care providers' understanding of health problems and the care their patients need (Winkelman 2009; Brown & Closser 2016).

Culture influences not only how individual health consumers perceive health conditions and appropriate treatments, it also influences the healthcare providers' perspectives. Cultural differences between healthcare providers and their patients can lead to cross-cultural misunderstandings and conflicts which ultimately impact on the quality of healthcare provision. There are plenty of examples of this misunderstanding and conflict in the literature and health practices. In order to avoid this misunderstanding and conflict and to improve healthcare, it is essential to consider the influences of culture on health conditions, concerns, beliefs and practices of individuals. It is suggested that healthcare can be more effective when it is responsive to the cultural needs of consumers. This means that healthcare providers should have knowledge of culture and possess competence in cross-cultural relationship skills (Winkelman 2009).

In this chapter, we focus on several important issues relevant to culture and health. First, we will discuss the concept of culture, the relevance of culture and health, illness and well-being, the explanatory model of illness (EM), culture-bound and culture-reactive syndromes, and cultural idioms of distress. We then look at the folk healing system and religion, health and healing. Last, we focus on cultural competence and its relevance to healthcare.

Conceptualising culture

Culture, according to Wiley and Allen (2017, p. 7), refers to 'patterns of behaviour' which are commonly shared by a group. Culture encompasses the traditions, beliefs, values and practices of a group. To Helman (2007, p. 2), culture is an 'inherited "lens"' through which individuals see and understand the world in which they live, and learn how to inhabit that world. Without such a shared perception of the world, the coherence and stability of any human group will be problematic. Culture determines health issues and concerns that prevail within the society as well as the means that people use for responding to health problems (Winkelman 2009). Culture also includes the social structures that impact on the lives of individuals (Brown & Closser 2016).

Culture
A system of shared ideas, attitudes and practices that defines the social system of its members. It is a way of life that is shared by group members.

It must be noted that culture is not static; it can change and adapt to new circumstances and situations (Helman 2007; Wiley & Allen 2017). This is very true with the migration process that we have witnessed. Thus, Helman suggests that culture is 'a fluid concept'. Additionally, culture is not the only factor that can influence health, illness and well-being. There are other significant factors that can have an impact on individuals' well-being. These include individual (age, gender, ethnicity, experience), educational, socio-economic (social class, poverty, occupation, social support) and environmental factors (Helman 2007; see also Chapter 1 in this volume).

Culture is an indispensable mechanism not only for responsive cross-cultural relations but also for avoiding intercultural conflicts between healthcare providers and their consumers. A crucial means for overcoming these conflicts is the **emic** perspective, or an insider's view, which refers to 'understandings that members of a culture have about themselves' (Wiley & Allen 2017, p. 7). This insider's view (a culture's perspective, worldview, values and assumptions) offers the ground for cross-cultural understandings. For example, instead of seeing eating dirt as a bizarre behaviour of illness, it can be perceived as 'an effective ethnomedical practice' within the cultural group (Winkelman 2009, p. 92).

Emic
An insider perspective of individuals within a culture.

The emic perspective is the basis for embracing **cultural relativism**. It is a term that requires an outsider (such as healthcare providers) to understand their consumers' behaviour in relation to their culture and the rational or meaningful context in which that behaviour occurs (Winkelman 2009). Cultural relativism requires 'reflective judgement' (Fitzgerald 2000) by the healthcare provider; their competence to determine their own expectations, re-assess the foundation for a position, and form new acceptances based on their consumers' perspective of culture (Winkelman 2009; see also 'Cultural competence' section below). Knowledge of cultural values and patterns permits healthcare providers to reconstruct problems and conflicts into consequential behaviour. This can help to avoid ethnocentrism in healthcare. **Ethnocentrism** refers to a profound 'sense of cultural superiority' which leads to a lack of understanding of cultural differences and ultimately damages relationships

Cultural relativism
Understanding other people's behaviour in relation to their culture and the rationale or meaningful context in which that behaviour occurs.

Ethnocentrism
A profound sense of cultural superiority, which leads to a lack of appreciation of cultural differences and damages relationships with other individuals/groups.

with other individuals or groups (Winkelman 2009, p. 88). Ethnocentrism may appear as a negative attitude, such as thinking that other people behave differently due to 'stupidity' or 'inferiority'. Others believe that their own cultural perspectives are legitimate and that other cultures are invalid. Some may not even recognise that they have their own cultural perspectives but see them as an objective system of evaluation. For example, healthcare providers may believe that only biomedicine is an effective means for treating illnesses, and reject other ethnomedical systems that can be efficacious for people in a particular culture. Such healthcare providers lack awareness of cultural differences and their relevance in healthcare (Winkelman 2009, p. 88).

Cultural sensitivity
A capability to build relationships with individuals from different cultures through culturally appropriate conduct and care. It involves recognition of cultural differences and the ability to accommodate them appropriately.

Ethnocentrism stands in stark contrast to **cultural sensitivity**. Cultural sensitivity requires healthcare providers to adapt to cultural differences. Such adaptations require healthcare providers to adjust their communication and behaviour to cultural differences so that they can interact with consumers from other cultures appropriately. Cultural sensitivity permits healthcare providers to question their own beliefs and replace them with expectations from other cultures in order to accurately interpret their behaviours and actions (Winkelman 2009).

Health, illness, well-being and culture

Health and illness are socially constructed. Thus, different cultures have different perceptions of health, illness and well-being (Fleming 2015; Brown & Closser 2016; Spector 2017; Wiley & Allen 2017). As we have pointed out, cultural understandings of health and illness operate as an important aspect in determining health and illness of individuals (Julian 2019). What embodies health, illness and well-being in one society can differ from another (Brown & Closser 2016). In some cultures, obesity is seen as unhealthy, but in others obese people are perceived to be healthy and thin people are viewed as sickly (Winkelman 2009). For example, the thin body ideal is seen as a symbol of health in the west. But in sub-Saharan Africa, it may signify malnutrition and illness (Brown & Closser 2016).

While health is well understood by most people in mainstream Australian society, within Indigenous Australian cultures, there is no single word for health (Fleming 2015). Concepts of health and well-being entail 'relationship with family, community and connectedness with traditional land or country rather than referring to an individual as a separate entity' (Taylor 2008, p. 6). Health, to Indigenous people, is 'about the totality of their environment' (Fleming 2015, p. 5). These collective approaches to health are held by many Indigenous people (Levin & Browner 2005; Fleming 2015; AIHW 2018). Within the Indigenous context, the concept of 'well-being' has a broader meaning than 'health' since it embraces wider relationships and connections with the environment and community (Taylor 2008; Fleming 2015; see also Chapter 8). Social determinants of health, for Australian Indigenous people, embrace 'cultural identity, family, participation in cultural activities, and access to traditional lands' (AIHW 2018, p. 335).

For Thai people, being in good health is understood as being normal and strong, and free of illness and disease (Mahanarongchai 2015). Within the Thai worldview, this understanding symbolises the characteristics of people's capability and is related to traditional understanding of *me ar-kaan crop sam-sib-song pra-garn* (having the complete 32 components of the body) in order to fulfil a person's normal routine such as eating, sleeping and working (Suwankhong 2011). Thai knowledge about the causes of good health and illness has been part of the culture for centuries. The causes include *kam* (bad karma), loss of soul, imbalance of bodily elements and supernatural beings (Muecke 1979; Liamputtong 2007; Lundberg & Kerdonfag 2010; Liamputtong et al. 2012; Liamputtong & Suwankhong 2015).

Hmong people, including the Hmong ethnic community in Australia, have a number of beliefs concerning supernatural beings that can cause illness and death. Health, for Hmong people, is seen as a combination of 'religion, lost souls and spirits, a balance of virtually all aspects of life' (Winkelman 2009, p. 4). Although they believe the primary cause of such misfortune is the loss of soul (see Case Example 3.1), they also see that some illnesses are due to natural or organic factors. The Hmong are conscious of the influence of natural forces on a person's good health or illness (Winkelman 2009). When a woman has just given birth, her body is believed to be in a state of disequilibrium with nature. She is therefore prohibited from participating in daily work for 30 days. During this period, she needs to rest and be mindful of 'cold' and 'wrong' food. Hot food, mainly chicken cooked with herbal medicines, is consumed for the entire period of 30 days. Failure to do this is believed to result in ill health later in life (Liamputtong Rice 2000).

Traditional healers, referred to as shamans, are an important part of Hmong life (Cha 2003; Symonds 2004; Liamputtong 2009). In Australia, there is at least one shaman in each state, and there are at least four shamans in Melbourne. The rituals of a shaman are mainly concerned with fertility, protection and curing (Cha 2003; Culhane-Pera et al. 2004; Liamputtong 2009; Winkelman 2009). The majority of Hmong in Australia continue to seek help from traditional healers despite the availability of care within the Australian healthcare system. This is most obvious when the Hmong are confronted with severe illnesses and health-related issues which are seen to be closely related to the Hmong cosmos (such as childhood illnesses, burns, bone fractures, infertility and childbirth).

Case Example 3.1

Childbirth and soul loss

The story of Mai

This case study is from Pranee's research with women from the Hmong ethnic community in Melbourne (Liamputtong Rice et al. 1994; Liamputtong 2010). Mai was 34 years old, married and had six children. Four children were born in a refugee camp in Thailand and two in Australia. Five of her children were born naturally. However, when Mai had her last child she was advised that she needed a caesarean operation since the baby was in a transverse lie. Mai refused the caesarean operation and insisted that she could give birth naturally. She was told that if she attempted a vaginal birth the baby might not survive. Because of the concern about the survival of her baby, Mai agreed to a caesarean operation. However, the caesarean operation was done under a general anaesthetic and she was alone in the operating theatre as her husband was not allowed to stay with her. Since the birth of her last child, Mai had been physically unwell. She had seen a number of specialists about her health, but they were not able to find anything wrong with her.

Mai believed that while she was unconscious under the general anaesthetic, one of her souls, which takes care of her well-being, left her body and was unable to re-enter. She believed that because she was moved out of the operating theatre and regained consciousness in a recovery room, her soul was left in the operating theatre. She strongly believed that the departure of this soul was the main cause of her ill health because she had frequent bad dreams in the last 10 months, occurring two or three times a week. Each time, after the dream, she felt very ill and experienced bad pains. In her dreams, she wandered to far-away places. She did not know where she was going since she had never seen those places before. It was as if she just had to keep walking and there was no ending. Mai believed this was a sign that her lost soul was wandering in another world.

Pranee asked if Mai had considered a soul-calling ceremony at the theatre where she had the operation, where the soul would be waiting. Mai's quick response was that this would not be possible—the hospital staff would not understand her customs and would refuse the request since the ceremony involved taking a live chicken into the operating theatre and burning an incense stick there. Her husband commented that since he was not able to accompany his wife into the operating theatre, it would be impossible to gain permission to perform a ceremony which is alien to western healthcare providers. If Mai were unable to perform a soul-calling ceremony, the family believed that the soul would transfer into another living thing as it had left Mai's body for a lengthy period of time. As a consequence, her health would continue to deteriorate.

Concerned about Mai's well-being, Pranee and colleagues contacted the hospital—the Deputy Chief Executive Officer agreed to the request. Her positive response was that 'the hospital is more than happy to do anything for the woman if this can help her', and she gave the name of a staff member to contact regarding arrangements.

Pranee was told that the operating theatre was busy during the week, so she suggested that Mai have the soul-calling ceremony done during a weekend. Since the date was not important, Mai agreed. At 8am one Sunday, Mai, her husband and a shaman met Pranee and her bi-cultural research assistant at the hospital. The charge nurses in the operating theatre were very helpful and supportive. They showed Mai where she was put to sleep and where she regained consciousness. They also showed Mai the path along which she was carried to the operating theatre because they wanted to ensure that the ceremony was performed with full knowledge. At 8.30am the shaman performed a soul-calling ritual in the operating theatre. It took him about 20 minutes to persuade Mai's soul to come back to her. To ensure that the soul was not confused with the body and where it belonged, the shaman also performed the ritual at the spot where Mai regained consciousness in the recovery room. This took only 10 minutes. Then the group went to Mai's house to perform a ceremony welcoming the soul back to its home.

Stop and Think

The positive aspects of this story are the hospital's agreement to allow Mai and her family to perform a soul-calling ceremony in the operating theatre, and the staff's concern for her well-being. This illustrates that mainstream health services can provide culturally sensitive care to consumers from different cultural backgrounds, if informed of those cultural beliefs and practices.

- Could this situation, involving the need for a soul-calling ceremony, have been prevented? How do you think it could have been avoided?
- If you were a healthcare provider where Mai gave birth, how would you respond to her case?
- What would you do to accommodate cultural differences among your clients?

Explanatory model of illness

In every culture, illness, the response to illness by the person experiencing it and treating it, and the social institutions relating to it are all interconnected (Kleinman 1980; Winkelman 2009). This means that a person's beliefs about their illness, the behaviours they display including their treatment expectations and the ways in which they are responded to by their family and treating health practitioners, all form their social reality (Kleinman 1980). These aspects of social reality, especially those relating to attitudes concerning the illness, combined with clinical relationships and healing activities, form a person's clinical reality (Kleinman 1980). Clinical realities are often viewed differently by clinicians and patients. Thus, it is important to understand a patient's clinical reality since discrepancies between views can lead to poor patient care and management (Kleinman 1978). One framework for understanding a patient's clinical reality is through understanding their **explanatory model of illness** (EM).

Explanatory model of illness
The perspective on the nature of illness concerns of an individual and healthcare providers, including its causes and the appropriate health-seeking strategy.

The EM refers to interpretive understandings that 'patients, families, and practitioners have about a specific illness episode' (Kleinman 1988, p. 121). Individuals, like clinicians, have culturally based models for interpreting or explaining their symptoms, and will use those models as a basis when seeking the most appropriate treatment for their symptoms (Kleinman 1980; Winkelman 2009).

According to Kleinman (1980), local healthcare systems include three structural components: professional, popular and folk. The professional sector represents the principles and practice of modern medicine, where knowledge and skills are based on scientific work through legally mandated education systems. Such professional practices are performed by modern health professionals authorised by licence. The popular sector includes non-professional and lay practices, including self-care. The majority of health problems and illness episodes are managed by this sector. The folk sector also falls into the category of non-professional practice. Folk knowledge and skills are gained outside education programs from traditional sources. Practitioners include sacred and secular healers who are folk healers, shamans and folk psychotherapists. The folk sector embraces a number of traditional cultural healing practices which are generally excluded from a professional healthcare system. These encompass 'natural and physical healers (herbalists, midwives and masseuses)', 'psychological healers (diviners, fortune-tellers)' and 'religious and spiritual healers' (Winkelman 2009, p. 165).

These different sectors serve differing health needs of individuals according to their cultural and social contexts. Individuals have their own criteria for selecting a healing model that best suits their condition and beliefs. They make healthcare choices according to their explanatory framework for health and illness (Suwankhong 2011).

The EM is a framework that can be used to understand an individual's health beliefs, illness behaviours and treatment expectations regardless of their cultural background. The five major questions that the EM seeks to explain include (1) the cause of the problem, (2) the time and mode of onset of symptoms, (3) the pathophysiological processes involved, (4) the course of sickness (nature and severity) and (5) the treatment for the condition (Kleinman 1980). As clinicians and patients tend to have different EMs, mutual understanding of each party's model is crucial in the development of an effective treatment plan (Katon & Kleinman 1981). This is particularly important when patients and clinicians come from different cultural and social backgrounds, since they are unlikely to share the same illness and treatment expectations (Katon & Kleinman 1981). As health, illness and healthcare are part of a person's cultural system, this means that a person's cultural beliefs play a role in shaping their EM, which in turn will strongly influence their perception of clinical reality and thus their behaviour (Kleinman et al. 2006). Therefore, it is only through understanding people's EM that treatment will become effective, as misunderstanding and miscommunications between clinician and patient EMs are minimised. For example, the EM theoretical framework can be used to explore older people's EM of falls, to gain insight into the reasons for older people's participation and adherence or non-adherence to an exercise program for falls prevention (Lam et al. 2015; Liamputtong et al. 2017), or reasons for HIV-positive individuals to adhere to medication regimes (Liamputtong et al. 2015).

Stop and Think

Recently, there was an outbreak of Ebola in the Democratic Republic of Congo. By May 2018, the outbreak had killed 27 people there. Health officials were extremely concerned by the disease's presence in Mbandaka, a city of some 10 million people and a crowded trading hub upstream from DR Congo's capital, Kinshasa. In late May, three patients infected with the deadly Ebola virus escaped from a hospital quarantine. The patients were taken out of the hospital by family members so that they could attend a religious ritual as part of the healing process. The family members did not want the patients to be kept in quarantine. Two patients died a day after their escape and healthcare workers had great concerns about the spread of the disease in the community.

- Using the EM discussed above, what can we say about the families' non-compliance with quarantine restrictions? Assuming that the need for quarantine had been explained to the families, why would they remove the patients?

Culture-bound and culture-reactive syndromes

Culture-bound syndrome refers to 'culturally specific systems' of emotional, psychological, cognitive and behavioural adversities which emanate from the interpersonal, psychological and social agitations of a specific culture (Winkelman 2009, p. 231). Often, they are termed 'culturally recognised illnesses' (Helman 2007). They are symbolised by markings of troubling individual experience or bizarre behaviour, which are seen as 'illnesses' within a culture. These aberrant behaviours have been given local names (Wiley & Allen 2017, p. 371). Essentially, culture-bound syndromes are 'folk illnesses' and are legitimate to the person who suffers from them (Wiley & Allen 2017). Some culture-bound syndromes have been incorporated into the DSM-5 as western psychiatric diseases, but many syndromes are excluded in biomedical (psychiatric) systems (Wiley & Allen 2017).

Culture-bound syndrome
A set of symptoms specific to a particular culture and generally not recognised by biomedicine.

Culture-bound syndromes, according to Helman (2007, p. 266), embrace a number of symbolic meanings (moral, psychological or social) for both the individual and those around them. Often, they connect the individual with wider social matters, for example, tensions in relationships with others and the community, with the natural environment and with supernatural beings. In many cases, the syndromes play a crucial role in deliberating and justifying 'anti-social emotions and social conflicts in a culturally patterned way'.

Culturally recognised illnesses include, for example, soul loss, spirit possession (in Africa and Asia), penis shrinkage (*koro* in China), extreme anxiety about loss of semen (*dhat* in India), magical fright (*susto* in Spain), startle-matching syndrome (*latah* in Malaysia), sudden violent attacks on people, animals and inanimate objects (*amok* in Malaysia), voodoo death (death following a curse from a sorcerer in the Caribbean), and nightmare attacks or deaths (*tsog tsuam* among the Hmong who migrated to the US and the Hmong in Laos) (Helman 2007; Winkelman 2009; Wiley & Allen 2017).

The traditional view of culture-bound syndromes implies that they are 'cultural illnesses' and only occur in a specific culture. As such, it signifies that the syndrome is a result of cultural and social causes (Winkelman 2009). This has been criticised by some anthropologists (Hahn 1995). A preferred alternative term is 'culture-reactive syndrome' (Hughes 1985). The concept of culture-reactive syndrome suggests that there is a possibility that a number of cultures may produce comparable psychological sufferings. The culture-reactive syndrome posits that 'social relations' or 'local cultural conditions' render members of the society susceptible to specific types of afflictions. For example, cultures which incite considerable sexual anxiety will bring about the 'psychological generation of anxiety', which appears as the 'genital retraction syndrome' (Winkelman 2009, p. 231). A culture-reactive syndrome concept underscores the importance of the socio-cultural factors that may lead to specific kinds of disorders. For instance, socio-cultural factors in industrialised societies may induce culture-bound syndromes in conditions such as premenstrual syndrome, agoraphobia (fear of leaving the house), driver anger, obesity and anorexia nervosa (Winkelman 2009).

Case Example 3.2

Hwabyung and Korean immigrant women

Hwabyung refers to a local psychiatric illness commonly found in Korean culture. The fourth edition of the Diagnostic Statistical Manual of Mental Disorder (DSM-IV), published in 1994, includes *hwabyung* as a Korean culture-bound syndrome caused by 'a prolonged suppression of anger'.

The literal meaning of *hwabyung* is 'fire illness', which is synonymously used with 'anger syndrome' (Lee 2015). The word *hwabyung* combines *hwa*, which refers to fire (anger) and *byung* (disease). *Hwabyung* is also referred to as *wol-hwabyung* which means 'suffocating anger illness' (Lee 2015). It is perceived as a culture-bound syndrome since it appears mainly among Korean women when they conceal hate, anger, frustration and other negative feelings regarding their family or significant others. If these feelings are suppressed for too long, some psychosomatic symptoms will result. These include anger, anxiety, panic, depression, palpitations, fatigue, loss of motivation for life, feelings of hopelessness, insomnia, aches and pains, stuffy feeling in the chest, or feelings of approaching destruction (Choi & Yeom 2011; Lee 2015).

Traditional Korean medicine suggests that *hwabyung* is caused by a neurotic fire (*hwa*) which occurs due to extreme distress that an individual suffers for a prolonged period (Lee 2013). The chronic stress causes an imbalance between *yang* (positive components) and *yin* (negative components). The neurotic fire (*hwa*) can accrue in the head, heart, chest, liver and stomach. Because of the deficiency of *yin*, the neurotic fire can become over-aroused, and this aggravates *hwabyung* (Min 2009).

Research has indicated that women are particularly susceptible to *hwabyung* because of the patriarchal norms of Korean culture (Khim & Lee 2003; Min 2009; Choi & Yeom 2011; Lee 2015). Research has linked *hwabyung* with life sufferings of Korean women including issues related to child-rearing, conjugal relationships, and unfair criticism from their in-laws. As such, *hwabyung* can be seen as a psychological phenomenon aggravated by the marginalised social position of Korean women.

Hwabyung has also been found to affect a large number of Korean immigrant women in US (Choi & Yeom 2011; Lee 2015). Due to their multiple roles as mothers, wives and wage-earners with few supportive resources, Korean immigrant women are particularly prone to *hwabyung*. Due to language and racial barriers, most Korean women work as dry-cleaners, assistants at restaurants and grocery stores in Korean ethnic communities. At home, the women are expected to perform their traditional obligations by having full responsibility for child-rearing and household chores. They encounter high levels of conflict with their husband when they ask for a more egalitarian conjugal relationship. The increased stress in their everyday lives manifests as *hwabyung* symptoms (Lee 2015).

Stop and Think

Generally, about 10 per cent of Korean men experience *hwabyung* symptoms. But after the financial crisis in 1997 which seriously affected the Korean economy, 30 per cent of men showed signs of *hwabyung* symptoms. It has been shown that *hwabyung* also affects a number of Korean immigrant men in the US.

- What do you think contributed to higher experiences of *hwabyung* among Korean men in Korea and in the US?

It has been suggested that the inability to fulfil the socially prescribed masculine role of family provider may provoke *hwabyung* symptoms among Korean men. It has also been suggested that challenges in life, including economic deprivation and difficulties relating to settlement in a new homeland, contribute to *hwabyung* symptoms among Korean male immigrants.

- What are your views about these suppositions? What can the social determinants of health explain about them?

Stop and Think

Littlewood and Lipsedge (1997) suggested that a number of conditions common in the contemporary UK could be perceived as western culture-bound syndromes. They identified one disorder, referred to as 'housewives' agoraphobia' or the 'housewives' disease'. They argue that housewives' agoraphobia can be perceived as 'a ritual display of (and a protest against) the cultural pressures' as well as 'injunctions on women, especially those that state that "a woman's place is in the home"'. By 'over-conforming' to this banality, the woman has an opportunity to 'dramatize the situation' and 'mobilize a caring family around herself'. Simultaneously, she can 'restrict her husband's movements by forcing him to stay at home and look after her' (Helman 2007, p. 267).

- What is your view about this western culture-bound syndrome?
- Are there other common illnesses that can be classified as western culture-bound syndromes?
- What about shoplifting committed by well-off, middle-aged women?
- What about anorexia nervosa and bulimia nervosa, which predominantly occur among white, middle-class girls who have access to abundant quantities of food? Should these be seen as western culture-bound syndromes?

Cultural idiom of distress

Cultural idiom of distress
A means for individuals to express their distress within the socio-cultural setting. It is often used as a culturally sanctioned way for an individual to express dissatisfaction with their position or role at a particular time.

Culture determines what idioms of distress are used to deliberate on an individual's suffering (Ventriglio et al. 2015; Wiley & Allen 2017). Idioms of distress refer to 'socially and culturally resonant means of experiencing and expressing distress in local worlds' (Nichter 1981, p. 405). Often, an idiom of distress is used as 'a culturally sanctioned way' for an individual to express dissatisfaction with their position or role at a particular time (Ventriglio et al. 2016, p. 3). **Cultural idioms of distress** are means for an individual to deliberate distress that may not have particular symptoms. They offer collective ways for people to discuss their shared experience and articulate personal or social matters (Tajan 2015; Toffle 2015).

An example of this is 'nerves', which can be linked to many health issues. A person having 'nerves' could be suffering from stress, anxiety, pre-menstrual syndrome, and so on. The idiom allows individuals to articulate a common experience that people from the same cultural group understand. It provides an opportunity for people to 'share and sympathise without knowing exactly what this problem is' (Toffle 2015, p. 450).

Idioms of distress are used as alternative ways of articulating difficulties, and link explanations of suffering to personal and cultural meanings. Distress may arise out of interpersonal struggles, cultural clashes and financial difficulties. These idioms of distress have social repercussions but they are understood and accepted by the family and others in the society (Desai & Chaturvedi 2017). For example, Cambodians often make sense of dizziness, palpitations, physical weakness and fears of death as *khyâl cap* or 'wind attacks' (Meyer et al. 2014; Hinton et al. 2015).

Khyâl cap is brought about by burdened thoughts, particular aromas that connect with bad recollections, and being in cramped areas (Toffle 2015).

There are several cultural idioms of distress that are well-known. *Hikikomori* in Japan is the social withdrawal phenomenon which has afflicted a large number of people. Individuals who experience *hikikomori* shut themselves in their room, often at their family's home, for many months or even years without participating in social functions or responsibilities (Tajan 2015). It has become a public health concern in Japan (De Luca 2017). There are over half a million individuals who suffer *hikikomori* in Japan. Notably, most of them are young men. According to Harding (2018), there are two main explanations for *hikikomori*. Socially, *hikikomori* reflects problems within contemporary Japanese society, including the nuclearisation of family, urbanisation and loss of community, the impact of the internet, problems with schools (academic pressures, bullying and so on), and instability of the job market for young people. Culturally, *hikikomori* is seen to be influenced by *amae*, a deep-rooted Japanese cultural value that an individual should be in harmony with others, often depending on and endlessly seeking affection and help from others. *Hikikomori* has been viewed sociologically as a behaviour of youths who transgress the 'Japanese cultural norm of strong determination and academic and professional achievement' among young people (De Luca 2017, p. e5). De Luca (2017, p. e4) suggests that the 'over-representation of males contributes to advocating a cultural and social determination in this syndrome' because 'boys undergo greater requirements and stronger pressure to succeed than do girls' in modern Japanese society.

However, the idiom of distress that appears to be common across cultural groups is that of excessive thinking—the 'thinking too much' idiom (Kaiser et al. 2015; Den Hertog et al. 2016). In their systematic review of the 'thinking too much' idiom, Kaiser and colleagues (2015, p. 178) found that typically 'thinking too much' contributed to worry and/or intrusive thoughts. The content of thoughts, however, differed widely both within and across settings. Common symptoms associated with the idiom included lack of interest, absentmindedness, loss of memory, poor concentration, tiredness, loss of appetite, depressed mood, sleep problems, impaired ability to function in work and family life, and social isolation/withdrawal. Perceived causes included financial difficulties, traumatic life events, illnesses, structural barriers and social relationships. Importantly, Kaiser and colleagues found that women were found to be more likely to experience 'thinking too much' and its consequences.

Among women in rural Haiti, *reflechi twòp* is the idiom of distress associated with 'thinking too much'. Thinking too much is a culturally acceptable response in Haiti to sadness or traumatic life events, and features social isolation, weight loss and sleeping problems. Kaiser and McLean (2015, p. 278) suggest that the essence of 'thinking too much' among these women is persistent thought, especially 'an unwavering focus on a singular problem, to the point of seeming detached or far away'. It is marked by thought which is not 'directed toward a solution' but only to the problem. Often, it occurs because of material hardship, such as lack of money or food. This can be heightened by lack of activities. Generally, these hardships are caused by external factors such as poor health, job loss or failed crops. *Reflechi twòp* is also embodied as 'failure to achieve one's goals or fulfil social expectations, which brings about shame'.

Table 3.1 presents the 'thinking too much' idioms of distress in several socio-cultural settings.

Table 3.1 'Thinking too much' idiom

Society	Idioms of distress
Thailand	*Khit maak*
Laos	*Khut lai*
Vietnam	*Nghi nhieu qua*
Cambodia	*Keut chreun, kut careen*
Malaysia	*Banyak fikir*
Indonesia	*Kepikiran, Ma-'tangna'-tangna'*
Timor-Leste	*Hanoin barak*
Papua New Guinea	*Tingting planti*
Haiti	*Reflechi twòp, Kalkile twòp*
Nicaragua	*Pensando mucho*
Mexico	*Anda pensando*
Zimbabwe	*Kufungisisa*
Uganda	*Alowooza nyo*
Kenya	*Jachir*
Ghana	*Taamebubasugbor*

Ethnomedicine and the folk healing system

Ethnomedicine
Healing practices commonly observed by members of a culture.

Folk healing
Cultural healing practices and practitioners prevalent in most traditional cultures, generally not part of the professional medical system.

Ethnomedicine refers to the healing traditions which can be found in every culture. Similar to herbs, which have contributed significantly to the development of the biomedical pharmacopoeia, ethnomedical practices can play an important role in healthcare (Winkelman 2009). Folk healing remains a significant contributor to local healthcare in most countries (Moore & McClean 2010; Shankar et al. 2012; Moe et al. 2014; Qamar 2015; Berdon et al. 2016; Zuma et al. 2016; Edae & Mulu 2017; Biswal et al. 2017; John 2017). Healing traditions often overlap with those of the professional and popular sectors. **Folk healing** can be the primary care model in societies where a professional sector does not exist, or can continue to play an effective role in community health alongside the professional sector.

The principles and practices of folk healing are related to natural, folk and spiritual remedies and involve the use of plants and herbs, physical manipulation, spiritual healing rituals and religious practices (Kayne 2010; Shankar et al. 2012; Qamar 2015; Berdon et al. 2016; Zuma et al. 2016; Edae & Mulu 2017; Biswal et al. 2017; John 2017). These principles are grounded in tradition and are continually practised by healers through the many healing traditions that link the historical circumstances, social contexts and cultural beliefs of local peoples.

The folk healing model gives priority to holistic healthcare (Winkelman 2009; Shankar et al. 2012; Zuma et al. 2016; Berdon et al. 2016; Biswal et al. 2017; John 2017). Snyder and Lindquist (2006, p. 6) contend that its healing method is 'considered physically, emotionally, mentally, and spiritually. The goal is to create harmony or balance within the person'. It defines healthy people as those with a balance between the physical, mental, social and spiritual dimensions. It provides people with a chance to obtain healthcare because of its philosophy, which focuses on personal responsibility for all healthcare decisions. The advantage of traditional healing is that it provides patients with choices that help them to understand the world and access holistic healthcare (Goldner 2004; Spector 2017).

The strategy of traditional healing is to bring about healing through the balance of all dimensions of experience within the body (Kleinman 1980; Helman 2007; John 2017). The treatment often includes religious ceremonies or spiritual rites alongside the primary treatment method. These comprehensive healing techniques are designed to return people to normal physical health and help them to achieve a balanced life-style after recovery (Golomb 1985; Helman 2007; Biswal et al. 2017; John 2017).

To provide such holistic healthcare, the healers involve family members, friends and relatives, who can participate informally in the healing process (Joe 2012; Suwankhong & Liamputtong 2014; Zuma et al. 2016). The healers provide personal care and spend as much time with patients as needed. This strategy strengthens relationships and reduces communication problems between healers and patients, creating a positive atmosphere that can help patients cope better with their health problems (Spector 2017). Folk healers adapt their services to suit patients' contexts, culture and life-styles. They do not separate the patient from family, friends and relatives. Patients' hopes for recovery are increased because they are with familiar people who share their sufferings and participate in the healing process, and decisions about treatments can be made in a familiar environment (Suwankhong & Liamputtong 2014).

In most traditional societies, folk healing was the dominant medical system before the introduction of western biomedicine. Its role continues in rural areas of developing countries because of the lack of access to modern healthcare facilities (Kulsomboon & Adthasit 2007; Shankar et al. 2012). But even as modern healthcare facilities and resources increase in local areas, people continue to seek alternative care from the folk sector (Helman 2007). People give many reasons for selecting folk healing over biomedical care. The most frequently mentioned reason is that biomedicine has failed to provide a satisfactory level of healing. The need to travel long distances to access western-oriented medical facilities is another disadvantage which makes people turn to alternative treatments. Folk treatments can reduce aggravated symptoms as well as produce fewer negative side-effects from prolonged treatment because it uses natural products (Kusinitz 1992; WHO 2002). Using readily available natural resources provides cost-efficient care, and folk products and methods are increasingly used in the mainstream health system (Kulsomboon & Adthasit 2007; Chokevivat et al. 2010).

People often consider that folk healing can cure illnesses they believe to be caused by social and spiritual circumstances (Helman 2007; see Case Example 3.1). These illnesses may not have clear physical symptoms, but are manifested through emotional signs. Folk medicine tends to be more effective in such cases because it operates within an individual's worldview, and thus provides better support in achieving holistic health among Indigenous peoples (Tantipidoke 2005; Chuengsatiansup 2007). Modern biomedicine may not be able to help because this kind of illness requires knowledge of the individual's social and cultural contexts (Helman 2007).

Folk healing thus plays a significant part in healthcare, highlighting traditional and alternative healing methods developed by local people using wisdom and local knowledge (Kulsomboon & Adthasit 2007; John 2017). Finding ways of using these resources has been recognised as a significant priority and a key direction of health policy development in many communities (BPS 2009).

Religion, health and healing

Religion
An organised system of beliefs, practices and rituals that have gradually developed within established traditions. It connects to health and well-being at myriad levels.

Symbolic healing
A healing method that involves the use of religious beliefs to arouse the healing response of an individual.

Religion refers to an organised system of beliefs, practices and rituals that have gradually developed within established traditions. Religion offers closeness to the transcendent (e.g. God, Allah, HaShem, Brahman, Buddha, Dao) and cultivates an understanding of responsibility and relationship in residing together in a community. Often, religion involves the mystical or supernatural, has a particular set of beliefs and rules for conduct within a social group, and has a belief system for what happens after death (Mahanarongchai 2015; Liamputtong 2017).

Religion has been shown to connect to health and well-being at myriad levels (Winkelman 2009; Sirikanchana 2015; John 2017; Spector 2017). It provides '**symbolic healing**' to individuals and communities (Kleinman 1973). It is particularly valuable in times of stress. During stressful life events, individuals often to turn to religion to deal with their stress and anxiety. Religion provides a sense of control and assists them in accommodating their adverse situations. In addition, religious beliefs and practices persuade individuals to engender better decisions, which can assist them in modifying their stressful situations. Religious activities may offer a greater sense of peace and hence reduce anxiety and stress. A number of clinical trials have shown that religious interventions reduced participants' anxiety levels. Recent research on eastern spiritual techniques, such as Buddhist mindfulness meditation, has also demonstrated a reduction in individuals' anxiety (Liamputtong 2017).

Religion functions as a resiliency factor between an individual's perceived stress and mental health. It plays a crucial role in the prevention and treatment of mental health problems. Generally, research has pointed to the beneficial effects of religion on mental health. Religious individuals tend to report better well-being, better mental health, higher quality of life and less perceived stress than non-religious individuals. They also report lower rates of anxiety, depression and suicide. For people with mental health disorders, religion functions as an important source of social support, which has been shown to mitigate emotional distress and emotional disorders. Involvement in religious groups offers protective and health-promoting influences on individuals' mental health. It also fosters hopefulness, which enhances individuals' resilience when dealing with stressful circumstances (Liamputtong 2017).

Religion is often a resource for coping with the emotional consequences of illness experiences. It provides both intrapersonal and interpersonal resources to deal with distress and promote positive adaptation to life (see Case Example 3.2). Religious beliefs, according to Winkelman (2009, p. 351), provide 'a sense of control' to individuals when they can stipulate their situation as 'known possibilities' and pay attention to coping behaviours that can reduce distress. When illness or misfortune occurs, people tend to ask why it happens and what can be done to alleviate the suffering and restore well-being. Winkelman (2009, p. 351) suggests that 'religion provides explanations, a worldview that makes maladies meaningful in the context of cultural life and may heal (whole) the individual by relieving emotional conflicts and distress'.

Thai Buddhists see HIV/AIDS as 'a disease of Karma (*rok khong khon mee kam*)' (Jirapaet 2001, p. 26). Research in Thailand revealed that people living with HIV/AIDS believed that their suffering was the consequence of their own *wen kam* (karma) (Klunklin & Greenwood 2005; Kobotani & Engstrom 2005; Ross et al. 2007a, 2007b; Liamputtong et al. 2012). Most women in Liamputtong and colleagues' study (2012) considered that their HIV status was brought about by their own *wen kam*. In Thai culture, *wen kam* refers to a bad or evil deed that the person has committed, which will result in disastrous consequences. The law of karma is that every action, be it good or bad, has its consequences (Chaiyasuj 2015; Sirikanchana 2015). The outcomes may happen immediately after an individual has performed the act, long afterward, or even in a subsequent life, but they are inescapable. From the strong belief in the law of karma among Buddhists, it follows that the state of an individual's present existence is the consequence of the karma accumulated in previous lives. The more good deeds are accumulated from a past life, the better and happier the state of being in the present one. This also holds true for bad deeds; usually, this results in the *wen kam* of an individual.

Many women used religious beliefs to cope with their health condition more positively. According to Plattner and Meiring (2006, p. 244), ascribing an HIV-positive status to religion and faith made the health status more meaningful. This ascription not only brings 'a purpose to their infection but also hope'. Attributing their HIV status to their karma can be a means of coping with difficulties in their lives when there is no other hope left. Religion performs a crucial role in the process of meaning-making. Ascribing health conditions to something beyond individual control, such as karma, is a mechanism that makes the reality of life more meaningful and comprehensible. In Liamputtong et al.'s study (2012), the women's belief that their HIV status was the result of their own *wen kam* was a beneficial rationale that allowed them to develop hope by doing good deeds. Hope allowed them to focus on their future and not give up on life.

Case Example 3.3

Religion as a therapeutic landscape of healing: women living with breast cancer

Breast cancer is an emotionally debilitating disease that affects the lives of women of all ages. Liamputtong and Suwankhong (2015) conducted qualitative research with women living with breast cancer in southern Thailand. Their findings offer a particular insight into the role of cultural beliefs and practices in forming therapeutic landscapes among those women. The therapeutic landscape concept embraces 'a holistic model of health' emphasising the complex interactions between the physical, emotional, spiritual, societal and environmental landscapes of well-being and healing (Milligan et al. 2004, p. 1783). These therapeutic landscapes provide individuals with physical and emotional healing and hence enliven hope. One important aspect of therapeutic landscapes found in Liamputtong and Suwankhong's study is the cultural landscape, which constitutes both the everyday and the extraordinary therapeutic landscapes. Culture here refers to a system of shared ideas, attitudes and practices that define the social system of its members; this includes religion and worldviews. The cultural landscape has a marked influence on how the women perceive and deal with their world as well as their understanding of health and well-being. Importantly, it assists the women in creating meanings in matters that 'seem uncontrollable', like the occurrence of breast cancer (Lopez-Class et al. 2011, p. 725). Within the cultural landscape, religious and spiritual practices are of particular importance. It has been affirmed that the connections between cultural beliefs/spiritual practices and places are crucial for healing and recovery (Panelli & Tipa 2007; Greeff & Loubser 2008; Leache et al. 2008; Williams 2010). The Thai women in this study adopted cultural beliefs and religious/spiritual practices commonly performed in their locality as their therapeutic landscapes for dealing with breast cancer, and relied on traditional medicines for healing and recovery. They used the Buddhist principles of life as a means to accept their illness. They practised meditation to ameliorate the effect of breast cancer, and gave alms and performed good deeds to cultivate merit so that their lives would improve. Religious beliefs and spiritual practices have been shown to enhance the functional and social well-being of individuals living with breast cancer (Tokgöz et al. 2008; Harandy et al. 2010; Cebeci et al. 2012). Doumit et al. (2007) suggested that a belief in religion and God were essential strategies for coping with the diagnosis of breast cancer. Similarly, Davey et al. (2012) showed that women with breast cancer relied on religiosity as a principal coping mechanism.

Cultural competence

A common concern among many healthcare professionals is how culture impacts on their relationships with individual clients. This concern can be effectively addressed through the concept of **cultural competence**, which requires healthcare providers and organisations to recognise and respond competently to the cultural and linguistic needs of patients (Winkelman 2009; Purnell 2013; Spector 2017). Cultural competence requires cultural knowledge and self-awareness. Knowledge about culture can assist health professionals to provide 'culturally sensitive, responsive, and competent healthcare' to clients from different cultural backgrounds (Winkelman 2009, p. xviii). **Cultural awareness** will lead to cultural sensitivity in response to differences, and will assist healthcare providers in providing culturally responsive care to people from different cultures through a knowledge of specific cultural information and the ability to address general barriers to effective cross-cultural relations (Winkelman 2009; Purnell 2013; Prentice 2014).

Cultural competence
Cultural competence involves the ability of healthcare providers and organisations to recognise and respond competently to the cultural and linguistic needs of patients. It requires cultural knowledge and self-awareness.

Cultural awareness
An awareness of the impacts of cultural differences on people's actions and healthcare-seeking. It involves awareness of one's own cultural values and the influences of those values on one's conduct.

Practically, according to Helman (2007, p. 15), there are several benefits from increasing the cultural competence of health professionals:

- improved communication between patient and health providers
- increased satisfaction and compliance among patients
- positive impacts on the diagnosis and treatment of ill-health
- improvement in the proper use of healthcare resources
- long-term reduction in disparities in health between minorities and the majority group.

Theoretically, cultural competence can lead to improved sensitivity to the cultural beliefs, practices and expectations of patients and their communities, among health professionals. For example, it will assist healthcare providers to appreciate and respond competently to different beliefs about the causes of illnesses, help-seeking patterns and the preference of some female patients to be examined by a female health professional. It also helps improve access to healthcare for cultural minority groups by eradicating structural barriers to quality healthcare—for example, through the provision of interpreter services and hospital foods which are congruent with religious or cultural beliefs. It can also reduce organisational barriers in healthcare, such as the low numbers of health professionals and policy-makers from minority communities, who could assist in the design and implementation of culturally appropriate healthcare to minority groups (Helman 2007, p. 15).

Acquiring cultural competence entails a number of personal attributes (Winkelman 2009, p. 87):

- awareness of personal cultural attributes and level of personal cultural competency development
- personal and interpersonal skills for engaging in intercultural relations
- knowledge of cultural systems and particular cultures.

For health professionals, cultural competence requires the ability to work competently with clients from different cultural backgrounds, based on a comprehension of cultural beliefs, values and behaviours. Culturally competent health providers can use knowledge of cultural patterns to understand the needs and concerns of clients, be responsive to individual and community priorities, convey acceptance and empathy, and work effectively with clients to develop culturally relevant healthcare (Spector 2017).

Generally, cultural competence is established through relationships with members of culture groups. This produces personal development and leads to a 'transformation of self-identification' (Winkelman 2009, p. 89). Reflexivity is a crucial part of cultural competence (Olson et al. 2016). This refers to the ability of healthcare providers to justly appraise their own cultural 'baggage'—for example, their personal beliefs or prejudices, which can hinder the success of healthcare delivery (Helman 2007, p. 16). One major area that can prevent cultural competence is ethnocentrism (discussed above). The ability to deal with cultural differences starts with overcoming one's ethnocentrism. Doing so can lead to the development of awareness and skills that are essential for adapting effectively to cultural differences and intercultural processes (Winkelman 2009; Spector 2017).

Case Example 3.4

'The spirit catches you and you fall down': cultural conflict and its consequence

The tragic consequences of conflicts between the cultures of patients and biomedicine is revealed through the work of Anne Fadiman (1997). This case shows the cultural conflicts that a Hmong family experienced with biomedicine. Fadiman (1997) documents an unfortunate story of interactions between a Hmong family and their daughter's doctors and illustrates why medicine needs cultural understanding about patients. 'Cultural conflicts and misunderstandings produced disastrous consequences—a brain-dead child in a permanent vegetative state' (Winkelman 2009, p. xxiv).

Lia had epilepsy and experienced seizures frequently from the age of three months. When Lia was that age, her sister slammed the front door and, a few moments later, Lia's arms jerked over her head, her eyes rolled up and she fainted. These symptoms are recognised by Hmong people as *qaug dab peg*, 'the spirit catches you and you fall down' (Fadiman 1977, p. 20). Seizures, to Hmong people, are a sign for the person to become a trance healer or shaman (Liamputtong 2000). The seizures signify that the person has the power to see things that other people cannot, as well as being a means of entering into trances (Fadiman 1977). Hmong individuals who have epilepsy often become shamans. Due to this belief, Lia's parents did not see her condition as an illness. They took her to hospital but always arrived after the seizure had finished. Because of the language issue and lack of an interpreter in the hospital, Lia's condition and its complications went uninvestigated for five months, leading to consequences that could have been avoided with earlier care. Additionally, Lia's parents tended to resist her treatment due to their lack of understanding about it. Importantly, they did not understand why the doctors often changed her medicine. The frequent changes made it difficult for the parents to medicate their daughter properly, and they were labelled as non-compliant. Thus, Lia continued to have seizures. The repeated visits to the emergency department evoked anger and frustration in Lia's doctors. This frustration led the doctors who dealt with Hmong people to have a standard joke that the best way to treat the Hmong was 'high-velocity transcortical lead therapy', meaning 'a bullet in the head' (Winkelman 2009, p. 4).

Eventually, Lia was removed from her family by court orders obtained by her doctor. She later returned home but suffered a major seizure which left her brain-dead at age three. Fadiman contends that Lia's life was destroyed by cross-cultural misunderstandings which could have been prevented by cultural knowledge and sensitivity about Hmong culture.

This case could have been managed better by providing culturally responsive care to Hmong people. It shows important cultural issues that hamper appropriate healthcare and the role of cultural knowledge that can help to manage healthcare more effectively. The presence of Hmong people in western societies like the US and Australia illustrates the important role of culture in accessing and providing appropriate health and healthcare for individuals from different cultural backgrounds.

Stop and Think

Fadiman (1997) contends that the EM could have helped to prevent the tragedy that occurred in the case of Lia. Understanding the cultural perspectives of Hmong people would lead to appreciation of the ways the family responded to treatment, and how the condition and treatment of Lia linked to their life. Embracing the cultural perspectives of the family could also help to resolve their non-compliance. Importantly, this would help to avoid the court order that removed Lia from her family.

- What is your view on this?
- Would the EM help to prevent this tragic case? If so, how?
- How can cultural competence be applicable to Lia's case?

Reflection Exercise

Although Vietnamese people have been settled in countries such as the US for more than three decades, misunderstanding about their cultural practices persists among healthcare providers. Vietnamese people tend to use the 'coin-rubbing' method (*cao gio*) to treat minor ailments like a common cold and fever. The method involves rubbing a coin or spoon on the affected parts such as the back, neck, head, shoulder and chest to get rid of the 'bad wind' in the body. The rubbing will leave red marks and bruises on the skin. Healthcare providers in the US do not understand this cultural practice. When Vietnamese children turned up at school with red marks on their body, it led to the belief that *cao gio* is a form of child abuse. Due to the perceived criticism of *cao gio*, many Vietnamese people do not have trust in their American healthcare providers. A better appreciation of the practice by those involved in the care of Vietnamese people is not only necessary but essential if the mislabelling and misinterpretation of cultural traditional practices as child abuse is to be avoided (Davis 2000).

Australia has a large number of Vietnamese migrants, many of whom continue to observe traditional beliefs and practices. The coin-rubbing therapy is also common among other south-east Asian peoples including Cambodians and Laotians. What are the implications of the case discussed above for Vietnamese and other south-east Asian peoples in Australia?

The chapter has illustrated that culture has significant implications for healthcare practice. It is crucial that healthcare providers understand and appreciate the cultural differences of consumers from culturally and linguistically diverse backgrounds, and how their culture impacts on their health beliefs and behaviours. Cultural differences, when misunderstood, can lead to mismanagement in healthcare, which ultimately impacts on the quality of care and healthcare access of people from different cultures. An appreciation of cultural differences is crucial if healthcare providers want to provide culturally appropriate healthcare to people from culturally diverse backgrounds.

Summary

Culture, a way of life that is shared by group members, determines the health, illness and well-being of an individual and communities. As we discussed in this chapter, each culture has its own set of beliefs and practices that influence members' behaviour, and different cultures have different ideas about health, illness and healthcare-seeking. Cultural beliefs and practices make sense to those who belong to the culture, but often these are different from those of healthcare providers who operate from the biomedical system. This can lead to cultural conflicts and mismanagement in healthcare. We contend that, to avoid cultural conflicts, healthcare providers must embrace cultural sensitivity which will lead to cultural competence in healthcare. This will result in culturally appropriate healthcare provision for people from different cultural backgrounds. This is crucial in multi-cultural societies such as the US, Europe, Canada and Australia, whose populations comprise people from diverse backgrounds.

Tutorial exercises

1. Form a group, then individually write down your understanding of culture and its influence on health and well-being. Share your thoughts with others in the group. Are there differences in how each person perceives culture? What might influence your understanding, to make it different from others? Discuss.
2. Locate some examples of cultural issues that have created conflict in the media, share with others in the class, and discuss its implications as a group.
3. Thomas (2018) found 'race-based discrimination' against patients in lactation care in the US: 'unequal care provided to patients of colour and overt racist remarks said in front of or behind patient's back'. Evidence has suggested that breastfeeding is linked with good health. Thus, all babies, regardless of their cultural background, should have equal access to breastfeeding. As African-born mothers have lower rates of breastfeeding initiation and duration, the reduction of disparities in lactation care is critical. The study revealed that lactation consultants, like other healthcare professionals, are 'prone to discriminatory beliefs and practices that affect the quantity and quality of care patients receive' (p. 1061).

As a group, discuss the finding of this study in relation to cultural sensitivity and cultural competence as outlined in this chapter.

Further reading

Brown, P.J., & Closser, S. (Eds) (2016). *Understanding and Applying Medical Anthropology: Biosocial and Cultural Approaches*, 3rd edn. Walnut Creek, CA: Left Coast Press.

Cockerham, W.C., Dingwall, R., & Quah, S.R. (Eds) (2014). *The Wiley-Blackwell Encyclopedia of Health, Illness, Behavior, and Society*. Hoboken, NJ: Wiley-Blackwell.

Eisenberg, L., & Kleinman, A. (Eds), *The Relevance of Social Science for Medicine*. Dordrecht: D. Reidel Publishing.

Fadiman, A. (1997). *The Spirit Catches You and You Fall Down: A Hmong Child, her American Doctors, and the Collision of Two Cultures*. New York: Farrar, Strauss & Giroux.

Hahn, R. (1995). *Sickness and Healing: An Anthropological Perspective*. New Haven: Yale University Press.

Helman, C.G. (2007). *Culture, Health and Illness*, 5th edn. London: Hodder Arnold.

Liamputtong, P., & Suwankhong, D. (2015). Therapeutic landscapes and living with breast cancer: the lived experiences of Thai women. *Social Science and Medicine*, 128, 263–271.

Liamputtong Rice, P., Ly, B., & Lumley, J. (1994). Soul loss and childbirth: the case of a Hmong woman. *Medical Journal of Australia*, 160, 577–578.

Singer, M.K., Dressler, W., George, S., & NIH Expert Panel (2016). Culture: the missing link in health research. *Social Science and Medicine*, 170, 237–246.

Spector, R.E. (2017). *Cultural Diversity in Health and Illness,* 9th edn. New Jersey: Pearson Prentice Hall.

Wiley, A.S., & Allen, J.S. (2017). *Medical Anthropology: A Biocultural Approach*, 3rd edn. New York: Oxford University Press.

Winkelman, M. (2009). *Culture and Health: Applying Medical Anthropology*. San Francisco: Jossey-Bass.

Websites

https://www.beyondintractability.org/essay/culture_conflict

This website provides some discussions about culture and conflicts.

https://www.kidsnewtocanada.ca/culture/influence

This website has been created by the Canadian Paediatric Society and introduces how culture influences health.

https://www2.palomar.edu/anthro/medical/med_4.htm

The website describes culture-specific diseases and how people manage in different cultural contexts.

https://www.euromedinfo.eu/how-culture-influences-health-beliefs.html/

This website provides some discussions regarding health beliefs which are influenced by cultures.

https://www.youtube.com/watch?v=fIAsZU-mleg

This video is an interview with Dr Albert Gaw about his early work on acupuncture and his landmark and methodical studies on culture-bound syndromes for DSM-IV. He describes his well-known work on *koro* (genital retraction syndrome), *amok* and possession syndrome.

https://www.youtube.com/watch?v=2GVPRbxgPQc

In this video anthropological theories are used to discuss different ways that cultures perceive sickness, health and medicine are presented. These perspectives are crucial for understanding uses of medicinal plants in healthcare.

https://www.youtube.com/watch?v=G87SfHPHj0A

This video discusses acupuncture and moxibustion, two forms of traditional Chinese medicine widely practised in China. They are also practised in regions of south-east Asia, Europe and the Americas.

https://www.youtube.com/watch?v=Dx4Ia-jatNQ&t=64s

In this video you will see examples of incompetent in contrast to competent cultural care. It raises questions such as how to deliver competent care based on a patient's cultural background, and how to avoid making cultural mistakes that may adversely affect the care being provided.

https://www.youtube.com/watch?v=dNLtAj0wy6I

This video discusses cultural competence for healthcare providers. It shows views of healthcare providers on cultural competence and highlights the importance of good personality of health personnel in aiding appropriate care for patients.

https://www.youtube.com/watch?v=c0TquroTHxo

This video is about culture, cultural competence and healthcare. Although it is common to speak of cultural awareness and cultural sensitivity, healthcare providers are increasingly recognising the importance of cultural competence and providing cultural safety to patients.

References

Adthasit, R., Kulsomboon, S., Chantraket, R., Suntananukan, S., & Jirasatienpong, P. (2007). The situation of knowledge management and research in the area of local wisdom in health care. In P. Petrakard & R. Chantraket (Eds), *The Report Situations of Thai Traditional Medicine, Indigenous Medicine and Alternative Medicine 2005–2007* (pp. 16–22). Nonthaburi: Mnat Films.

AIHW (Australian Institute of Health and Welfare) (2018). *Australia's Health 2018*. Canberra: Australian Institute of Health and Welfare. Retrieved from https://www.aihw.gov.au/getmedia/7c42913d-295f-4bc9-9c24-4e44eff4a04a/aihw-aus-221.pdf.aspx?inline=true

Berdon, Z.J.S., Ragosta, E.L., Inocian, R.B., Manalag, C., & Lozano, E.B. (2016). Unveiling Cebuano traditional healing practices. *Asia Pacific Journal of Multidisciplinary Research*, 4(1), 51–59.

Biswal, R., Subudhi, C., & Acharya, S.K. (2017). Healers and healing practices of mental illness in India: the role of proposed eclectic healing model. *Journal of Health Research and Reviews in Developing Countries*, 4, 89–95.

BPS (Bureau of Policy and Strategy) (2009). *Health Policy in Thailand 2009*. Ministry of Public Health. Retrieved from http://whothailand.healthrepository.org/handle/123456789/589

Brown, P.J., & Closser, S. (2016). Medical anthropology: an introduction. In P.J. Brown & S. Closser (Eds), *Understanding and Applying Medical Anthropology: Biosocial and Cultural Approaches*, 3rd edn (pp. 13–24). Walnut Creek, CA: Left Coast Press.

Cebeci, F., Balcı Yangın, H., & Tekeli, A. (2012). Life experiences of women with breast cancer in south-western Turkey: a qualitative study. *European Journal of Oncology Nursing* 16, 406–412.

Cha, D. (2003). *Hmong American Concepts of Health, Healing and Conventional Medicine*. New York: Routledge.

Chaiyasuj, A. (2015). Thai traditional medicine in Thailand health system. In F. Lan & F.G. Wallner (Eds), *The Concepts of Health and Disease* (pp. 293–307). Nordhausen: Verlag Traugott Bautz GmbH.

Choi, M., & Yeom, H-A. (2011). Identifying and treating the culture-bound syndrome of *hwa-byung* among older Korean immigrant women: recommendations for practitioners. *Journal of the American Academy of Nurse Practitioners*, 23, 226–232.

Chokevivat, V., Wibulpolprasert, S., & Petrakard (Eds) (2010). *Thai Traditional Health Profile 2009–2010.* Bangkok: War Veterans Organization.

Chrisman, N., & Zimmer, P. (2000). Cultural competence in primary care. In P. Meredith & N. Horan (Eds), *Adult Primary Care* (pp. 65–75). Philadelphia: Saunders.

Chuengsatiansup, K. (2007). Indigenous health system in rural Thailand. In K. Chuengsatiansup & Y. Tantipidoke (Eds), *Thai Health, Thai Culture* (pp. 113–144). Bangkok: Nungsurdeeone.

Culhane-Pera, K.A., Cha, D., & Kunstadter, P. (2004). Hmong in Laos and the United States. In C.R. Ember & M. Ember (Eds), *Encyclopedia of Medical Anthropology: Health and Illness in the World's Cultures,* pp. 729–743. New York: Kluwer Academic/Plenum.

Davey, M.P., Niño, A., Kissil, K., & Ingram, M. (2012). African American parents' experiences navigating breast cancer while caring for their children. *Qualitative Health Research*, 22(9), 1260–1270.

Davis, R.E. (2000). Cultural health care or child abuse? The south-east Asian practice of *cao gio*. *Journal of the American Academy of Nurse Practitioners*, 12(3), 89–95.

De Luca, M. (2017). *Hikikomori*: cultural idiom of present-day expression of the distress engendered by the transition from adolescents to adulthood. *L'Evolution Psychiatrique*, 82, e1–e15. http://doi.org/10.1016/j.evopsy.2016.11.005

Den Hertog, T.N., de Jong, M., van der Ham, A.J., Hinton, D., & Reis, R. (2016). 'Thinking a lot' among the Khwe of South Africa: a key idiom of personal and interpersonal distress. *Culture, Medicine and Psychiatry*, 40, 383–403.

Desai, G., & Chaturvedi, S.K. (2017). Idioms of distress. *Journal of Neurosciences in Rural Practice*, 8(1), 94–97.

Doumit, M., Abu-SaadHuijer, H., & Kelley, J. (2007). The lived experience of Lebanese oncology patients receiving palliative care. *European Journal of Oncology Nursing*, 11, 309–319.

Edae, M., & Mulu, F. (2017). Indigenous wisdom and folk healing practices among urban Oromo of the Gibe region in Ethiopia: a case study of Jimma and Agoro towns. *International Journal of Multicultural and Multireligious Understanding*, 4(2), 1–23.

Fadiman, A. (1997). *The Spirit Catches You and You Fall Down: A Hmong Child, her American Doctors, and the Collision of Two Cultures*. New York: Farrar, Strauss & Giroux.

Fitzgerald, M. (2000). Establishing cultural competency for health professionals. In V. Skultans & J. Cox (Eds), *Anthropological Approaches to Psychological Medicine* (pp. 149–200). London: Jessica Kingsley.

Fleming, M.L. (2015). Defining health and public health. In M.L. Fleming & E. Parker (Eds), *Introduction to Public Health*, 2nd edn (pp. 3–43). Sydney: Churchill Livingstone.

Goldner, M. (2004). Consumption as activism: an examination of CAM as part of the consumer movement in health. In P. Tovey, G. Easthope & J. Adams (Eds), *The Mainstreaming of Complementary and Alternative Medicine: Studies in Social Context* (pp. 11–24). London: Routledge.

Golomb, L. (1985). *An Anthropology of Curing in Multiethnic Thailand*. Urbana: University of Illinois Press.

Greeff, A.P., & Loubser, K. (2008). Spirituality as a resiliency quality in Xhosa-speaking families in South Africa. *Journal of Religious Health* 47, 288–301.

Hahn, R. (1995). *Sickness and Healing: An Anthropological Perspective*. New Haven: Yale University Press.

Harandy, T.F., Ghofranipour, F., Montazeri, A., Anoosheh, M., Bazargan, M., Mohammadi, E., Ahmadi, F., & Niknamia, S. (2010). Muslim breast cancer survivor spirituality: coping strategy or health-seeking behavior hindrance? *Health Care for Women International*, 31, 88–98.

Harding, C. (2018). Hikikomori. *Lancet Psychiatry*, 5(1), 28–29.

Helman, C.G. (2007). *Culture, Health and Illness*, 5th edn. London: Hodder Arnold.

Hinton, D.E., & Lewis-Fernandez, R. (2010). Idioms of distress among trauma survivors: subtype and clinical utility. *Culture, Medicine and Psychiatry*, 34, 209–218.

Hinton, D.E., Pich, V., Marques, L., Nickerson, A., & Pollack, M.H. (2010). *Khyâl* attacks: a key idiom of distress among traumatized Cambodian refugees. *Culture, Medicine and Psychiatry*, 34, 244–278.

Hinton, D.E., Reiss, R., & de Jong, J. (2015). The 'thinking a lot' idiom of distress and PTSD: an examination of their relationship among traumatized Cambodian refugees using the 'thinking a lot' questionnaire. *Medical Anthropology Quarterly*, 29, 357–380.

Hughes, C. (1985). Culture-bound or construct bound? In R. Simons & C. Hughes (Eds), *The Culture-bound Syndromes: Folk Illnesses of Psychiatric and Anthropological Interest* (pp. 3–24). Dordrecht: Reidel.

Hunt, M. (2007). Taking culture seriously: considerations for physiotherapists. *Physiotherapy*, 93(3), 229–232.

Idler, E.L. (2014). Health and religion. In W.C. Cockerham, R. Dingwall, & S.R. Quah (Eds), *The Wiley-Blackwell Encyclopedia of Health, Illness, Behavior, and Society* (Vol. 4, pp. 1095–1099). Hoboken, NJ: Wiley-Blackwell.

Jirapaet, V. (2001). Factors affecting maternal role attainment among low-income, Thai, HIV-positive mothers. *Journal of Transcultural Nursing*, 12(1), 25–33.

Joe, J.R. (2012). The struggle with the devastation of diabetes. In J.R. Joe & F.C. Gachupin (Eds), *Health and Social Issues of Native American Women* (pp. 133–151). Santa Barbara: Praeger.

John, S.S. (2017). Traditional healing rituals of Tamil Nadu. *Oriental Anthropologist*, 17(2), 377–393.

Jones, K., & Creedy, D. (2012). *Health and Human Behaviour*, 3rd edn. Melbourne: Oxford University Press.

Julian, R. (2019). Ethnicity, health, and multiculturalism. In J. Germov (Ed.), *Second Opinion: An Introduction to Health Sociology*, 6th edn, pp. 180–204. Melbourne: Oxford University Press.

Kaiser, B.N., McLean, K.E., Kohrt, B.A., Hagaman, A., Wagenaar, B., Khoury, N., & Keys, H. (2014). *Reflechi twòp*—thinking too much: description of a cultural syndrome in Haiti's Centre Plateau. *Culture, Medicine and Psychiatry*, 38(3), 472–488.

Kaiser, B.N., & McLean, K.E. (2015). 'Thinking too much' in the Central Plateau: an apprenticeship approach to treating local distress in Haiti. In B.A. Kohrt & E. Mendenhall (Eds), *Global Mental Health: Anthropological Perspectives* (pp. 277–290). Walnut Creek, CA: Left Coast Press.

Kaiser, B.N., Haroz, E.E., Kohrt, B.A., Bolton, P.A., Bass, J.K., & Hinton, D.E. (2015). 'Thinking too much': a systematic review of a common idiom of distress. *Social Science and Medicine*, 147, 170–183.

Katon, W., & Kleinman, A. (1981). Doctor–patient negotiation and other social science strategies in patient care. In L. Eisenberg & A. Kleinman (Eds), *The Relevance of Social Science for Medicine* (pp. 253–279). Dordrecht: D. Reidel Publishing.

Kayne, S.B. (2010). *Traditional Medicine: A Global Perspective*. London: Pharmaceutical Press.

Keys, H.M., Kaiser, B.N., Kohrt, B.A., Khoury, N.M., & Brewster, A-R.T. (2012). Idioms of distress, ethnopsychology and the clinical encounter in Haiti's Central Plateau. *Social Science and Medicine*, 75, 555–564.

Khim, S.Y., & Lee, C.S. (2003). Exploring the nature of 'hwa-byung' using pragmatics. *Journal of Korean Academy of Nursing*, 33(1), 104–112.

Kleinman, A. (1973). Medicine's symbolic reality: on a central problem in the philosophy of medicine. *Inquiry*, 16, 206–213.

Kleinman, A. (1978). Concepts and a model for the comparison of medical systems as cultural systems. *Social Science and Medicine*, 12, 85–93.

Kleinman, A. (1980). *Patients and Healers in the Context of Culture: An Exploration of the Borderland between Anthropology, Medicine, and Psychiatry*. Berkeley: University of California Press.

Kleinman, A. (1988). *The Illness Narratives: Suffering, Healing, and the Human Condition*. New York: Basic Books.

Kleinman, A., Eisenberg, L., & Good, B. (2006). Culture, illness, and care: clinical lessons from anthropologic and cross-cultural research. *Focus*, 4(1), 140–149.

Klunklin, A., & Greenwood, J. (2005). Buddhism, the status of women and the spread of HIV/AIDS in Thailand. *Health Care for Women International*, 26(1), 46–61.

Kobotani, T., & Engstrom, D. (2005). The roles of Buddhist temples in the treatment of HIV/AIDS in Thailand. *Journal of Sociology and Social Welfare*, 6, XXXII(4), 5–21.

Kohrt, B.A., & Hruschka, D.J. (2010). Nepali concepts of psychological trauma: the role of idioms of distress, ethnopsychology and ethnophysiology in alleviating suffering and preventing stigma. *Culture, Medicine and Psychiatry*, 34, 322–352.

Kohrt, B.A., Rasmussen, A., Kaiser, B., Haroz, E., Maharjan, S., Mutamba-Byamah, B., et al. (2014). Cultural concepts of distress and psychiatric disorders: literature review and research recommendations for global mental health epidemiology. *International Journal of Epidemiology*, 43(3), 365–406.

Kulsomboon, S., & Adthasit, R. (2007). *The Status and Trend of Research in Local Wisdom for Health*. Bangkok: War Veterans Organization.

Kusinitz, M. (1992). *Folk Medicine*. New York: Chelsea House.

Lam, J., Liamputtong, P., & Hill, K. (2015). Perceptions of the role of physiotherapist and falls prevention among Australian and Italian-born older people. *Journal of Cross-Cultural Gerontology*, 30, 233–249.

Leache, M., Fairhead, J., Millimouno, D., & Diallo, A. (2008). New therapeutic landscapes in Africa: parental categories and practices in seeking infant health in the Republic of Guinea. *Social Science and Medicine* 66, 2157–2167.

Lee, J. (2013). Factors contributing to *hwabyung* symptoms among Korean immigrants. *Journal of Ethnic and Cultural Diversity in Social Work*, 22(1), 17–39.

Lee, J. (2015). *Hwabyung* and depressive symptoms among Korean immigrants. *Social Work in Mental Health*, 13, 159–185.

Levin, B.W., & Browner, C.H. (2005). The social construction of health: critical contributions from evolutionary, biological and cultural anthropology. *Social Science and Medicine*, 61(4), 745–750.

Liamputtong, P. (2007). *The Journey of becoming a Mother amongst Women in Northern Thailand*. Lanham, MD: Lexington Books.

Liamputtong, P. (2009). Treating the afflicted body: perceptions of infertility and ethnomedicine among fertile Hmong women in Australia. In L. Culley, N. Hudson & F. van Rooij (Eds), *Marginalized Reproduction: Ethnicity, Infertility and Reproductive Technologies*, pp. 151–164. Oxford: Earthscan Publishing.

Liamputtong, P. (2010). *Performing Qualitative Cross-cultural Research*. Cambridge: Cambridge University Press.

Liamputtong, P. (2017). Spirituality/religion and anxiety, stress, and health. In A. Wenzel (Ed.), *The Sage Encyclopedia of Abnormal and Clinical Psychology*. Thousand Oaks, CA: Sage.

Liamputtong, P., Haritavorn, N., & Kiatying-Angsulee, N. (2012). Living positively: the experiences of Thai women in central Thailand. *Qualitative Health Research*, 22(4), 441–451.

Liamputtong, P., Haritavorn, N., & Kiatying-Angsulee, N. (2015). Local discourse on antiretrovirals and the lived experience of women living with HIV/AIDS in Thailand. *Qualitative Health Research*, 25(2), 253–263.

Liamputtong, P., Lam, J., & Hill, K. (2017). Exercise for falls prevention: decision-making and uptake among Australian-born and Italian-born older people. *Activities, Adaptations and Aging*. doi:https://doi.org/10.1080/01924788.2017.1398036

Liamputtong, P., & Suwankhong, D. (2015). Therapeutic landscapes and living with breast cancer: the lived experiences of Thai women. *Social Science and Medicine*, 128, 263–271.

Liamputtong Rice, P. (2000). *Hmong Women and Reproduction*. Westport, CT: Bergin & Garvey.

Liamputtong Rice, P., Ly, B., & Lumley, J. (1994). Soul loss and childbirth: the case of a Hmong woman. *Medical Journal of Australia*, 160, 577–578.

Littlewood, R., & Lipsedge, M. (1997). *Aliens and Alienists*, 3rd edn. Abingdon: Routledge.

Lopez-Class, M., Perret-Gentil, M., Kreling, B., Caicedo, L., Mandelblatt, J., & Graves, K.D. (2011). Quality of life among immigrant Latina breast cancer survivors: realities of culture and enhancing cancer care. *Journal of Cancer Education*, 26, 724–733.

Lundberg, P.C., & Kerdonfag, P. (2010). Spiritual care provided by Thai nurses in intensive care units. *Journal of Clinical Nursing*, 19, 1121–1128.

Mahanarongchai, S. (2015). The wheel of life and Buddhist understanding of health. In F. Lan & F.G. Wallner (Eds), *The Concepts of Health and Disease* (pp. 265–281). Nordhausen: Verlag Traugott Bautz GmbH.

Meyer, S.R., Robinson, W.C., Chhim, S., & Bass, J.K. (2014). Labor migration and mental health in Cambodia: a qualitative study. *Journal of Nervous and Mental Disorders*, 202, 200–208.

Milligan, C., Gatrell, A., & Bingley, A. (2004). 'Cultivating health': therapeutic landscapes and older people in northern England. *Social Science and Medicine*, 58, 1781–1793.

Min, S.K. (2009). *Hwabyung* in Korea: culture and dynamic analysis. *World Cultural Psychiatry Research Review*, 4(1), 12–21.

Moe, T., Al Obaidly, F.A., Al Khoder, R., & Schmid, D. (2014). Folk healing and integrative healing in West Africa: analysis of historical and modern practice and perceptions. Avicenna, 1. doi:http://dx.doi.org/10.5339/avi.2014.1

Moore, R., & McClean, S. (Eds) (2010). *Folk Healing and Health Care Practices in Britain and Ireland: Stethoscopes, Wands and Crystals*. Oxford: Berghahn Books.

Muecke, M. (1979). An explanation of 'wind illness' in northern Thailand. *Culture, Medicine and Psychiatry*, 3, 267–300.

Nichter, M. (1981). Idioms of distress: alternatives in the expression of psychological distress. A case study from South India. *Culture, Medicine and Psychiatry*, 5, 379–408.

Nichter, M. (2010). Idioms of distress revisited. *Culture, Medicine and Psychiatry*, 34, 401–416.

Olson, R., Bidewell, J., Dune, T., & Lessey, N. (2016). Developing cultural competence through self-reflection in interprofessional education in Australia. *Journal of Interprofessional Care*, 30(3), 347–354.

Panelli, R., & Tipa, G. (2007). Place well-being: a Maori case study of cultural and environmental specificity. *EcoHealth* 4, 445–460.

Park, Y.C. (2004). *Hwabyung*: symptoms and diagnosis. *Psychiatry Investigation*, 1(1), 25–28.

Plattner, I.E., & Meiring, N. (2006). Living with HIV: the psychological relevance of meaning making. *AIDS Care*, 18(3), 241–245.

Prentice, R. (2014). Health, cultural competence in. In C. Cockerham, R. Dingwell & S. Quah (Eds), *The Wiley-Blackwell Encyclopedia of Health, Illness, Behavior and Society*. Chichester, West Sussex: Wiley-Blackwell.

Purnell, L.D. (2013). *Transcultural Health Care: A Culturally Competent Approach*, 4th edn. Philadelphia: F.A. Davis.

Qamar, A.H. (2015). Tona, the folk healing practices in rural Punjab, Pakistan. *Journal of Ethnology and Folkloristics*, 9(2), 59–74.

Ross, R., Sawatphanit, W., Draucker, C.B., & Suwansujarid, T. (2007a). The lived experiences of HIV-positive, pregnant women in Thailand. *Health Care for Women International*, 28(8), 731–744.

Ross, R., Sawatphanit, W., & Suwansujarid, T. (2007b). Finding peace (*kwam sa-ngob jai*): a Buddhist way to live with HIV. *Journal of Holistic Nursing*, 25(4), 228–235.

Shankar, R., Lavekar, G.S., Deb, S., & Sharma, B.K. (2012). Traditional healing practice and folk medicines used by Mishing community of north-east India. *Journal of Ayurveda and Integrative Medicine*, 3(3), 124–129.

Singer, M.K., Dressler, W., George, S., & NIH Expert Panel (2016). Culture: the missing link in health research. *Social Science and Medicine*, 170, 237–246.

Sirikanchana, P. (2015). Thai Buddhism on health. In F. Lan & F.G. Wallner (Eds), *The Concepts of Health and Disease* (pp. 283–292). Nordhausen: Verlag Traugott Bautz GmbH.

Snyder, M., & Lindquist, R. (2006). An overview of complementary/alternative therapies. In M. Snyder & R. Lindquist (Eds), *Complementary/alternative Therapies in Nursing*, 5th edn (pp. 3–13). New York: Springer Publishing.

Spector, R.E. (2017). *Cultural Diversity in Health and Illness*, 9th edn. New Jersey: Pearson Prentice Hall.

Suwankhong, D. (2011). Traditional healers (*mor pheun baan*) in southern Thailand: a contribution towards Thai health. Unpublished PhD thesis. School of Public Health, La Trobe University, Melbourne.

Suwankhong, D., & Liamputtong, P. (2014). Traditional health services utilization among indigenous peoples. In C. Cockerham, R. Dingwell & S. Quah (Eds), *The Wiley-Blackwell Encyclopedia of Health, Illness, Behavior and Society*. Chichester, West Sussex: Wiley-Blackwell.

Symonds, P.V. (2004). *Gender and the Cycle of Life: Calling in the Soul in a Hmong Village*. Seattle: University of Washington Press.

Tajan, N. (2015). Social withdrawal and psychiatry: a comprehensive review of *hikikomori*. *Neuropsychiatrie de l'enfance et de l'adolescence*, 63, 324–331.

Tantipidoke, Y. (2005). *Network of Traditional Healers and their Social Space in Thai Health Care System*. Bangkok: Desire.

Taylor, S.D. (2008). The concept of health. In S. Taylor, M. Foster & J. Fleming (Eds), *Health Care Practice in Australia*, pp. 3–21. Melbourne: Oxford University Press.

Thomas, E.V. (2018). 'Why even bother; they are not going to do it': the structure roots of racism and discrimination in lactation care. *Qualitative Health Research*, 28(7), 1050–1064.

Toffle, M.E. (2015). 'Mal d'Afrique' in Italy: translating African 'cultural idioms of distress' for more effective treatment. *Procedia: Social and Behavioral Sciences*, 205, 445–456.

Tokgöz, G., Yalug, I., Özdemir, S., Yazıcı, A., Uygun, K., & Aker, T. (2008). The prevalence of post-traumatic stress disorder in patients with cancer and post-traumatic growth. *New Symposium Journal*, 46(2), 51–61.

Turnock, B.J. (2016). *Public Health: What it is and How it Works*, 6th edn. Burlington, MA: Jones & Bartlett Learning.

Ventriglio, A., Ayonrinde, O., & Bhugra. D. (2015). Relevance of culture-bound syndromes in the 21st century. *Psychiatry and Clinical Neurosciences*, 70, 3–6.

WHO (World Health Organization) (2002). *WHO Traditional Medicine Strategy 2002–2005*. Retrieved from http://whqlibdoc.who.int/hq/2002/WHO_EDM_TRM_2002.1.pdf

Wiley, A.S., & Allen, J.S. (2017). *Medical Anthropology: A Biocultural Approach*, 3rd edn. New York: Oxford University Press.

Williams, A. (2010). Spiritual therapeutic landscapes and healing: a case study of St Anne de Beaupre, Quebec, Canada. *Social Science and Medicine*, 70, 1633–1640.

Winkelman, M. (2009). *Culture and Health: Applying Medical Anthropology*. San Francisco: Jossey-Bass.

Zuma, T., Wight, D., Rochat, T., & Moshabela, M. (2016). The role of traditional health practitioners in rural KwaZulu-Natal South Africa: generic or mode specific? *BMC Complementary and Alternative Medicine*, 16, 304. doi:10.1186/s12906-016-1293-8

Chapter 4

Deviance, Difference and Stigma as Social Determinants of Health

Pranee Liamputtong and Somsri Kitisriworapan

Topics covered

This chapter covers the following topics:

- definitions of deviance, difference, stigma and discrimination
- impact of deviance and stigma on health
- stigma and HIV/AIDS
- what has been done to combat HIV-related stigma

Key terms

deviance
difference
discrimination
gender
HIV/AIDS
labelling theory
moral career
social class
social determinants of health
social exclusion
social norms
stigma
stigmatisation

Introduction

Sociologist Emile Durkheim (1895/1982) suggested that deviance is a universal feature of all societies because it expresses the values and norms of a culture. Moral interpretation exists in all societies, and some qualities and conduct are perceived as more desirable than others. As such, deviance is always present in every society (Goode 2015; Worthen 2016). By identifying what is deviant, societies also identify what is not. This in turn creates 'shared standards' within the society (Clinard & Meier 2016).

Often, deviance leads to the notion that some people are different and this leads to stigma, which refers to certain traits and behaviours which are disvalued by others (Goffman 1963). The word 'stigma' is derived from Ancient Greek, meaning 'mark'. Marks were impressed on slaves as a way to identify their position in the social structure and suggest that they were of lesser value (Goffman 1963; Whitehead et al. 2001a; Sherman 2007; Link & Stuart 2016). Although deviance, difference and stigma are socially constructed concepts, they have a negative impact on the life and well-being of the individuals and groups who are so labelled (Link & Stuart 2016). As such, deviance, difference and stigma form an important component of the **social determinants of health** (see also Chapter 1 in this volume).

Social determinants of health
A range of individual, social, economic, environmental and cultural conditions that have the potential to contribute to or detract from the health of individuals, communities or whole populations.

In this chapter, we will discuss several important issues relevant to deviance, difference and stigma. We first introduce notions of deviance, difference and stigma, then discuss the impact of deviance and stigma on the health and well-being of those who are stigmatised. We also discuss stigma and HIV/AIDS, and what has been done to combat HIV-related stigma as a case example.

Deviance and difference

Deviance
Behaviour which transgresses social expectations and is likely to attract sanctions from other members of a society.

Deviance constitutes a universal aspect of our everyday social life (Goode 2015, 2016; Roach Anleu 2006, 2019). Indeed, the ideas of conformity, rule observation and correct conduct can only be comprehended because of the existence of deviance. Even a simple question like 'Why did you do it?' could suggest that the person has violated some social rules. Questions like this usually elicit some unease or awkwardness and may eventually discourage individuals from violating specific social norms. As such, it is a type of informal social control that stops individuals from engaging in 'deviant' behaviour (Roach Anleu 2006, 2019).

Difference
When an individual possesses characteristics which are dissimilar to, or behaves differently from, the majority of people within a society.

At the simplest level, Clinard and Meier (2016) suggest, deviance marks out those who are '**different**'. Deviant people behave differently, and hence they are different from 'us'. However, the concept of deviance goes beyond a simple examination of differences between individuals and their behaviour. Often, when we refer to the notion of deviance, we tend to think about some things we disvalue or evaluate negatively (Clinard & Meier 2016; Goode 2015). A common definition of deviance refers to 'behaviour which violates social norms' (Roach Anleu 2019,

p. 282; see also Goode 2015; Thompson & Gibbs 2016). Deviance symbolises 'non-confomity' to a norm or set of norms which is approved of or observed by the majority of people in a particular society or culture (Scambler 2003; Thompson & Gibbs 2016). Deviant behaviour signifies behaviour which, 'once it has become public knowledge, is routinely subject to sanctions—to punishment, correction or treatment' (Scambler 2003, p. 192). According to Goode (2015, p. 3), deviance has been defined by sociologists as 'behavior, beliefs and characteristics that violate society's or a collective's norms, the violation of which tends to attract reactions from audiences. Such negative reactions include contempt, punishment, hostility, condemnation, criticism, denigration, condescension, stigma, pity, and/or scorn'.

Social norms are rules or standards that guide or constrain individuals' actions or behaviour (Stuber et al. 2008; Goode 2015; Roach Anleu 2006, 2019). Norms are 'established standards of behaviour and beliefs' that have been observed by a specific social group (Worthen 2016, p. 15). A norm is a social rule indicating what individuals ought to or ought not to say, think or do in given situations (Goode 2015). Transgression of norms usually elicits negative responses or sanctions from others in the society (Goode 2015; Thompson & Gibbs 2016). These responses or sanctions put pressure on people to conform to social norms (Clinard & Meier 2016). Relevant to the concept of normatic deviance is 'social control'. This involves the use of strategies which attempt to compel comformity, or at least to deal with or deflect deviant behaviour (Roach Anleu 2006, 2019; Deflem 2015; Goode 2015).

Social norms
Rules or standards which guide or constrain individuals' actions or behaviours.

Although norms are shaped, encouraged and sustained by the social and situational contexts within a society (Becker 1963a, b), most deviant concepts are usually created by some segments of society who strive to enforce their positions about what is proper and improper and what is right and wrong into norms (Clinard & Meier 2016). They tend to be those who have more power because of their social status due to **social class**, age and **gender** (Roach Anleu 2019; see also Chapters 1, 7 & 9 in this volume). When these groups sense threats to their interests from particular conditions or acts, they might try to advance those interests by convincing others of the authority behind their concern (Clinard & Meier 2016). These processes have shaped criteria for many forms of deviance, for example, single motherhood, drink driving, consumption of illegal drugs, abortion, prostitution and homosexuality.

Social class
The position of a person in a system of structured inequality, grounded in unequal distribution of income, wealth, status and power.

Gender
Socially and culturally constructed categories reflecting what it means to be 'masculine' and 'feminine', and associated expectations of roles and behaviours of men and women.

Stop and Think

Emma, who is in her late 30s, has a great career path. She does not have any children, and has recently gotten a divorce. Due to a promotion, she has moved to Melbourne. As she meets new colleagues and friends, Emma starts to feel that she is somehow being treated differently. In a number of conversations, it becomes clear to her that some of her new network regard her 'family situation' as unusual. Emma begins to feel that she is excluded from social gatherings where couples with children are welcomed. This makes Emma think that she is in some sense deviant. But is she? (adapted from Clinard & Meier 2016).

Stop and Think

Consider the case of Emma presented above.

Nowadays, more couples choose not to have children and divorce is common. There are no 'absolute standards' which dictate that adults should have children or that people should not be divorced. But Emma feels uncomfortable within her social network because she is excluded from social occasions due to her social status (being divorced and childless). But why would her colleagues and new friends see her as deviant? Clinard and Meier (2016) contend that an answer might be that the group norms imply that couples and parents are the valued statuses. Emma might be feeling deviant because those in her new social network groups who have partners and children think that this is the way things *should* be in our society.

- What is your view about this theory?
- Is there any other theory that you can use to explain this case?

Concepts of deviance ebb and flow over time and can change in different situations (Roach Anleu 2006; Clinard & Meier 2016; Worthen 2016). Durkheim (1964, p. 71) said this clearly a long time ago: 'Today's deviance can become tomorrow's morality'. For example, in most western societies, there is no longer much moral disapproval of premarital sexual intercourse. Hence, it is no longer seen as deviant behaviour. Masturbation has also been increasingly accepted, and some even perceive the practice as an essential part of 'normal sexual development' (Clinard & Meier 2016). Interracial marriage was treated as a criminal act in the US until 1967, when the illegality of interracial marriage was repealed. Over time, there was a shift in the perception of interracial marriage as deviant (Worthen 2016). Homosexuality was once perceived as an extremely deviant and morally wrong behaviour. It is now tolerated by many people, and seen as an example of difference (Roach Anleu 2006; Goode 2016; Worthen 2016). According to Goode (2015), the most astonishing shift in attitude toward homosexuality has been the acceptance of same-sex marriage in many western societies—for example, New Zealand, Ireland and Australia (see also Chapter 9).

The daily newspapers in Australia reveal that the kinds of deviance requiring social control nowadays tend to include abortion, domestic violence, bottle-feeding practices, homelessness, drug trafficking, juvenile delinquency, sex work, environmental pollution and tobacco consumption. These activities have always occurred in Australian society, but they have not always been labelled as deviant (Roach Anleu 2006). Cohen (1974) uses the term 'elasticity of evil' to suggest that activities and behaviour which are interpreted as deviance are always evolving. Hence, what is deviant at one point in time or situation might not be perceived as such in another (Roach Anleu 2006).

As we have suggested, particular groups in society have more power to elicit, change and sustain specific concepts of deviance. Constantly, there are movements to abandon some perceived deviant practices such as personal drug comsumption, public drunkenness and prostitution. There have also been attempts to make some activities deviant and sanction them by law. A good example of this is the deviantisation of cigarette smoking, which has occurred in a number of nations including Australia and US. Up to the 1970s, smoking was an acceptable behaviour. Nowadays, it is viewed as deviant, as shown in the 'no smoking' signs in numerous public places including restaurants, planes and, in Australia, all Commonwealth government offices and buildings. Smoking is forbidden by law in these locations and there are penalites if this statute is violated (Roach Anleu 2006).

What is deviant in one culture may be normal or acceptable in another (Curra 2014; Worthen 2016). For example, in many western societies, smoking marijuana is deviant but consuming alcohol is not. In some Middle Eastern cultures, however, the reverse is true (Scambler 2003). Making a loud noise when consuming food is acceptable in Japanese or Chinese culture (it is a form of food appreciation), but is seen as 'deviant' by most people in Australia. Traditional practices regarding painful initiation ceremonies, arranged marriages or the confinement of women during childbirth and menstruation, for instance, may seem highly deviant, if not barbaric, to Australian and other western societies. However, these practices are normal in some cultures and form an important part of their way of life (Roach Anleu 2006).

Case Example 4.1

Breast- and bottle-feeding: moral and deviant mothers

Notions of deviance always elicit a strong moral stance. Even everyday conduct can have this moral tone. The argument on whether mothers should breastfeed or bottle-feed babies embodies a moral attitude of this kind. Murphy's (1999) study of first-time mothers in England and Liamputtong and Kitisriworapan's research with working mothers in Thailand (2011) reveal that whether the mothers intend to breastfeed or bottle-feed, they face tremendous challenges from those who disagree with their decision. Clinard and Meier (2011, p. 5) put it succinctly, that 'not even the time-honoured institution of motherhood is immune from allegations of deviance'.

The dominant idea that 'breast is best' is pervasive in literature on infant feeding patterns and in policy and health promotion material which attempts to educate women about infant feeding practices. Within the lay population, this idea is also promulgated (Liamputtong 2011; Sulaiman et al. 2016; Joseph 2018). Due to societal perception of the superiority of breastfeeding, mothers' intention not to breastfeed their babies may tarnish the 'moral status' of motherhood (Murphy 1999, p. 187). By choosing to bottle-feed, a mother is subjected to the accusation that she is a 'bad' mother who 'places her own needs, preferences or conveniences above her baby's welfare' (Murphy 1999, p. 187). The 'good mother' is 'deemed to be one who prioritises her child's needs, even (or perhaps especially) where this entails personal inconvenience or distress' (Murphy 1999, pp. 187–188), such as trying to breastfeed despite many obstacles.

Motherhood is 'often represented as the ultimate expression of womanhood while breast-feeding is represented as the ultimate experience of motherhood' (Nadesan & Sotirin 1998, p. 221). Because of this, the decision to bottle-feed likely 'leaves women open to the charge of being a poor mother, in short, of maternal deviance' (Murphy 1999, p. 188). The intention to formula-feed threatens women's claims to qualities such as selflessness, wisdom, responsibility and far-sightedness, all of which are widely seen as evidence of being a 'good mother' (Murphy 1999, p. 188).

The discourses on motherhood have created this moral image of breastfeeding (Guttman & Zimmerman 2000). In Earle's study (2000, p. 327) with women in Coventry, England, women perceived breastfeeding as natural. A woman who did not breastfeed was considered 'a horrible mother'. Women who intended to bottle-feed their infant opened themselves to being perceived as deviant or 'immoral mothers' (Liamputtong 2006; Liamputtong & Kitisriworapan 2011).

Deviance, according to Murphy (1999, p. 189), 'involves a charge that public morality is being violated'—in the case of infant feeding, mothers break the 'rules' of infant feeding. But more than that, 'the moral mother is not simply one who follows the rules. Rather, she is one who follows the rules *knowingly*' (Murphy 1999, p. 188). Hence, simply breaking the rules does not make the mother deviant. Rather, 'her deviance rests upon a judgement that she has broken the rules *knowingly*' (McHugh 1970, p. 188, original emphasis). In the case of infant feeding, mothers who choose not to breastfeed despite knowing the likely impact of the practice on the infant's health, are potentially subject to the charge of deviance or being stigmatised as 'immoral mothers'.

However, there appear to be some possibilities for women who intend to bottle-feed to 'challenge or resist the interpretation of their behaviour as morally sanctionable' (Murphy 1999, pp. 189–190). They must prove that, while their behaviour breaks the 'rule', it is nonetheless justified. When the decision to formula-feed her baby is questioned, a mother must justify that her intention is 'non-conventional'; that is, 'she could not have done otherwise' (Murphy 1999, p. 190). Her intention is justified and therefore should not be sanctioned. When breastfeeding is socially valued in societies, women choosing not to breastfeed may use socially and culturally acceptable grounds for their actions, such as the need to work in paid employment or having insufficient milk. This will help them avoid being seen as 'bad mothers'.

Stigma, stigmatisation and discrimination

Stigma
An attribute or characteristic that separates people from one another. It is used by individuals to interpret specific attributes of others as 'discreditable' or 'unworthy', which results in the stigmatised person becoming devalued.

Closely related to the concept of deviance is **stigma** (Thompson & Gibbs 2016). The foundation of stigma lies in 'differences'. These can be in physical appearance, personality, age, gender, sexuality, illness, disability or specific behaviours which evoke discontent, abhorrence, panic or sympathy from others (Mason et al. 2001; Goode 2016).

Stigma, according to Goffman (1963, p. 3) is a 'devaluation' process that links with stereotyping and prejudice. It is used by individuals to interpret specific traits of others as 'discreditable or unworthy', which results in the stigmatised person becoming 'discounted' or 'tainted' (Thomas 2006, p. 3175). Those who are stigmatised are 'disqualified from full social acceptance' (Goffman 1963, preface). Following Goffman's theory of stigma as an attribute, Jones et al. (1984) coined the term 'mark' to mean stigma which would eventually lead to the definition of the person as 'flawed' or 'spoiled' (Yang et al. 2007, p. 1525). On the basis of a social position which dictates that some individuals are 'tainted' and 'less than', stigma is a mark that separates people from one another (Pescosolido et al. 2008; Goode 2015; Major et al. 2018).

According to Mason and colleagues (2001, p. 4), the main element of the stigmatising strategies is to create the 'them and us' principle (see also Foucault 1973). Its aim is to lay a foundation which could separate individuals who are perceived as 'good and in favour' from those who are 'bad and out of favour' within a given social norm (Foucault 1973). Once this principle is initiated, **stigmatisation** and **social exclusion** are permitted. This process is established and confirmed by the prejudiced position which accentuates the difference; that is, the 'them and us'. As Sontag (1991) suggests, HIV/AIDS symbolises 'sin' and 'evil'. Hence, people living with HIV/AIDS are perceived as discredited individuals who have '[im]moral characters'. As a consequence, they are socially conditioned as not 'one of us' (Mason et al. 2001, p. 4). Often, this leads to **discrimination** against the discredited persons (Krupchanka & Thornicroft 2016; Sheehan et al. 2016; Malik & Dixit 2017).

Stigmatisation
The process of stigmatising a person.

Social exclusion
The exclusion of individuals from social networks and resources because of their different and stigmatised statuses.

Discrimination
The idea that someone is of less value and should be excluded from social networks and the benefits of society.

Goffman (1963) suggests that there are three kinds of stigmatising condition. The first is 'tribal identity', which includes such identities as gender, race, religion and nationality. Second is 'blemishes of individual character', which may include having mental illness, a history of addiction or incarceration, and living with HIV/AIDS. Third is 'abominations of the body', which include such bodily conditions as deformities and physical disabilities (LeBel 2008, p. 411). Based on Goffman's stigmatising conditions, there are many individuals who would be stigmatised in many societies due to their social and health statuses. However, Falk (2001) proposes two types of stigmatising states which are based on the 'cause' of stigma. First, 'existential stigma', which occurs when an individual does not create the stigma or has very little control over it. This includes being old, race and ethnicity and having mental illness. Second is 'achieved stigma', which happens when an individual has acquired a stigma due to their own action and behaviour and/or because they have personally cultivated it. This may include such actions as becoming a refugee, immigrant, prisoner or homeless, and living with HIV/AIDS (LeBel 2008).

Similar to the concept of deviance presented above, stigma theorists have focused more on the position of **social norms** in the process of constructing stigma (Stuber et al. 2008). Goffman (1963), for instance, contends that because deviations from social rules are inescapable, stigmatisation is a common characteristic of any society. Others suggest that stigmatisation is a characteristic of all socio-cultural groups. It is employed to elicit conformity with the social standings of society so

Social norms
Rules or standards which guide or constrain individuals' actions or behaviour.

that law and order can be enforced. Based on this perspective, stigmatisation is the result of deviating from social rules which attempt to make the deviant individual conform. It is also used to illustrate to other group members the behaviours which are not condoned, and the effects that will be felt by those who engage in such actions. However, it can only be used in these ways to enforce conformity around voluntary behaviours—for example, illicit drug consumption and cigarette smoking (Stuber et al. 2008). Stigma has also been defined by scholars in terms of a person's social identity, and the essence of unique social contexts has been emphasised. According to Crocker et al. (1998), the central feature of social stigma suggests that stigmatised persons have, or are believed to have, some characteristics which are associated with a disvalued social identity in a particular social situation (see also Major et al. 2018).

How does stigma occur? Stigma is a process which is grounded within the 'construction of social identity' (Yang et al. 2007, p. 1527). Stigma eventuates through what Goffman (1963, p. 32) refers to as a '**moral career**'. A stigmatised individual initially makes sense of their social position in society and later acquires a set idea of what it would be like to have a specific stigma. The person will then pass from a 'normal' to 'discreditable' status. Through social interaction, they eventually obtain a 'discredited' status and 'damaged identity' (Curra 2014; Finzen 2016). When an individual's new identity is 'assumed through interaction (i.e., "re-identifying") with socially constructed categories', stigma will occur (Yang et al. 2007, p. 1527). A good example is the case of mental illness. A person with mental illness (a non-visible stigma) passes from a 'normal' status to 'discredible' one. Their 'discredited' status is gained when they disclose the mental illness condition to others.

Moral career
A process when a stigmatised individual initially makes sense of the social position of him/herself within the society and later acquires a set idea of what it would be like to hold a specific characteristic.

Stigma also occurs through the process of 'labelling' (Curra 2014; Goode 2015). Scheff (1966) posits a '**labelling theory**' and applies it to the case of mental illness. He suggests that when an individual living with mental illness is given a deviant label, it will eventually lead the person to change their self-perception and social opportunity (Yang et al. 2007; Link & Stuart 2016). Scheff argues that individuals learn about the stereotypes of mental illness through the process of socialisation and daily reinforcement. Due to its highly discrediting status, once the stereotype is fully formed, the person's 'patient' role will become a 'master status' (Markowitz 2005). Consistent reactions from others, particularly the application of social exclusion, will prevent the person from recliaming their former ('normal') social functions (Yang et al. 2007; Goode 2015; Link & Stuart 2016).

Labelling theory
The process of labelling a person with stigma. Through the process of social interaction, this eventually leads the person to change their self-perception and lose social opportunity.

Impact of deviance and stigma on health

For the stigmatized, stigma compounds suffering (Yang et al. 2007, p. 1528).

The most widespread suffering inflicted by stigma in modern times involves 'ethnic cleansing'. A mass killing of harmless people occurs simply because they are of different race, ethnicity, religion or culture, or merely because they are different. This is proof of what humans can do to others if reactions to stigma are not taken seriously (Whitehead et al. 2001b).

Health and illness conditions which tend to produce stigma are those which are connected with negative characteristics, have uncertain or unknown causes and limited treatment, and produce intense reactions such as fear and disgust (Sontag 1991; LeBel 2008). Historically, leprosy and tuberculosis were met with revulsion; later, we witnessed the same emotional responses toward cancer, mental illness and HIV/AIDS (Sontag 1991; LeBel 2008; Liamputtong 2013a; Malik & Dixit 2017; Gaebel et al. 2017) (see later section on stigma and HIV/AIDS). Numerous health-related issues still attract stigma, for example, abortion, infertility, being overweight, obesity, bottle-feeding practices and cigarette smoking. Those who belong to stigmatised classifications (or 'deviants', as outlined earlier)—such as poor people; homeless people; gay, lesbians and transgender individuals; refugees; Indigenous people and ethnic minority groups—are also likely to have to deal with the negative repercussions of stigma-related health issues (Pescosolido et al. 2008).

The effect of stigma on the stigmatised individuals can differ in its manifestation and magnitude (Link & Phelan 2001; Mason et al. 2001; Corrigan et al. 2003a, b; Link & Stuart 2017; Major et al. 2018). Often, stigma generates negative credibilities; these are termed stereotypes. It then gives legitimacy to the negative credibilities; this is referred to as prejudice. Prejudice leads to a wish to shun individuals who possess stigmatised statuses. This is called discrimination (Pescosolido et al. 2008, p. 431; see also Link & Phelan 2001; Williams et al. 2008; Krupchanka & Thornicroft 2016; Sheehan et al. 2016; Major et al. 2018). Any form of discrimination and prejudice may lead to social exclusion, as it functions to disconnect stigmatised persons from society and prohibit them from societal benefits, such as access to services like education, housing, social support and healthcare (Mason et al. 2001; LeBel 2008; Krupchanka & Thornicroft 2016; Major et al. 2018).

Individually, the effects of stigma and social exclusion can be destructive. They can result in isolation, low self-esteem, depression, self-harm, poor academic achievement and social relationships, poor physical and mental health, and suicide (Mason et al. 2001; Major & O'Brien, 2005; Yang et al. 2007; Krupchanka & Thornicroft 2016; Ferlatte et al. 2017; Major et al. 2018). For stigmatised individuals with major health problems, stigma can 'intensify the sense that life is uncertain, dangerous, and hazardous' (Yang et al. 2007, p. 1528). It is clear that stigma and discrimination have a negative impact on the quality of life of stigmatised persons (Pescosolido et al. 2008; Major et al. 2018).

Importantly, an emphasis on the association between a person's behaviour and health has created a 'new morality' (Becker 1993, p. 4). 'Being ill' is reinterpreted as 'being guilty'. For example, people with obesity are stigmatised because they 'let themselves go' and smokers are stigmatised because they 'have no willpower' to stop (Bayer 2008, p. 468). Guilt is used as a prompter, and it might be successful in certain situations. However, guilt itself has a tremendous ability to produce negative physical and emotional health outcomes (Becker 1993). It may be worth noting that health conditions, poverty, non-standard life-styles and so forth have long been considered a failure of will and evidence of lack of moral fibre. The reconstruction of alcoholism as a disease, for example, was an attempt to shift the attitude from a moral problem to a physiological condition.

The impact of stigma on public health is huge (Hatzenbuehler et al. 2013; Pausé 2017; Major et al. 2018). Herek (2002, p. 604) states bluntly that 'stigma and discrimination are the enemies of public health'. The fact that stigma has a damaging effect on individuals' health has led public health officials and advocates to notice the powerfully negative results of stigmatisation for public health. In the area of HIV/AIDS, for example, it is clear that the stigmatisation of certain groups such as commercial sex workers, injecting drug users and gay men only increases their susceptibility to HIV infection and pushes them away those who attempt to help them to modify the risky behaviours (Stuber et al. 2008; Ferlatte et al. 2017).

Within healthcare settings, Whitehead and colleagues (2001b, p. 29) contend, perceptions of difference may 'become professionalised'. Within a medical framework, it may be acceptable to treat someone differently because they are seen, in some ways, to be too 'dis-ordered'. For example, due to the lack of an interpreter, healthcare providers might be reluctant or refuse to provide care to individuals from ethnic minorities who are living with mental illness. This is simply because healthcare providers think that such people cannot or do not speak English and, due to both the language inadequacy and the illness, would not understand what they are told. This means that those individuals could be excluded from healthcare services to which others have access. This is 'social exclusion', which can have a negative impact on the lives of many marginalised people.

Stop and Think

- An injecting drug user who has no history of HIV infection is not allowed to donate blood at a local blood donation event. What do you think may explain this?
- A new mother who has been living in an area for a number of years is told not to bring her newborn baby to a play group in that area because the baby has a visible physical malformation. What impact will this have on her and her newborn?

Stigma, discrimination and HIV/AIDS

HIV/AIDS

Human Immunodeficiency Virus (HIV) and Acquired Immunodeficiency Syndrome (AIDS) emerged as a major public health issue in 1981 in North America. It has affected gay men, injecting drug users, women and newborn babies in many parts of the world. It is a highly stigmatised illness as it is seen to be associated with individuals who engage in deviant sexual behaviour or anti-social behaviour of other kinds.

Globally and locally, the **HIV/AIDS** epidemic has offered the circumstance for a powerful argument that connects stigmatisation and public health (Parker & Aggleton 2003; Bayer & Stuber 2006; Liamputtong 2013a, 2016; Malik & Dixit 2017). From the onset of the epidemic, HIV/AIDS has been seen not only as a medical condition, but also as a stigmatised state (Herek & Glunt 1993; Letteney & LaPorte 2004). Scambler (2003, p. 199) states clearly that HIV/AIDS 'has been both medicalized as "disease" and moralized as "stigma"'. HIV/AIDS was first recognised in 1981 and since then has provoked forceful reactions as it uniquely combines 'sex, drugs, death and contagion' (Scambler 2003, p. 199). This unique combination made HIV/AIDS a powerfully stigmatising disease that is prevalent among those who are already members of stigmatised groups, such as gay men and injecting drug users (Scambler 2003; Parker & Aggleton 2003). In countries where HIV/AIDS is predominantly heterosexually transmitted, stigmatisation and discrimination remain pervasive. Those from marginalised groups such as poor people, women, mothers, sex workers and injecting drug users bear the brunt of the impact of HIV/AIDS (Liamputtong 2013a, 2013b, 2016; Ferlatte et al. 2017; Malik & Dixit 2017; Le et al. 2018; see also Chapter 14). Some have suggested that the stigmatisation and discrimination of these people have violated their human rights (see Chapter 5). Mann and Tarantola (1998, pp. 4–5) put it succinctly: 'Those who—before the arrival of HIV/AIDS—were societally marginalized, stigmatized or discriminated against, were found gradually and increasingly to bear the brunt of the HIV/AIDS epidemic. Human rights violations are now recognized to be primordial root causes of vulnerability to the epidemic'.

Despite the fact that society now has better understanding about the causes and impacts of HIV/AIDS, the burden of prejudice continues (Carlisle 2001; Liamputtong et al. 2009; Vlassoff & Ali 2011; Liamputtong 2013a, 2016). Goffman (1963, p. 70) warned that 'familiarity need not reduce contempt'. Research continues to reveal the ways in which society neglects the need for healthcare for those living with HIV/AIDS (Carlisle 2001; Deng et al. 2007; Anderson et al. 2008).

It is suggested that HIV and AIDS have particular traits which initiate a high level of stigma (Parker & Aggleton 2003). As stigma is socially constructed and attributable to cultural, social, historical and situational factors, stigmatised individuals are subject to 'feelings of shame and guilt'. As discussed earlier, a major consequence of stigmatisation is discrimination, which occurs when an individual 'is treated unfairly and unjustly' due to the perception that they are deviant from others (Deng et al. 2007, p. 1561). The HIV/AIDS stigma is perceived as 'an individual's deviance from socially accepted standards of normality', including such deviance as 'immorality', 'promiscuity', 'perversion', 'contagiousness' and 'death'. Hence, people living with HIV/AIDS (PLWHA) are socially constructed as the 'other' who are 'disgracefully different from and threatening to the general public' (Zhou 2007, p. 2856).

HIV/AIDS stigmas continue to increase class, race, and gender inequalities (Parker & Aggleton 2003; Reidpath & Chan 2005; Simbayi et al. 2007; Wyrod 2013; Malik & Dixit 2017). Those who are seen to be associated with sexual promiscuity, homosexuality and drug use are particularly vulnerable to stigma. Women are more vulnerable to the stigma associated with HIV/AIDS as a sexually transmitted disease (Lawless et al. 1996; Cullinane 2007; Ndinda et al. 2007; Paudel & Baral 2015; Cuca & Rose 2016; Malik & Dixit 2017). In African and Asian countries, women living with HIV/AIDS are frequently referred to as 'vectors', 'diseased' and 'prostitutes', but these terms are seldom used about infected men (Ndinda et al. 2007, p. 93). Clearly, discrimination against PLWHA is not simply about HIV/AIDS as a disease. Rather, it intersects with other social prejudices including homophobia, racism and sexism (Parker & Aggleton 2003). Hence, when women living with HIV/AIDS feel stigma, it is not 'only their internalization of the AIDS stigma, but also an effect of their interactions with others or actual experiences with public attitudes through which AIDS-related social standards are manifested' (Zhou 2007, p. 2856; see also Liamputtong 2013a, 2016; Paudal & Baral 2015; Malik & Dixit 2017; Le et al. 2018).

Often, stigma is multi-dimensional. There are three broad types of HIV/AIDS-related stigma. First is self-stigma, which occurs through 'self-blame and self-deprecation' of those living with HIV/AIDS. Second is perceived stigma, which is related to fear that if an individual discloses their HIV-positive status, they may be stigmatised. Third is enacted stigma, which occurs when individuals are actually discriminated against because of their HIV status—actual or perceived (Thomas 2006, p. 3175).

Stigma may be manifested in actions such as gossip, verbal abuse and distancing from individuals living with HIV/AIDS. It ranges from subtle actions to 'extreme degradation, rejection and abandonment' (Thomas 2006, p. 3175). These manifestations may change over time (Thomas 2006). Ignorance, lack of accurate information about HIV and AIDS, and misunderstanding about HIV transmission are common sources of HIV/AIDS stigma (Apinundecha et al. 2007; Zhou 2007; Vlassoff & Ali 2011).

However, as Parker and Aggleton (2003, p. 17) warn, it is crucial to recognise that stigma occurs 'within specific contexts of culture and power'. They also suggest that 'discrimination is characterized by cross-cultural diversity and complexity' (p. 14). Hence, socio-cultural beliefs, values and morals within local contexts have played a major role in constructing stigma and discrimination (Zhou 2007). Stigma also changes over time. What was stigmatised in previous times may not be seen as a strong stigma now. The HIV/AIDS stigma may appear transparent to some groups of people, but not so to others (Reidpath & Chan 2005; LeBel 2008; Liamputtong 2013a, 2013b, 2016). Some individuals or groups are more likely to be perceived by society as 'innocent victims of HIV' (Sontag 1991)—for example, infants who contracted it through maternal transmittion or infected blood (Liamputtong 2016). The label of 'innocence' is applied because they are perceived as 'blameless' (Katz 1981). Those who contracted HIV/AIDS through homosexual activities and drug use tend to face an extra stigma because of their 'deviant behavior' (LeBel 2008, p. 411).

Case Example 4.2

Stigma and Thai women living with HIV/AIDS

There is a high prevalence of HIV and AIDS among Thai women. Despite the fact that Thailand has a progressive national approach to dealing with HIV and AIDS, the stigma of HIV/AIDS and the fear of infection remains. Liamputtong et al. (2009, 2012) suggest that fear, stigma and discrimination toward PLWHA in Thailand, as experienced by the women in their study, still exists, although it is less marked than previously. Fear is created by the AIDS campaigns in Thailand. Although the initial mass media campaigns in Thailand were an 'effective buffer against high rates of transmission' (Lyttleton 2000, p. 224), the campaigns also created fear of AIDS among Thai people. The aggressive campaigns created a continuing sense of stigma attached to HIV and AIDS. Although there is more local acceptance in some parts of Thailand, such as the north and in rural areas due to the commonness of the disease (Lyttleton 2004; VanLandingham et al. 2005; Suwankhong & Liamputtong 2017), PLWHA are still rejected by their families, close kin and particularly others in the community (Lyttleton 2004; Maneesriwongul et al. 2004; Sringernyuang et al. 2005; Apinundecha et al. 2007). The advancement of HIV treatments such as antiretroviral vaccines has prolonged the lives of many PLWHA as well as reducing AIDS to a manageable chronic condition (Lyttleton et al. 2007; Liamputtong et al. 2015). This has led to increased disclosure of HIV/AIDS, and many affected individuals are now subjected to stigma and discrimination in the community (Apinundecha et al. 2007; Liamputtong & Haritavorn 2016).

What has been done to manage stigma

According to LeBel (2008), in order to entirely reshape public perceptions and reactions toward stigmatised people, we need more organised and structural attempts that include both policy and legal action. The results may produce a long-term effect on our anti-stigma efforts (Link et al. 2002; Parker & Aggleton 2003; Puhl & Brownell 2003; Heijnders & Van Der Miej 2006). It has been suggested that through contact with stigmatised persons and educational campaigns, the stigmatising attitudes of the public could be improved. It has been shown that when the general public have direct interaction with individuals from stigmatised groups, their attitudes toward the stigmatised have improved (Brown et al. 2003). Similarly, involving stigmatised individuals as speakers in educational sessions for the general public is effective in promoting positive perceptions and responses in the target audiences, as these individuals can provide accurate information and debunk many misconceptions about them (Corrigan et al. 2002; Couture & Penn 2003).

Additionally, LeBel (2008) suggests that protest and advocacy can work effectively as a strategy to reduce stigma. Collective tactics such as 'social activism' have proved to be valuable (Colvin 2014; Gaebel et al. 2016; Rodier 2017; Daftary et al. 2018). Thus far, collective responses from several stigmatised groups including gays/lesbians/transgender persons, individuals with physical disabilities, people living with mental illness, and other stigmatised groups have been successful in changing official policies and laws. It is argued that this strategy is the most powerful and long-lasting means for the reduction and eradication of prejudice and discrimination for many stigmatised groups (Major et al. 2000; see also Sayce 2000; Corrigan & Lundin 2001; Parker & Aggleton 2003; Shih 2004; Liamputtong et al. 2009).

The motive and ability to resist or deny the label of deviance among stigmatised groups is an interesting aspect of stigma-related reduction and eradication. In Foucault's words (1981), these people employ 'reverse discourse' to resist the label of deviance and hence avoid being stigmatised. This discourse allows individuals and groups to 'present a positive affirmation of their identity and perspectives rather than a deviance designation' (Roach Anleu 2006, p. 422). Collectively, the stigmatised groups can generate a strategy to reject the standard social values and norms (Anspach 1979; Liamputtong et al. 2009; Major et al. 2018). In HIV/AIDS, there have been many strategies that individuals and groups have used to combat and abolish stigma. Gay men have adopted such symbols as the pink triangle, which the Nazis used in the Holocaust to mark out homosexuals before slaughtering them, to counteract their stigmatisation (Gilmore & Somerville 1994). Two UK voluntary organisations, 'Gay Men Fighting AIDS' and 'ACT UP' (AIDS Coalition to Unleash Power) are good examples of political activism which make use of power to combat stigma (Taylor 2001, pp. 795–796). Case Example 4.3 discusses a stance adopted by Thai women living with HIV/AIDS as a way to resist the stigmatisation of their condition.

Case Example 4.3

AIDS support group and women living with HIV/AIDS in Thailand

Many PLWHA attempt to find strategies to deal with or to fight against stigma and discrimination. Liamputtong and colleagues' study (2009) revealed that joining AIDS support groups was a strategy used by some Thai women to counteract the stigma of their conditions and lives. As Lyttleton and colleagues (2007, p. S49) contend, PLWHA support groups act as 'a panacea for stigma and alienation', hence it is not surprising to see many women participating in group activities regardless of their physical condition.

Support groups offer women more knowledge about the illness and how to deal with it better. As Foucault (1980) theorises, with more knowledge, individuals feel that they have more power to deal with their situations. Support groups also provide women with a sense of belonging. The Thai women learnt more about others who were in the same situation as themselves. Joining the group made them realise that they were not alone in living with HIV/AIDS. With more knowledge and an increased sense of belonging from the support groups, the women attained greater emotional strength to deal with their health condition and the stigma associated with it. Joining support groups created collective power for all women, which allowed the women to defend their conditions and deal with their situations in a more positive light.

The most powerful way to fight stigma and discrimination against HIV/AIDS occurs when communities are able to mobilise themselves to do so (Parker & Aggleton 2003). Several studies have clearly demonstrated empowerment and social mobilisation in response to HIV and AIDS in various societies (Daniel & Parker 1993; Altman 1994; Epstein 1996; Parker 1996; Liamputtong et al. 2009).

Parker and Aggleton (2003) argue that it is time for us to begin thinking more seriously about using new models for advocacy and social change in response to HIV/AIDS-related stigma and discrimination—building community strength is one of these models. The development of AIDS support groups in Thailand and elsewhere is a good example of community strength (Liamputtong et al. 2009; Mburu et al 2013; Oosterhoff & Bach 2013; Snyder et al. 2014; Bacigalupe et al. 2016; Persson et al. 2016).

Reflection Exercise

Consider whether you see the following as questionable.

- A nurse refuses to provide care to a female patient with HIV/AIDS because of her own ideas about the cause of HIV/AIDS. The nurse believes that the woman acquired the disease through promiscuity, which she does not approve of.
- The mother of an autistic boy has difficulty placing him in the local school because the school thinks that he would not be able to learn or fit in with others, and his condition may lead to discrimination against him.
- An overweight young woman who works at a local business office is told to lose a substantial amount of weight or be sacked, even though to sack her would be illegal.

What does this tell you about our societal values? How do the concepts of deviance and differences discussed in this chapter apply to these values? How do these concepts link with the concepts of stigma and discrimination?

An in-depth understanding of these concepts, how they occur and what can be done about them will lead to more sensitive healthcare and social care among people who are labelled as deviant. This would lead to the eradication of stigma and discrimination toward people who are seen as different, and ultimately to a more equitable society.

Summary

Deviance is a common characteristic of all societies because it signifies the values and norms of a culture. Deviance is based on the idea that some individuals are different, and this often leads to stigma. Although deviance and stigma are socially constructed, they can impact on the lived experiences of many individuals and groups, particularly those who are already vulnerable to ill health, such as individuals with mental health concerns or HIV/AIDS. In order to eradicate deviance and stigma, we agree with Scambler (2003, p. 201) who contends that there should be no sanction that 'marks' some individuals as deviant, stigmatises and treats them as 'outsiders'. Instead of treating difference as a basis for discrimination and rejection, it should be 'a source of celebration'. As primary deliverers of healthcare, health professionals are in the best position to embark on local and global dialogue which can influence the creation of new policies and laws to improve the experiences of stigmatised individuals and groups. This will enhance their health and well-being and improve the lives of marginalised and vulnerable people in many ways.

Tutorial exercises

1. Watch the Australian film *The Black Balloon* (Film Finance Corporation Australia 2007), which portrays the lives of the parents and brother of an autistic child. It is accessible in most university libraries and online. How does the film help you make sense of the concepts in this chapter, particularly in terms of difference, deviance and stigma?
2. Gay and bisexual men and injecting drug users have been labelled 'guilty HIV/AIDS carriers' by the media (Scambler 2003). What is your opinion about this accusation? How has this label come about? What can we explain about this accusation?
3. Cigarette smoking used to be a norm in society. However, it has become 'deviant behaviour'. As a result, there are bans on smoking in offices and public places such as restaurants. What are the main reasons for this change in societal norms? What arguments have been used to make the behaviour deviant? Is there any benefit in making cigarette smoking a deviant behaviour?

Further reading

Bayer, R. (2008). Stigma and the ethics of public health: not can we but should we. *Social Science and Medicine*, 67, 463–472.

Becker, H.S. (1963). *Outsiders: Studies in the Sociology of Deviance*. New York: Free Press.

Clinard, M.B., & Meier, R.F. (2016). *Sociology of Deviant Behavior*, 15th edn. Boston: Cengage Learning.

Falk, G. (2001). *Stigma: How we Treat Outsiders*. Amherst, NY: Prometheus Books.

Goffman, E. (1990). *Stigma: Notes on the Management of Spoiled Identity*. Harmondsworth: Penguin.

Goode, E. (2016). *Deviant Behavior*, 11th edn. New York: Routledge.

Liamputtong, P. (2013). *Stigma, Discrimination and Living with HIV/AIDS: A Cross-cultural Perspective*. Dordrecht: Springer.

Liamputtong, P., Haritavorn, N., & Kiatying-Angsulee, N. (2009). HIV and AIDS, stigma and AIDS support groups: perspectives from women living with HIV and AIDS in central Thailand. *Social Science and Medicine*, special issue on Women, Motherhood and AIDS Care in Resource-poor Settings, 69(6), 862–868.

Link, B.G., & Phelan, J.C. (2001). Conceptualizing stigma. *Annual Review of Sociology*, 27, 363–385.

Major, B., Dovidio, J.F., & Link, B.G. (Eds) (2018). *The Oxford Handbook of Stigma, Discrimination and Health*. Oxford: Oxford University Press.

Mason, T., Carlisle, C., Watkins, C., & Whitehead, E. (Eds) (2001). *Stigma and Social Exclusion in Health Care*. London: Routledge.

Roach Anleu, S.L. (2006). *Deviance, Conformity and Control*, 4th edn. Sydney: Pearson Education Australia.

Websites

http://community-2.webtv.net/stigmanet/LINKSAntiStigma/

This website is maintained by the National Stigma Clearinghouse. It provides information on anti-stigma programs, resources and research.

www.sdsmt.edu/online-courses/is/soc00/Deviance.htm

This website includes a collection of different sites which discuss issues relevant to deviance and criminology.

http://www.avert.org/hiv-aids-stigma.htm

The website provides good discussions on the impact of stigma and discrimination against people living with HIV/AIDS.

http://www.stampoutstigma.org/

This is a good website that provides information on news, research and other material. It aims to provide information about how to combat and eradicate HIV/AIDS-related stigma.

http://nortonbooks.typepad.com/everydaysociology/2010/03/rethinking-nudity-and-deviance.html

This is an interesting blog that discusses deviance in the context of cosmetic surgery, which has been a popular trend among celebrities, movie stars and many others.

www.positivedeviance.org/

This website explores the notion of positive deviance, an interesting concept that readers might like to explore further.

References

Altman, D. (1994). *Power and Community: Organizational and Cultural Responses to AIDS*. London: Taylor & Francis.

Anderson, M., Elam, G., Gerver, S., Solarin, I., Fenton, K., & Easterbrook, P. (2008). HIV/AIDS-related stigma and discrimination: accounts of HIV-positive Caribbean people in the United Kingdom. *Social Science and Medicine*, 67(5), 790–798.

Anspach, R. (1979). From stigma to identity politics: political activism among the physically disabled and former mental patients. *Social Science and Medicine*, 13, 765–773.

Apinundecha, C., Laohasiriwong, W., Cameron, M.P., & Lim, S. (2007). A community participation intervention to reduce HIV/AIDS stigma, Nakhon Ratchasima province, northeast Thailand. *AIDS Care*, 19(9), 1157–1165.

Bacigalupe, G., Cantrell, K., & Chickerella, R. (2016). The power of online patient communities for HIV youth. In P. Liamputtong (Ed.), *Children and Young People Living with HIV/AIDS: A Cross-cultural Perspective* (pp. 339–358). Dordrecht: Springer.

Bayer, R. (2008). Stigma and the ethics of public health: not can we but should we. *Social Science and Medicine*, 67, 463–472.

Bayer, R., & Stuber, J. (2006). Tobacco control, stigma, and public health: rethinking the relations. *American Journal of Public Health*, 96, 47–50.

Becker, H.S. (1963a). *Perspectives on Deviance: The Other Side*. Toronto: Macmillan.

Becker, H.S. (1963b). *Outsiders: Studies in the Sociology of Deviance*. New York: Free Press.

Becker, M.H. (1993). A medical sociologist looks at health promotion. *Journal of Health and Social Behavior*, 34, 1–6.

Brown, L., Macintyre, K., & Trujillo, L. (2003). Interventions to reduce HIV/AIDS stigma: what have we learned? *AIDS Education and Prevention*, 15, 49–69.

Carlisle, C. (2001). HIV and AIDS. In T. Mason, C. Carlisle, C. Watkins & E. Whitehead (Eds), *Stigma and Social Exclusion in Health Care* (pp. 117–125). London: Routledge.

Le, B.C., Do, M.H., Nguyen, M.H., & Nguyen, D.A. (2018). Linkage between HIV diagnosis and care: understanding the role of gender in a northern province in Vietnam. *Health Care for Women International*, 39(4), 429–441.

Clinard, M.B., & Meier, R.F. (2011). *Sociology of Deviant Behavior*, 14th edn. Belmont, CA: Thomson Wadsworth.

Clinard, M.B., & Meier, R.F. (2016). *Sociology of Deviant Behavior*, 15th edn. Boston: Cengage Learning.

Cohen, A.K. (1974). *The Elasticity of Evil: Changes in the Social Definition of Deviance*. Oxford: Blackwell.

Colvin, C.J. (2014). Evidence and AIDS activism: HIV scale-up and the contemporary politics of knowledge in global public health. *Global Public Health*, 9, 57–72.

Corrigan, P.W., & Lundin, R. (2001). *Don't Call me Nuts! Coping with the Stigma of Mental Illness*. Tinley Park, IL: Recovery Press.

Corrigan, P.W., Markowitz, F.E., Watson, A., Rowan, D., & Kubiak, M.A. (2003a). An attribution model of public discrimination towards persons with mental illness. *Journal of Health and Social Behavior*, 44, 162–179.

Corrigan, P.W., Rowan, D., Green, A., Lundin, R., River, L.P., Uphoff-Wasowski, K., White, K., & Kubiak, M.A. (2002). Challenging two mental illness stigmas: personal responsibility and dangerousness. *Schizophrenia Bulletin*, 28, 293–309.

Corrigan, P.W., Thompson, V., Lambert, D., Sangster, Y., Noel, J.G., & Campbell, J. (2003b). Perceptions of discrimination among persons with serious mental illness. *Psychiatric Services*, 54, 1105–1110.

Crocker, J., Major, B., & Steele, C. (1998). Social stigma. In D. Gilbert, S. Fiske & G. Lindzey (Eds), *Handbook of Social Psychology*, 4th edn, vol. 2 (pp. 504–553). Boston: McGraw-Hill.

Couture, S.M., & Penn, D.L. (2003). Interpersonal contact and the stigma of mental illness: a review of the literature. *Journal of Mental Health*, 12, 291–305.

Cullinane, J. (2007). The domestication of AIDS: stigma, gender, and the body politic in Japan. *Medical Anthropology*, 26(3), 255–292.

Curra, J. (2014). *The Relativity of Deviance*, 3rd edn. Thousand Oaks, CA: Sage.

Daftary, A., Frick, M., Venkatesan, N., & Pai, M. (2018). Fighting TB stigma: we need to apply lessons learnt from NHIV activism. *BMJ Global Health*, 2, e000515. doi:10.1136/bmjgh-2017-000515

Daniel, H., & Parker, R.G. (1993). *Sexuality, Politics and AIDS in Brazil*. London: Falmer Press.

Deflem, M. (2015). Deviance and social control. In E. Goode (Ed.), *The Handbook of Deviance* (pp. 30–44). Malden, MA: Wiley-Blackwell.

Deng, R., Li, J., Sringernyuang, L., & Zhang, K. (2007). Drug abuse, HIV/AIDS and stigmatization in a Dai community in Yunnan, China. *Social Science and Medicine*, 64, 1560–1571.

Downes, D., Rock, P., & McLaughlin, E. (2016). *Understanding Deviance*, 7th edn. Oxford: Oxford University Press.

Durkheim, E. (1895/1982). *The Rules of Sociological Method*. New York: Free Press.

Durkheim, E. (1964). *The Elementary Forms of Religious Life*. New York: Free Press.

Earle, S. (2000). Why some women do not breast feed: bottle feeding and father's role. *Midwifery*, 16, 323–330.

Epstein, S. (1996). *Impure Science: AIDS, Activism and the Politics of Knowledge*. Berkeley: University of California Press.

Falk, G. (2001). *Stigma: How we treat Outsiders*. Amherst, NY: Prometheus Books.

Ferlatte, O., Salway, T., Oliffe, J.L., & Trussler, T. (2017). Stigma and suicide among gay and bisexual men living with HIV. *AIDS Care*, 29(1), 1346–1350.

Finzen, A. (2016). Stigma amd stigmatization within and beyond psychiatry. In W. Gaebel, W. Rössler & N. Sartorius (Eds), *The Stigma of Mental Illness: End of the Story?* (pp. 29–42). Dordrecht: Springer.

Foucault, M. (1973). *The Birth of the Clinic*. London: Tavistock.

Foucault, M. (1980). The politics of health in the eighteenth century. In C. Gordon (Ed.), *Power/Knowledge: Selected Interviews and Other Writings, 1972–1977* (pp. 166–182). Brighton, US: Harvest Press.

Foucault, M. (1981). *The History of Sexuality: An Introduction*, trans. Harmondsworth: Penguin.

Gaebel, W., Rössler, W., & Sartorius, N. (Eds) (2016). *The Stigma of Mental Illness: End of the Story?* Dordrecht: Springer.

Gilmore, N., & Somerville, M.A. (1994). Stigmatisation, scapegoating and discrimination in sexually transmitted diseases: overcoming 'them' and 'us'. *Social Science and Medicine*, 39(9), 1339–1358.

Goffman, E. (1963). *Stigma: On the Management of Spoiled Identity*. Englewood Cliffs, NJ: Prentice-Hall.

Goode, E. (2015). The sociology of deviance: an introduction. In E. Goode (Ed.), *The Handbook of Deviance* (pp. 3–29). Malden, MA: Wiley-Blackwell.

Guttman, N., & Zimmerman, D.R. (2000). Low-income mothers' views on breastfeeding. *Social Science and Medicine*, 50(10), 1457-1473.

Hatzenbuehler, M.L., Phelan, J.C., & Link, B.G. (2013). Stigma as a fundamental cause of population health inequalities. *American Journal of Public Health*, 103(5), 813–821.

Heijnders, M., & Van Der Meij, S. (2006). The fight against stigma: an overview of stigma-reduction strategies and interventions. *Psychology, Health, and Medicine*, 11, 353–363.

Herek, G.M. (2002). Thinking about AIDS and stigma: a psychologist's perspective. *Journal of Law, Medicine, and Ethics*, 30, 594–607.

Herek, G.M., & Glunt, E.K. (1993). Public reactions to AIDS in the United States: a second decade of stigma. *American Journal of Public Health*, 83(4), 573–577.

Jones, E.E., Farina, A., Hastort, A.H., Markus, H., & Miller, D.T. et al. (1984). *Social Stigma: The Psychology of Marked Relationships*. New York: W.H. Freeman.

Joseph, J. (2018). Feeding an infant in a foreign land: the experiences of refugee mothers from Vietnam and Myanmar. Unpublished PhD thesis. University of Queensland, Brisbane.

Katz, I. (1981). *Stigma: A Social Psychological Analysis*. Hillsdale, NJ: Erlbaum.

Krupchanka, D., & Thornicroft, G. (2016). Discrimination and stigma. In W. Gaebel, W. Rössler & N. Sartorius (Eds), *The Stigma of Mental Illness: End of the Story?* (pp. 129–139). Dordrecht: Springer.

Lawless, S., Kippax, S., & Crawford, J. (1996). Dirty, diseased and undeserving: the positioning of HIV-positive women. *Social Science and Medicine*, 43(9), 1371–1377.

LeBel, T.P. (2008). Perceptions of and responses to stigma. *Sociology Compass*, 2(2), 409–432.

Letteney, S., & LaPorte, H.H. (2004). Deconstructing stigma: perceptions of HIV-seropositive mothers and their disclosure to children. *Social Work in Health Care*, 38, 105–123.

Liamputtong, P. (Ed.) (2011). *Infant Feeding Practices: A Cross-cultural Perspective*. New York: Springer.

Liamputtong, P. (2013a). *Stigma, Discrimination and Living with HIV/AIDS: A Cross-cultural Perspective*. Dordrecht: Springer.

Liamputtong, P. (2013b). *Women, Motherhood and Living with HIV/AIDS: A Cross-cultural Perspective*. Dordrecht: Springer.

Liamputtong, P. (Ed.) (2016). *Children, Young People and HIV/AIDS: A Cross-cultural Perspective*. Dordrecht: Springer.

Liamputtong, P., & Haritavorn, N. (2016) To tell or not to tell: disclosure and women living with HIV/AIDS in Thailand. *Health Promotion International*, 31(1), 23–32.

Liamputtong, P., Haritavorn, N., & Kiatying-Angsulee, N. (2009). HIV and AIDS, stigma and AIDS support groups: perspectives from women living with HIV and AIDS in central Thailand. *Social Science and Medicine*, Special Issue: Women, Mothers and HIV Care in Resource-poor Settings, 69(6), 862–868.

Liamputtong, P., Haritavorn, N., & Kiatying-Angsulee, N. (2012). Living positively: the experiences of Thai women in central Thailand. *Qualitative Health Research*, 22(4), 441–451.

Liamputtong, P., & Kitisriworapan, S. (2011). Good mother, infant feeding and social change in northern Thailand. In P. Liamputtong (Ed.), *Infant Feeding Practices: A Cross-cultural Perspective* (pp. 141–159). New York: Springer.

Link, B.G., & Phelan, J.C. (2001). Conceptualizing stigma. *Annual Review of Sociology*, 27, 363–385.

Link, B.G., Struening, E.L., Neese-Todd, S., Asmussen, S., & Phelan, J.C. (2002). On describing and seeking to change the experience of stigma. *Psychiatric Rehabilitation Skills*, 6, 201–231.

Link, B., & Stuart, H. (2016). On revisiting some origins of the stigma concept as it applies to mental illnesses. In W. Gaebel, W. Rössler & N. Sartorius (Eds), *The Stigma of Mental Illness: End of the Story?* (pp. 3–28). Dordrecht: Springer.

Lyttleton, C. (2000). *Endangered Relations: Negotiating Sex and AIDS in Thailand*. Amsterdam: Harwood Academic Press.

Lyttleton, C. (2004). Fleeing the fire: transformation and gendered belonging in Thai HIV/AIDS support groups. *Medical Anthropology*, 23, 1–40.

Lyttleton, C., Beesey, A., & Sitthikriengkrai, M. (2007). Expanding community through ARV provision in Thailand. *AIDS Care*, 19(Supplement 1), S44–S53.

Major, B., Dovidio, J.F., & Link, B.G. (Eds) (2018). *The Oxford Handbook of Stigma, Discrimination and Health*. Oxford: Oxford University Press.

Major, B., Quinton, W.J., McCoy, S.K., & Schmader, T. (2000). Reducing prejudice: the target's perspective. In S. Oskamp (Ed.), *Reducing Prejudice and Discrimination* (pp. 211–237). Mahwah, NJ: Lawrence Erlbaum Associates.

Major, B., & O'Brien, L.T. (2005). The social psychology of stigma. *Annual Review of Psychology*, 56, 393–421.

Malik, A., & Dixit, S. (2017). Women living with HIV/AIDS: psychosocial challenges in the Indian context. *Journal of Health Management*, 19(3), 474–494.

Maneesriwongul, W., Panutat, S., Putwatana, P., Srirapo-ngam, Y., Ounprasertpong, L., & Williams, A.B. (2004). Educational needs of family caregivers of persons living with HIV/AIDS in Thailand. *Journal of the Association of Nurses in AIDS Care*, 15(3), 27–36.

Mann, J., & Tarantola, D. (1998). Responding to HIV/AIDS: a historical perspective. *Health and Human Rights: An International Journal*, 2(4), 5–8.

Markowitz, F.E. (2005). Sociological models of mental illness stigma. In P.W. Corrigan (Ed.), *On the Stigma of Mental Illness: Practical Strategies for Research and Social Change* (pp. 129–144). Washington, DC: American Psychological Association.

Mason, T., Carlisle, C., Watkins, C., & Whitehead, E. (2001). Introduction. In T. Mason, C. Carlisle, C. Watkins, & E. Whitehead (Eds), *Stigma and Social Exclusion in Health Care* (pp. 1–13). London: Routledge.

Mburu, G., Ram, M., Skovdal, M., Bitira, D., Hodgson, I., Mwai, G.W., Stegling, C., & Seeley, J. (2013). Resisting and challenging stigma in Uganda: the role of support groups of people living with HIV. *Journal of the International AIDS Society*, 16(Supplement 2), 18636. doi:10.7448/IAS.16.3.18636

McHugh, P. (1970). A commonsense conception of deviance. In J.D. Douglas (Ed.), *Deviance and Responsibility: The Social Construction of Moral Meanings* (pp. 61–88). New York: Basic Books.

Murphy, E. (1999). 'Breast is best': infant feeding decisions and maternal deviance. *Sociology of Health and Illness*, 21, 187–208.

Nadesan, M.H., & Sotirin, P. (1998). The romance and science of 'breast is best': discursive contradictions and contexts of breast-feeding choices. *Text and Performance Quarterly*, 18, 217–232.

Ndinda, C., Chimbwete, C., McGrath, N., Pool, R., & MDP Group (2007). Community attitudes towards individuals living with HIV in rural Kwa-Zulu Natal, South Africa. *AIDS Care*, 19(1), 92–101.

Oosterhoff, P., & Bach, T.X. (2013). The effect of collective action on the confidence of individual HIV-positive women in Vietnam. In P. Liamputtong (Ed.), *Women, Motherhood and Living with HIV/AIDS: A Cross-cultural Perspective* (pp. 215–229). Dordrecht: Springer.

Parker, R., & Aggleton, P. (2003). HIV and AIDS-related stigma and discrimination: a conceptual framework and implications for action. *Social Science and Medicine*, 57(1), 13–24.

Parker, R.G. (1996). *Empowerment, Community Mobilization, and Social Change in the Face of HIV/AIDS. AIDS* 10(Suppl.3), S27–S31.

Paudel, V., & Baral, K.P. (2015). Women living with HIV/AIDS (WLHA), battling stigma, discrimination and denial and the role of support group as a coping strategy: a review of literature. *Reproductive Health*, 12(53). doi:10.1186/s12978-015-0032-9

Pausé, C. (2017). Borderline: the ethics of fat stigma in public health. *Journal of Law, Medicine and Ethics*, 45, 510–517.

Persson, A., Newman, C.E., & Miller, A. (2016). 'There's more to you than just this virus': young people growing up with perinatally acquired HIV in Australia. In P. Liamputtong (Ed.), *Children and Young People Living with HIV/AIDS: A Cross-cultural Perspective* (pp. 107–124). Dordrecht: Springer.

Pescosolido, B.A., Martin, J.K., Lang, A., & Olafsdottir, S. (2008). Rethinking theoretical approaches to stigma: a framework integrating normative influences on stigma (FINIS). *Social Science and Medicine*, 67(3), 431–440.

Puhl, R., & Brownell, K.D. (2003). Ways of coping with obesity stigma: review and conceptual analysis. *Eating Behaviors*, 4, 53–78.

Reidpath, D.D., & Chan, K.Y.A. (2005). A method for the quantitative analysis of the layering of HIV-related stigma. *AIDS Care*, 17(4), 425–432.

Roach Anleu, S.L. (2006). *Deviance, Conformity and Control*, 4th edn. Sydney: Pearson Education Australia.

Roach Anleu, S.L. (2019). The medicalisation of deviance. In J. Germov (Ed.), *Second Opinion: An Introduction to Health Sociology*, 6th edn. Melbourne: Oxford University Press.

Rodier, D. (2017). *The Legacy of the HIV/AIDS Fight in Canada*. Retrieved from http://policyoptions.irpp.org/magazines/january-2017/the-legacy-of-the-hivaids-fight-in-canada/

Sayce, L. (2000). *From Psychiatric Patient to Citizen: Overcoming Discrimination and Social Exclusion*. New York: St Martin's Press.

Scambler, G. (2003). Deviance, sick role and stigma. In G. Scambler (Ed.), *Sociology as Applied to Medicine* (pp. 192–202). Edinburgh: Saunders.

Scheff, T. (1966). *Being Mentally Ill: A Sociological Theory*. Chicago: Aldine Publishing.

Sheehan, L., Nieweglowski, K., & Corrigan, P.W. (2016). Structures and types of stigma. In W. Gaebel, W. Rössler & N. Sartorius (Eds), *The Stigma of Mental Illness: End of the Story?* (pp. 43–66). Dordrecht: Springer.

Sherman, P. (2007). *Stigma, Mental Illness, and Culture*. http://www.scribd.com/doc/11731670/The-Stigma-of-Mental-Illness.

Shih, M. (2004). Positive stigma: examining resilience and empowerment in overcoming stigma. *Annals of the American Academy of Political and Social Science*, 591(1), 175–185.

Simbayi, L.C., Kalichman, S., Strebel, A., Cloete, A., Henda, N., & Mqeketo, A. (2007). Internalized stigma, discrimination, and depression among men and women living with HIV/AIDS in Cape Town, South Africa. *Social Science and Medicine*, 64(9), 1823–1831.

Snyder, K., Wallace, M., Duby, Z., Aquino, L.D.H., Stafford, S., Hosek, S., Futterman, D., & Bekker, L-G. (2014). Preliminary results from *Hlanganani* (Coming Together): a structured support group for HIV-infected adolescents piloted in Cape Town, South Africa. *Children and Youth Services Review*, 45, 114–121. doi:10.1016/j.childyouth.2014.03.027

Sontag, S. (1991). *Illness as Metaphor: AIDS and its Metaphors*. London: Penguin Books.

Sringernyuang, L., Thaweesit, S., & Nakapiew, S. (2005). A situational analysis of HIV/AIDS-related discrimination in Bangkok, Thailand. *AIDS Care*, 17(Suppl.2), S165–S174.

Stuber, J., Galea, S., & Link, B.G. (2008). Smoking and the emergence of a stigmatized social status. *Social Science and Medicine*, 67, 420–430.

Sulaiman Z., Liamputtong, P., & Amir, L. (2016). Infant feeding practices: challenges among women working in urban Malaysia. *Australian Journal of Advanced Nursing*, 72(4), 825–835. doi:10.1111/jan.12884

Suwankhong, D., & Liamputtong, P. (2018). 'I was told not to do it, but …': infant feeding practices among HIV-positive women in southern Thailand. *Midwifery*, 48, 69–74.

Thomas, F. (2006). Stigma, fatigue and social breakdown: exploring the impacts of HIV/AIDS on patient and carer well-being in the Caprivi Region, Namibia. *Social Science and Medicine*, 63(12), 3174–3187.

Thompson, W.E., & Gibbs, J.C. (2016). *Deviance and Deviants: A Sociological Approach*. Chichester, West Sussex: Wiley-Blackwell.

VanLandingham, M., Im-em, W., & Saengtienchai, C. (2005). Community reaction to persons with HIV/AIDS and their parents: an analysis of recent evidence from Thailand. *Journal of Health and Social Behavior*, 46, 392–410.

Vlassoff, C., & Ali, F. (2011). HIV-related stigma among South Asians in Toronto. *Ethnicity and Health*, 16(1), 25–42.

Whitehead, E., Carlisle, C., Watkins, C., & Mason, T. (2001a). Historical developments. In T. Mason, C. Carlisle, C. Watkins, & E. Whitehead (Eds), *Stigma and Social Exclusion in Health Care* (pp. 11–28).

Whitehead, E., Mason, T., Carlisle, C., & Watkins, C. (2001b). The changing dynamic of stigma. In T. Mason, C. Carlisle, C. Watkins, & E. Whitehead (eds), *Stigma and Social Exclusion in Health Care* (pp. 29–39). London: Routledge.

Williams, D.R., Gonzalez, H.M., Williams, S., Mohammed, S.A., Moomal, H., & Stein, D.J. (2008). Perceived discrimination, race and health in South Africa. *Social Science and Medicine*, 67(3), 441–452.

Worthen, M.G.F. (2016). *Sexual Deviance and Society: A Sociological Examination*. London: Routledge.

Wyrod, R. (2013). Gender and AIDS stigma. In P. Liamputtong (Ed.), *Stigma, Discrimination and Living with HIV/AIDS: A Cross-cultural Perspective* (pp. 39–51). Dordrecht: Springer.

Yang, L.H., Kleinman, A., Link, B.G., Phelan, J.C., Lee, S., & Good, B. (2007). Culture and stigma: adding moral experience to stigma theory. *Social Science and Medicine*, 64, 1524–1535.

Zhou, Y.R. (2007). 'If you get AIDS … you have to endure it alone': understanding the social constructions of HIV/AIDS in China. *Social Science and Medicine*, 65(2), 284–295.

Chapter 5

Social Justice, Human Rights and Social Determinants of Health

Debra Miles

Topics covered

This chapter covers the following topics:

- definitions of human rights and social justice
- impact of social injustice and human rights violations on health
- human rights and the health of vulnerable groups
- principles of human rights-based approaches to addressing social determinants of health

Key terms

health equity
human rights
human rights-based approaches
social determinants of health
social justice
structural disadvantage
vulnerable and marginalised people

Introduction

> In countries at all levels of income, health and illness follow a social gradient: the lower the socioeconomic position, the worse the health. It does not have to be this way and it is not right that it should be like this. … Putting right these inequities — the huge and remediable differences in health between and within countries — is a matter of social justice…. Social injustice is killing people on a grand scale (CSDH 2008, p. 1)

Social justice
Systemic and structural social arrangements that improve equality. They include the fair distribution of resources, equal access to opportunities and rights, and protection of the marginalised and vulnerable.

Social determinants of health
A number of factors, including social, cultural, economic and political, which can impact on the health of individuals.

Structural disadvantage
The disadvantage experienced by some individuals, families, groups or communities because of the way society functions. These disadvantages are systematically rooted in the normal operations of dominant social institutions such as markets, militaries, employment systems, social networks, health and education and taxation systems. They impact how resources are distributed, how people relate to each other, who has power, who makes decisions and how institutions are organised.

In 2005 the World Health Organization (WHO) established the Commission on Social Determinants of Health, which released its report in 2008. Charged with the responsibility of developing a pathway to global health equity, the Commission clearly and unequivocally pointed to **social justice** as an essential element that allows people to live healthy lives uninhibited by illness and premature death (CSDH 2008). The final report of the Commission drew together decades of evidence establishing the link between an individual's health status, no matter where they live in the world, and a much larger context described as 'social determinants'. **Social determinants** refer to the social, political, economic, environmental and cultural factors that affect health status, the circumstances of people's lives such as educational attainment, work conditions and housing as well as structural aspects such as the distribution of power and income and the experience of discrimination and racism (NRHA 2013; see also Chapters 1, 13 & 14 in this volume). In confirming the significant impact of these social determinants on the health of individuals and populations, the Commission highlighted the differential and unequal distribution of both health status and the conditions that contribute to that status.

The report emphasised global and national inequality in the distribution of power, income, goods and services as the cause of 'poor health of the poor, the social gradient of health within countries and the marked health inequities between countries' (CSDH 2008, p. 2). Such inequities are not natural, unavoidable or unamenable, and therefore their existence is unfair and unjust. The social inequalities observable in the health of marginalised people reflect injustices apparent in the basic structures of society that disadvantage the poor and benefit better-off groups: they are the product of inherent **structural disadvantage** and unjust economic and social policies (Chapman 2015).

Poverty, discrimination and marginalisation are structural contributors to health and health disparities, and are particularly unjust. However, such injustices have proved particularly resistant to historical policy approaches. In this chapter, I explore the relevance and usefulness of human rights-based approaches in guiding action to address health inequities and to improve the underlying social determinants of health (Stronks et al. 2016). A conceptual framework informed by human rights principles offers sustainable opportunities to create positive change and develop successful local and global initiatives that improve social determinants of health, well-being and equity (Mariner & Annas 2016).

I will discuss the nature of social justice and human rights concepts as they are relevant to understanding and influencing social determinants of health. In later sections, I highlight direct links between human rights violations, social injustice and health disparities, and explore the possibilities offered by policy and practice approaches informed by human rights.

Health and social justice

Concepts of social justice are integral to understanding social determinants of health and the imperatives to improve them (Taket 2019). However, while the term 'social justice' is popular among a variety of policy-makers to justify a range of decisions, it is rarely clearly defined (Reisch 2002). In this discussion, social justice is understood as those systemic and structural social arrangements that improve equality and ensure individuals and groups who need to actively claim their human rights have the capacity to do so (NPBRC 2011).

Developing and sustaining socially just arrangements of this type requires the fair distribution of resources, equal access to opportunities and rights, and protection of **vulnerable and marginalised people** in a manner that ensures their ability to take up opportunities and exercise their rights. These principles focus on eliminating inequity by promoting inclusiveness and diversity, seeking an equality of outcomes that goes beyond equal opportunity. Social justice, from this perspective, focuses attention on the environments where people live and work and on the social conditions that impact the ability of individuals and groups to make real choices about their everyday lives (Taket 2019).

The connections between **health equity** and social justice are well established in international literature. For example, the Helsinki statement on Health in All Policies (WHO 2014) recognises equity in health as both an outcome of socially just arrangements and a facilitative condition of a socially just society: 'Good health enhances quality of life, increases capacity for learning, strengthens families and communities and improves workforce productivity. Likewise, action aimed at promoting equity significantly contributes to health, poverty reduction, social inclusion and security' (WHO 2014, p. 1). Much of the international literature identifies the responsibility of governments to create the conditions that provide all people with equal chances to lead a healthy life (Stronks et al. 2016). Connecting the realisation of social justice principles with the capacity of individuals and groups to attain and sustain good health requires governments to acknowledge the diverse policy areas which influence people's lives and livelihoods, and ultimately their health, and to bring this awareness to political and economic decision-making.

Vulnerable and marginalised people
Distanced from economic, political and social power and resources, because they are perceived as undesirable or without function. This distancing works to exclude marginalised people from systems of protection and integration, increasing their susceptibility to adverse circumstances and harm.

Health equity
Providing everyone with the resources they individually need to enjoy full and healthy lives. It differs from equality, which provides the same resources to everyone regardless of need.

Stop and Think

Homelessness is one of the most severe forms of marginalisation and exclusion that a person can experience. Homelessness makes it difficult to engage in employment, education or training, and directly contributes to an individual's vulnerability to chronic ill-health and violence. Research has consistently identified that homelessness is the consequence of diverse and complex problems, including discrimination, a chronic shortage of affordable housing, domestic and family violence, intergenerational poverty, and severe and persistent mental illness. Common health problems for people who are homeless include poor nutrition, poor dental health, substance misuse and mental health problems (Steen 2018).

Consider the definition of vulnerable and marginalised people provided in the margin note. Think about specific examples of how Australians experiencing homelessness are excluded from participating in social, recreational, cultural and economic opportunities in their community.

- What might be some common health problems experienced by homeless people?
- What 'protective systems' are homeless people unable to access, therefore making them more vulnerable to the health issues described above?

Health and human rights

Human rights
An internationally agreed set of principles and standards by which to assess and redress inequality, and to advocate for, and even enforce, a fairer distribution of resources in the world.

While undoubtedly contested and difficult to define, human rights are something everyone is born with, derived from our humanity. They are an aspect of the human tradition. By their very nature **human rights** are:

- universal (part of all people everywhere)
- inalienable (unable to be taken away)
- indivisible (not to be compromised for other rights)
- interdependent (Ife 2012).

This conception of human rights is enshrined in the Universal Declaration of Human Rights and subsequent covenants. It provides an internationally agreed set of principles and standards by which to assess and redress inequality, and to advocate for, and even enforce, a fairer distribution of resources in the world (NPBRC 2014). This perception of human rights has several implications. Like social justice principles, it imposes obligations on governments to protect and formally pursue methods of realising the human rights of their citizens. For example, the right to education, enshrined as article 26 of the Declaration, requires governments to provide education facilities and services. However, this understanding of human rights as natural and universal also positions 'rights' as a special kind of claim on other people aside from government—a claim that acknowledges human dignity as an end in itself. Human rights emerge from our shared and negotiated understandings of how we should treat others and how we can expect to be treated by others (Ife 2012). With this awareness, human rights should always be considered within a framework of social justice as it is, ironically, those most vulnerable and disadvantaged who continue to have their most basic human rights violated, are most likely to have their innate humanness contested, and are least able to access the systems established to protect human rights. There is, therefore, a need to commit to social justice to facilitate such access and to affirm every individual's dignity (Taket 2019).

Historically, two types of human rights have been distinguished: civil and political rights (such as life, privacy and freedom of expression) and economic, social and cultural rights (health, food, education and housing). Ife (2012) argues that these rights have in some quarters been treated hierarchically, with civil and political rights afforded higher status as first-generation rights, and economic, social and cultural rights considered as second-generation rights and thus more likely to be modified and diluted. However, if human rights are interdependent and interrelated by their very nature, as suggested above, then a hierarchical listing makes little sense. All the rights support and reinforce each other and rights to life, to privacy and information, and to bodily integrity are as important as the rights to education, food and housing in protecting the health of individuals.

The right to health is specifically enshrined in various international legal documents, including the Universal Declaration of Human Rights and the International Covenant on Economic, Social and Cultural Rights. Article 25 of the Declaration states:

> Everyone has the right to a standard of living adequate for the health and well-being of himself and of his family, including food, clothing, housing and medical care and necessary social services, and the right to security in the event of unemployment, sickness, disability, widowhood, old age or other lack of livelihood in circumstances beyond his control (UN General Assembly 1948).

The Covenant, Article 12, recognises 'the right of everyone to the enjoyment of the highest attainable standard of physical and mental health' (UN General Assembly 1966). It requires states to provide the conditions and care necessary to protect the health of their populations as much as possible. However, perhaps reflective of arguments that prioritise civil and political rights over others, significant debate emerged challenging the notion that health, especially the provision of healthcare, could be considered a human right (Barlow 1999). In 2000 the UN adopted General Comment No. 14 to discuss the right to the highest attainable standard of health as described in Article 12 of the Covenant. General comments are documents released by the UN to explicitly clarify the meaning and implications of certain aspects of conventions, treaties and declarations so as to assist states in fulfilling their obligations (Stronks et al. 2016). The General Comment on the Right to Health took a broad approach to defining health as a human right. For example, it recognised that 'the highest attainable standard of physical and mental health' is not confined to the right to primary healthcare, and that the right to health embraces a wide range of socio-economic factors that promote the conditions that facilitate people's capacity to lead a healthy life. The Comment explicitly includes the underlying social determinants of health, such as food and nutrition, housing, access to safe water supplies and adequate sanitation, safe and healthy working conditions, and a healthy environment as integral to the human right to health (Stronks et al. 2016). In so doing, the UN inextricably linked the protection of basic human rights to action that addresses and improves social determinants of health (Taket 2019).

Of course, not all states fully respect human rights (Mariner & Annas 2016; Ramos 2018) and even if they do, the negotiated nature of human rights often impedes the full realisation of human rights for marginalised and disenfranchised groups. It is only when human rights are understood in conjunction with the concept of social justice that the complexities of ensuring the realisation of universal human rights for vulnerable and marginalised populations are fully illuminated. Differences in social determinants such as access to education, employment, housing, social and economic opportunities and political voice, among different classes, races, ethnicities and genders have significant effects on health, despite rhetorical and even sincere government commitments to the human right to health (Mariner 2016). Increased health resources alone are not sufficient to avoid significant health disparities and inequity, suggesting that the political empowerment of disadvantaged groups, embedded in respect for universal human rights, is more likely to see improvement in diverse social determinants of health (Mariner & Annas 2016).

Stop and Think

Indigenous children in Australia are twice as likely to die and twice as likely to be hospitalised than non-Indigenous children. They have ear infection rates that are three times the rates identified internationally as constituting a major public health issue. The causes of these health problems are consistently linked to poor nourishment, poor housing and unsatisfactory water and sanitation services in communities (McDonald et al. 2017). Indigenous children also experience discrimination, racism, a lack of access to basic health and education facilities, and culturally inappropriate interventions in their lives—all human rights violations.

Think about the nature of these causes and compare them with the International Declaration on the Rights of the Child. Highlight the areas where basic human rights are denied, thus resulting in significant health discrepancies between Indigenous children and other children in Australia.

Health consequences of human rights violations and social injustice

The discussion to date has proceeded on the assumption that social justice and fully recognised human rights are good for people's health by equitably distributing the social conditions that create opportunities for good health. Can such an assumption be justified? There is certainly literature which argues that individual behaviour and life-style choices have a substantial influence on health and many other social conditions (Balia & Jones 2008; Whelan & Wright 2013). However, most international commentators, including the members of the Commission on Social Determinants of Health, point to the legion of examples of fundamental social and environmental circumstances which filter through multiple pathways to expose individuals to health risks, to influence behaviour and choice, to affect access to healthcare and other supports, and to ultimately either mitigate or enhance the effects of subsequent health outcomes:

> Wealth enables a good education, which in turn facilitates well-paying employment and well-constructed housing in a safe community, free from pollutants, with access to good nutrition. In contrast, young children living in poverty may be exposed to poor nutrition, violence, or toxic substances, such as lead, risking brain damage that impedes their development and educational opportunities (Mariner 2016, p. 289).

The connections between poor health and poverty permeate most discussion of social determinants of health. Basic visible issues such as the cost of doctors' fees, medications or transport to health facilities impact on poor people, even those within wealthy countries, denying them possibilities for timely treatment and positive outcomes. Overcrowded and poor living conditions expose people to communicable diseases that are mostly eradicated in high-income countries, and a lack of food, clean water and sanitation either kills or weakens vulnerable people across the world every day (Davis 2013; see also Chapters 3, 11 & 14).

Case Example 5.1

Dying of poverty

In 2012 the local media reported that a four-year-old Aboriginal girl, Layla, was taken to hospital in a community in the Northern Territory with symptoms of coughing, wheezing and high temperature. She had been active and apparently healthy that morning but within a few hours she was coughing up blood and specialist services were called. However, she died before they arrived, from undiagnosed acute rheumatic heart fever. Rheumatic fever is an illness caused by bacterial infection, commonly called the strep bacteria. It is a disease that declined dramatically throughout the 20th century due to improved living conditions, better access to health services, and the introduction of penicillin. In Australia, Aboriginal people are 69 times more likely than non-Aboriginal people to develop rheumatic fever and 64 times more likely to have rheumatic heart disease. Between 2007 and 2009, 897 deaths were attributed to rheumatic heart disease and children under five were at greatest risk. An Indigenous person living in the Northern Territory is 54.8 times as likely to die from complications of rheumatic heart disease than a non-Indigenous person. The state coroner reported that Layla 'died of a disease of poverty'.

- Consider the human rights violations that led to Layla's death. Could a human rights approach have changed this situation?

Adapted from https://www.sbs.com.au/news/aboriginal-kids-die-from-poverty-diseases

Exclusion and discrimination based on gender, race or age restrict opportunities for targeted populations in education, employment and housing, undermining health and access to the treatment that is needed as a result. The cultural and social barriers faced by marginalised groups mean they use health services less, with serious consequences for their health (Mitrou et al. 2014).

Stop and Think

Tobacco use kills more than 7 million people worldwide each year (WHO 2018) and the rate continues to increase. The health consequences of smoking include premature death, chronic obstructive pulmonary disease and asthma, and the prohibitive cost of tobacco seriously impacts smokers and their families financially. Empirical evidence demonstrates that these health burdens are disproportionately experienced by those in low-income countries and by the poor in developed countries (Voigt 2010). Smoking is most prevalent in poor countries and among poor people. However, smoking is an individual choice 'freely made'; such health issues are said to result from poor decision-making and poor life-style choices. But are they? Consider issues such as the purposefully high prevalence of tobacco advertising in marginalised neighbourhoods, the limited access in low-income countries to accurate information about the health impacts of smoking, the different perceptions and social meanings associated with smoking among the poor, and the high cost, and subsequent limited access, to nicotine replacement therapies for poor people and poor countries (Voigt 2010).

- Is smoking really a purely individual choice? Or do the poor bear an unfair and avoidable health burden, to maintain tobacco company profits?

Human rights and social determinants of health in Australia

Despite Australia's ratification of international human rights documents such as the Declaration and the Covenant, there is no Commonwealth legislation which explicitly enshrines the right to health in domestic law. There are, however, pieces of legislation that impact Australia's approach in implementing a commitment to the right to health (Attorney-General's Department 2018).

The *Health Insurance Act 1973* underpins the Medicare scheme which provides financial assistance for medical expenses and free in-hospital services in public hospitals (see also Chapter 13). While current Medicare provisions may fall short of its original objectives—universal health insurance coverage for all Australians, provided in a manner that fairly distributes costs and ensures equitable access for all—this legislation is still an important foundation in Australia's attempts to realise individuals' right to health. The *Aged Care Act 1997* legislates the quality of care and accommodation for recipients of aged care services and, at least rhetorically, includes a commitment to the human rights of all older Australians in receipt of aged care services. The *Disability Services Act 1986* was intended to ensure that people with disability receive necessary services in a manner that reflects their human dignity and enables their full participation as members of the community. The *Australian Institute of Health and Welfare Act 1987* established the Australian Institute of Health and Welfare, whose functions are to collect and provide information and statistics on Australia's health and welfare. The Institute aims to improve the health and well-being of Australians through better health and welfare information and statistics. The legislation mentioned here by no means forms a comprehensive list. Instead, it illustrates the particular approach taken by the Australian government to meet its international obligations to its citizens.

In addition to specific legislation, the Australian government commissioned a Senate Inquiry to explore and report on Australia's response to the Commission on Social Determinants of Health 2008 report (CARC 2013a). The core recommendation of that Inquiry was that Australia adopt a 'Health in All Policies' (HiAP) approach to government action on social determinants of health. A HiAP strategy incorporates good health as a shared goal across all areas of government and encourages diverse policy portfolios to work collaboratively on complex health inequities. This approach acknowledges that while specific health portfolios are important, they cannot address social determinants of health alone, and that other government departments such as transport, agriculture, employment and education must also accept these determinants of health and well-being as their business. The Senate committee recommended a social determinants approach be taken across government, in particular in social, economic and employment policy decisions that affect social determinants (such as employment status, levels of welfare benefit and access to education) (CARC 2013a). This approach is already embedded in Australian policy-making, where all new legislation must be considered in terms of compatibility with human rights. Extending this process to social determinants of health both brings an appropriate broad vision of health to the policy landscape and embeds human rights as core components of such a vision.

Human rights and social determinants of health: vulnerable groups in Australia

Despite the legislative protections and policy approaches described above, there is little doubt that vulnerable and marginalised groups in Australia continue to experience a range of socially unjust conditions which simultaneously negatively impact their physical and mental health and overall well-being, and demonstrate a denial of the most basic human rights. This section discusses three vulnerable groups in detail. Issues regarding Indigenous people are covered in Chapter 8 and hence will not be included here.

Asylum seeker/refugee health and human rights

In 1951 the UN adopted the Convention Relating to the Status of Refugees (the Refugee Convention). Australia ratified this agreement in 1954, committing to the fundamental principles, most notably non-discrimination, non-penalisation and non-refoulement (not forcing a return to a country where the individual fears persecution). However, Australia falls significantly short of its international obligations to protect the human rights of all asylum seekers and refugees who arrive in Australia, regardless of how or where they arrive and whether they arrive with or without a visa (https://www.refugeecouncil.org.au/ and https://www.humanrights.gov.au/our-work/asylum-seekers-and-refugees).

Once in Australian territory, asylum seekers and refugees have the rights not to be arbitrarily detained and not to be sent back to a country where their life or freedom would be threatened. However, these rights are not protected—Australia maintains one of the most restrictive immigration detention systems in the world. Detention is mandatory, not time-limited, and people are not given access to a court of law in which to challenge the need for their detention. Even when released into the community, the denial of work rights to asylum seekers on bridging visas may force individuals and families into poverty and lead to breaches of multiple human rights.

The health issues confronting asylum seekers who experience these human rights abuses are well documented (Robertshaw et al. 2017; Sundram & Ventevogel 2017). However, the situation of children requires particular comment. In 2015 the Australian Human Rights Commission released a report on the health and well-being of children being held in detention centres:

> The children interviewed, most of whom had spent several months in Nauru, are amongst the most traumatised children the paediatricians have ever seen. There was an evident lack of understanding by centre staff of the relationship between prolonged detention and post-traumatic stress disorder and the cumulative impact of one episode of trauma upon another. For example, some children had witnessed atrocities at home, survived a traumatic boat trip, had been moved between several onshore to offshore detention centres, were traumatised by the presence of uniformed guards and actions such as head counts and had palpable anticipatory trauma at mention of return to Nauru (Elliott & Gunasekera 2015, p. 3).

This is a significant human rights travesty that attracts significant worldwide condemnation.

People with disabilities

Around 20 per cent of Australians have a disability and most experience significant barriers to good health, meaningful work and simply taking part in everyday activities. Australia has a number of legislative protections aimed at ensuring that the human rights of people with disabilities are realised. The *Disability Discrimination Act 1992* makes disability discrimination unlawful and promotes equal rights, equal opportunity and equal access for people with disabilities. The Convention on the Rights of Persons with Disabilities was ratified in 2008 and the Commonwealth government developed the National Disability Strategy 2010–2020 as a plan of action to progressively implement the Convention. This strategy specifically identifies that health and access to healthcare are essential to ensuring people with disabilities have equal opportunities to acquire and maintain 'the highest attainable standard of physical and mental health'. Issues of choice, control and participation are highlighted as important in realising the basic human rights of people with disabilities.

Despite these protections and the advances made in recognising the rights of people with disabilities, the overall health of people with disabilities is much worse than that of the general population. Though by definition people with disabilities must have a health condition or impairment, the health inequities extend to areas that have no biological connection to the condition associated with a person's disability and significant connection to disadvantage and marginalisation. Statistics consistently demonstrate that people with disabilities and their carers are among the most socially and economically marginalised groups in Australia. Disability is both a consequence and a cause of exclusion and disadvantage, in that people with a disability are more likely to experience disadvantage, and those who experience disadvantage are more likely to become disabled (AIHW 2017; Iacono & Bigby 2019).

Equally as concerning is the level of discrimination and oppression experienced by people with disabilities. Research demonstrates that virtually every Australian with a disability encounters human rights violations at some point in their lives, and very many experience them every day of their lives (VicHealth 2012). For example, unlike in most developed countries, Australian people with disabilities have no legislative rights to equipment such as wheelchairs, hoists and communication devices essential for daily living. Over a million people with disabilities have reported difficulty using public transport. Despite legislation to protect people with disabilities from forced sterilisation, available data indicates the numbers of sterilisations far exceed those lawfully approved, with the majority performed on females with an intellectual disability (WWDA 2013).

Violence against women

The UN Declaration on the Elimination of Violence against Women defines violence against women as any act of gender-based violence that results in, or is likely to result in, physical, sexual or psychological harm or suffering to women. In practice, the term 'violence against women' encompasses an array of abuses targeted at women and girls, ranging from sex-selective abortion to the abuse of older women. It includes geographically or culturally specific forms of abuse such as female genital mutilation, dowry deaths, acid-throwing and honour killings (the murder of women who have allegedly brought shame to their family), as well as forms of violence that are prevalent worldwide, such as domestic violence and rape (AHRC 2017b).

International literature identifies violence against women as both a violation of human rights and a serious public health concern around the globe. According to WHO estimates, 35 per cent of women globally have experienced physical and/or sexual violence at some point in their lives (WHO 2017). Violence against women is a violation of women's rights and freedoms. It impacts their entitlements to equality, liberty, integrity and dignity in political, social, economic, cultural and civic life and as such constitutes a significant abuse of human rights. Violence also has major harmful effects on women's health and well-being, including on their sexual and reproductive and their mental health (AASW 2015). A fundamental cause of violence against women is ongoing and entrenched gender inequality, which is reflected across all aspects of a woman's life and results in a range of disadvantages and poor health and well-being outcomes across the life-span.

Research on violence against women has commonly focused on individual determinants associated with violent acts, and has ignored how patterns of violence are connected to structural violence perpetrated by social systems and social institutions. Structural violence is marked by deeply unequal access to the social determinants of health, such as education, housing and employment, which shape the nature of women's vulnerable social position and create conditions where interpersonal violence can happen. For instance, interpersonal violence is more likely to occur in relationships where a relatively large income gap exists between the partners (Stephanie & Thurston 2015).

A recent report by the Australian Sex Discrimination Commissioner highlights that there are several gaps in how Australia is addressing the number of social determinants which contribute to ongoing violence against women:

> Despite Australia ranking as first for educational attainment for women in the World Economic Forum Global Gender Index, our overall ranking in gender equality has regressed from 15th in 2006 to 46th in 2016. Australia ranks 42nd in women's economic participation and opportunity, 72nd in health and survival and 61st in political empowerment (AHRC 2017b, no page number).

Case Example 5.2

Forced sterilisation of women with intellectual disabilities

In 2013 the Royal Australian and New Zealand College of Obstetricians and Gynaecologists submitted the following argument to the Senate Committee Inquiry into the coerced sterilisation of people with disabilities.

- Some disabled girls or women may still have their best interests served by hysterectomy or sterilisation.
- Sterilisation is a way both to prevent conception and to deal with menstrual issues.
- Sterilisation is sometimes the best option when other methods of menstrual regulation fail.
- People with disabilities are more susceptible to sexual assault.

The College shared the following example: a mute woman with an intellectual disability had seven children, all of whom were given to her ageing parents for care. Her parents begged the health facility to sterilise her, but it did not happen and she had another baby. A few months later she fell pregnant again, to a new and violent partner who killed her during the pregnancy.

Advocate organisation Women with Disabilities Australia (WWDA 2013, p. 48) included the following quote from a woman with an intellectual disability, in its submission:

> I got sterilised at 18, my mum said I had to. She said that if I ever had a child, she'd probably have to help look after it. She said: 'I went through hell bringing you up and I will not do it again'. It's more than 30 years now since I was sterilised and the pain is still unspeakable. It is the biggest regret of my life.

Consider the social attitudes and structures behind these two different submissions.

- Which human rights could be considered?
- How could a human rights-based approach inform decision-making?

Adapted from CARC (2013b)

Practice implications of using human rights and social justice to address social determinants of health

The Commission on Social Determinants of Health made three overarching recommendations for addressing the health inequities that impact the lives of those at the bottom of global and national social gradients. The second of those recommendations calls on all social institutions, including governments and civil society, to 'tackle the inequitable distribution of power, money and resources' (CSDH 2008, p. 10). The Commission acknowledged that in essence it was calling for action on 'the way society is organised' (CSDH 2008, p. 2). Using human rights as an organising principle provides the framework to both understand and act to eliminate the social inequities embedded within the organisational structures of society. Practice approaches informed by human rights and social justice can inform the way in which government and non-government organisations work towards addressing social determinants of health. The synergy described in this chapter between good health and fulfilment of human rights makes it clear that clinical intervention and medical care are not the only, or even the most important, contributors to good health. So, any action that protects basic human rights will inherently positively impact population health (Mariner & Annas 2016).

A basic tenet of human rights approaches to practice is the consideration that all rights are interdependent and intertwined. Similarly, a social determinants approach to health requires an understanding of the interconnection between wide-ranging issues such as income levels, unemployment, experiences of racism, and

Human rights-based approaches
Frameworks for action that are based on international human rights standards and are operationally focused on promoting and protecting human rights through principles of participation, accountability, non-discrimination, empowerment and legality.

education attainment, and the health of individuals and groups. A **human rights-based approach** to health draws attention to the following elements:

- the accountability of governments to address inequities in socio-economic outcomes
- the application of non-discriminatory principles that provide for equitable availability and access
- the establishment of distinct and specific programs and services that meet the needs and aspirations of particular cultural groups
- the endorsement of an intricate combination of responses that respect, protect and fulfil the right to health
- the commitment to the process of achieving improvements in social determinants—that is, ensuring that people have the opportunity to contribute and participate and that the single-minded pursuit of health goals does not infringe other basic human rights
- the establishment of criteria based on the internationally sanctioned principles of availability, accessibility, affordability and quality against which specific health policies, practices and services are assessed
- the commitment to internationally recognised principles of participation that are essential to a human rights-based approach such as:
    - people as key actors in their own development, rather than passive recipients of commodities and services
    - participation as both a means and a goal
    - empowering, not disempowering, strategies
    - active engagement of all stakeholders.

Case Example 5.3

Applying a human rights approach

Pregnant Indigenous women in a regional town were required to attend antenatal clinics in the wards of the local hospital, which was located in an area poorly served by public transport. Women often spent many hours in sterile hospital environments and, as most staff were non-Indigenous, there was little understanding of cultural protocols. Unsurprisingly, attendance was low, with many pregnant Indigenous women accessing significantly less antenatal care than their non-Indigenous counterparts. This contributed at least in part to higher rates of preterm birth, low birthweight and perinatal mortality.

A new program was established with the following features:

- a daily community-based clinic held in the premises of an Aboriginal-controlled community medical service
- an integrated team which included Aboriginal health workers, Indigenous outreach workers, female doctors, midwives and child health nurses

- a family-oriented environment including a playground, educational toys and playgroups
- a pregnancy register which included monthly recalls and a daily walk-in clinic
- comprehensive care plans, developed with patient and family
- brief intervention for associated risk factors such as smoking cessation, nutrition, antenatal education and breastfeeding
- a transport service.

Consider the features of a human rights-based approach to health, and identify aspects of the new program that respond to basic human rights which have an influence on the women's health.

Adapted from Panaretto et al. (2005)

Reflection Exercise

This chapter has argued strongly that human rights and social justice are not only core social determinants of health in and of themselves, but that policy and practice approaches informed by human rights instruments and social justice principles provide real opportunities to respond to and address the complex social determinants that adversely affect the health of marginalised people. However, the actual implementation of human rights-based approaches is sometimes seen as too hard or too ambiguous for healthcare and social care front-line practitioners. Reflect on the following issues that affect homeless people, and consider the implications of a rights-based approach to homelessness as opposed to welfare-oriented approaches.

Understanding homelessness as a dynamic process that exists on a continuum of exclusions and rights violations is crucial to a human rights approach to homelessness. The relationship between the right to housing and other rights is profound—decent housing is a primary means of protecting health and well-being by offering a space to cook food hygienically, to shelter from weather, and to store clothing and other possessions connected with well-being. Safe and appropriate housing safeguards rights to privacy and self-determination, enables freedom of speech and of religious practice, and provides some security from cruel, inhumane or degrading treatment.

The experience of homelessness is a cause of marginalisation, social injustice and human rights abuse. Homeless people are criminalised in a variety of ways for carrying out life-sustaining activities in public even though they have no other option. For example, a homeless person's right to equality before the law is infringed by the selective enforcement of public space laws that penalise and even incarcerate them for minor offending behaviour such as sleeping out, storing belongings in public and urinating in public—all of which are directly related to being homeless (Walsh 2006). Many organisations that work with homeless people provide services aimed at finding and sustaining housing, however, the human rights violations experienced by homeless people do not necessarily abate through the provision of such services.

What would a rights-based approach look like? Committing to a human rights approach requires a different mindset—just recognising that homelessness impacts on a person's ability to enjoy a range of basic rights and freedoms has important consequences for the way practitioners perceive, treat and work with homeless people. Rather than delivering welfare services, a practitioner informed by a human rights approach may look to meaningfully involve people experiencing homelessness in the development of solutions, or focus on ensuring homeless people are informed and educated about their human rights and what that means. Defending the rights of homeless people to 'exist and survive' in public spaces—for example, by advocating for 'safe zones' or negotiating for permission to distribute food on the streets—may be more reflective of a rights-based approach than advocating for more beds in shelters or negotiating short-term admissions to hospital (Kenna & Fernández Evangelista 2013).

Reflect back on the material in this chapter and consider some of the specific strategies that organisations and practitioners can use to develop a human rights-based approach to homelessness as both a social determinant of health and a human rights violation.

- What do you think about these ideas?
- What barriers to the use of such an approach can you see?

Summary

Attention to principles of social justice and human rights can enhance the value and effect of any efforts to address social determinants of health. The respect, protection and fulfilment of human rights—including civil, political, economic, social and cultural rights—is necessary not only because they are moral and legal obligations of governments but because they are essential for the improved health status of individuals and groups. The unique nature of a human rights approach is especially relevant to addressing social determinants of health for marginalised groups because the indivisibility of human rights links civil and political rights to socio-economic rights, including the right to health. Human rights approaches assume and draw upon the active agency of those most vulnerable to human rights violations. They draw attention to the structural causes of health inequities and ensure the active participation of those most affected. Finally, a human rights approach establishes clear accountability to provide protections and freedoms, not only on governments but on all of society: what we expect and are prepared to accept.

> The policies needed to realise human rights lay the foundation for improving population health, well-being and equity … As better policies are adopted, the public might come to enjoy and expect health, well-being, and equity, regardless of the priority placed on health itself (Mariner & Amos 2016, p. 2003).

Tutorial exercises

1. Our Rights Continuum

Create a space where participants can stand in a line from one end of the room to the other (a continuum), showing how strongly they agree or disagree with a statement. It is useful to explain that the statements tend to produce strong feelings and reactions and that the purpose is to consider their own view and to listen to the views of others. Read a statement from the list below or create your own. Ask participants to stand along the invisible continuum depending on whether they disagree or agree with the statement. Once positions have been selected, ask participants to share their reasons for their position. Encourage respectful discussion from both ends of the continuum.

Possible statements:

- Human rights are ideals. They cannot be practically applied in health settings.
- In countries like Australia, good health is an issue of choice not rights.
- Men have more rights than women and this is reflected in their health.
- The human right to health is a luxury that few countries can afford.

Further questions to promote learning:

- Which statements were easy to agree on?
- Why was it difficult to find agreement on some statements?
- Do participants feel more strongly about some of the issues than about others? Why?

2. Rotating Think Tanks

Divide the tutorial into equal-sized groups. Write four or five issues or questions onto separate large pieces of paper. For example:

- How does a focus on health as a human right, improve quality of life?
- What can practitioners outside the health sector do to promote a human rights approach to health?
- How can improving the education options of Indigenous children impact their individual health outcomes?
- How could a 'Health in all Policies' approach be integrated into a child welfare organisation?

Give one sheet of paper to each group. Each group writes its responses to the question on its sheet. After five to six minutes, ask each group to rotate to another sheet. Each new group should spend some time considering the ideas already recorded and then add their own. After all the groups have contributed to each sheet, the tutorial as a whole can discuss the different ideas and opinions reflected in the responses to each issue.

3. Needs, Wants and Rights

Ask participants, working in small groups, to create a list of 10–20 items that they think human beings need in order to be healthy. Each group exchanges its list with another group. The group then rewrites the new list into the following categories: NEEDS (e.g. things essential for survival); WANTS (e.g. desirable but not essential for survival); and NEITHER.

Ask the whole tutorial to combine the lists on a whiteboard. Discuss some of these questions.

- Is it easy to differentiate between wants and needs?
- What happens to someone when their wants are not fulfilled?

- What happens to someone when their basic needs are not met?
- What happens to a community when many people's basic needs are not met?
- Are there people who don't have their basic needs met in Australia? In your community?
- What actions can be taken to help meet the basic needs of others in Australia? In the community?
- What is the relationship between human needs and human rights?
- Are there situations where 'wants' conflict with 'needs'?
- Are there situations where a person's 'wants' conflict with the 'needs' of others? Are these situations to do with rights? For example, do future generations have a right to a clean planet on which to maintain health? What implications does that have for our wants and/or needs now?

4. Rights, Health and Equality

Select six participants from the group. Assign each one of the following roles. Encourage them to consider these roles for a few minutes to build their view of what the character might be like:

- you are a single woman (35) with three school-age children, receiving Newstart benefits
- you are the daughter of a wealthy local family, studying economics at university
- you are the son of a Chinese immigrant who runs a successful business, where you are employed
- you are a young man and a wheelchair-user and live in a group home
- you are a 17-year-old Aboriginal woman from a remote community who has not completed secondary school
- you are the 19-year-old son of a farmer living in a rural country area and working the family farm.

Ask the participants to line up beside each other (like a starting line). Tell them you are going to read out a list of situations or events. Every time that a participant can answer 'yes' to a statement, they should take a step forward. Otherwise, they should stay where they are. Tell them the answers will depend on the details they have determined about their role.

Read out the following statements one at a time:

- you have never encountered any serious financial difficulty
- you have decent housing with phone, internet, a computer and a television
- you feel that your language, religion and culture are respected in Australia
- you are not afraid of being stopped by the police
- you know where to turn for help and advice if you need it
- you have never felt discriminated against
- you have private health insurance
- you can go away on holiday once a year, or more
- you can invite friends for dinner at home
- you can meet friends out for coffee, drinks or other social events
- you can study and follow the profession of your choice
- you are not afraid of being harassed or attacked on the street, or in the media
- you can buy new clothes when you want or need them.

Pause for a while between each statement to allow people to step forward (or not), and to look around and note their positions in relation to each other. When all the situations have been read out, invite everyone to take note of their final position and to announce their role to the rest of the group. Now ask the whole group to consider what might be the impact for each character if they were to

- have a stroke
- have asthma
- have a diagnosis of leukaemia.
- How far forward in the line did a character have to be to have a positive outcome from any of these health issues? Encourage the group to consider what situations made a difference to the health outcomes.

5. Human Rights in Practice

Divide the tutorial into small groups and assign each group the description of an organisation. For example, you may choose:

- a medium-size non-government organisation that recruits, trains and support foster carers. Four per cent of the carers and 37 per cent of the children being cared for are Indigenous
- a small non-government organisation that provides lunch, housing assistance and emergency financial relief to disadvantaged people. Eighty per cent of clients are male and 45 per cent are Indigenous
- a women's refuge with capacity for six women and 15 children. Usually full, with most residents from non-English-speaking backgrounds.

Ask each group to develop a policy and practice framework to address the health needs for the client group of their organisation, informed by a human rights approach to health as described in the chapter.

Further reading

Bustreo, F., & Hunt, P. (2013). *Women's and Children's Health: Evidence of Impact of Human Rights.* Geneva: World Health Organization. Retrieved from http://www.who.int/maternal_child_adolescent/documents/women_children_human_rights/en/

Chapman, A. (2016). *Global Health, Human Rights, and the Challenge of Neoliberal Policies.* Cambridge: Cambridge University Press.

Kenyon, K.H., & Garcia, R. (2016). Exploring human rights-based activism as a social determinant of health: insights from Brazil and South Africa. *Journal of Human Rights Practice*, 8(2), 198–218. doi.org/10.1093/jhuman/huw008

Stronks, K., Toebes, B., Hendriks, A., Ikram, U., & Venkatapuram, S. (2016). *Social Justice and Human Rights as a Framework for addressing Social Determinants of Health.* Final Report of the Task Group on Equity, Equality and Human Rights. Review of the Social Determinants of Health and the Health Divide in the WHO European Region. Geneva: World Health Organization. Retrieved from http://www.euro.who.int/__data/assets/pdf_file/0006/334356/HR-task-report.pdf?ua=1

Taket, A. (2012). *Health Equity, Social Justice and Human Rights.* London: Routledge.

Websites

http://www.who.int/topics/human_rights/en/

The World Health Organization is instrumental in promoting the worldwide realisation of the highest standard of health as a basic and core human right. It produces a number of resources and publications aimed at supporting states and organisations to take deliberate steps towards the full realisation of 'the right to health'. This website is particularly relevant to issues addressed in this chapter.

https://www.amnesty.org.au/

Amnesty International is a non-government organisation which focuses on human rights, with a vision that every person in the world will one day enjoy the full array of rights enshrined in the Universal Declaration of Human Rights. It runs local and global campaigns to expose human rights abuses and to promote the human rights of the most disadvantaged. Many of its campaigns are particularly relevant to resolving inequities in social determinants of health.

http://www.ohchr.org/EN/pages/home.aspx

The Office of the UN High Commissioner for Human Rights is a UN agency that works to promote and protect human rights. It was established by the UN General Assembly on 20 December 1993 in the wake of the 1993 World Conference on Human Rights. This website has a rich array of resources on a range of topics including health.

https://www.humanrights.gov.au/

The Australian Human Rights Commission has responsibility for investigating human rights breaches by Commonwealth agencies, and the website has a range of important resources relevant to the work of the AHRC. Specific health-related campaigns include the Close the Gap campaign, which examines access to health services for people with disability, and human rights and mental illness.

http://www.abc.net.au/radionational/programs/boyerlectures/series/2016-boyer-lectures/7802472

The Boyer Lecture series involves prominent speakers who deliver stimulating and thought-provoking lectures on a wide range of topics. In 2016 Sir Michael Marmot presented a series titled 'Fair Australia: Social Justice and the Health Gap'. This website takes you to the podcasts of this series.

References

AASW (Australian Association of Social Workers) (2015). *Position Statement: Violence against Women*. Retrieved from https://www.aasw.asn.au/document/item/7652

AHRC (Australian Human Rights Commission) (2017a). *Asylum Seekers, Refugees and Human Rights. Snapshot Report*, 2nd edn. Retrieved from https://www.humanrights.gov.au/sites/default/files/document/publication/AHRC_Snapshot%20report_2nd%20edition_2017_WEB.pdf

AHRC (Australian Human Rights Commission) (2017b). *Unleashing the Power of Gender Equality*. Retrieved from https://www.humanrights.gov.au/our-work/sex-discrimination/publications/unleashing-power-gender-equality-2017

AIHW (Australian Institute of Health and Welfare) (2017). *Australia's Welfare 2017: In Brief*. Cat. No. AUS 215. Canberra: Australian Institute of Health and Welfare.

Attorney-General's Department (2018). *Right to Health*. Retrieved from https://www.ag.gov.au/RightsAndProtections/HumanRights/Human-rights-scrutiny/PublicSectorGuidanceSheets/Pages/Righttohealth.aspx

Balia, S., & Jones, A. (2008). Mortality, lifestyle and socio-economic status. *Journal of Health Economics*, 27(1), 1–26.

Barlow, P. (1999). Health care is not a human right. *British Medical Journal*, 319(7205), 321.

Bustreo, F., & Hunt, P. (2013). *Women's and Children's Health: Evidence of Impact of Human Rights.* Geneva: World Health Organization. Retrieved from http://www.who.int/maternal_child_adolescent/documents/women_children_human_rights/en/

CARC (Community Affairs References Committee) (2013a). *Australia's Domestic Response to the World Health Organization's (WHO) Commission on Social Determinants of Health Report 'Closing the Gap in a Generation'*. Canberra: Parliament of Australia. Retrieved from https://www.aph.gov.au/Parliamentary_Business/Committees/Senate/Community_Affairs/Completed_inquiries/2010-13/socialdeterminantsofhealth/report/index

CARC (Community Affairs References Committee) (2013b). *Involuntary or Coerced Sterilisation of People with Disabilities in Australia.* Canberra: Parliament of Australia. Retrieved from https://www.aph.gov.au/Parliamentary_Business/Committees/Senate/Community_Affairs/Involuntary_Sterilisation

Chapman, A. (2015). The social determinants of health: why we should care. *American Journal of Bioethics*, 15(3), 46–47. doi:10.1080/15265161.2014.998375

Chapman, A. (2016). *Global Health, Human Rights, and the Challenge of Neoliberal Policies*. Cambridge: Cambridge University Press.

CSDH (Commission on Social Determinants of Health) (2008). *Closing the Gap in a Generation: Health Equity through Action on the Social Determinants of Health.* Final Report of the Commission on Social Determinants of Health. Geneva: World Health Organization. Retrieved from http://www.who.int/social_determinants/final_report/csdh_finalreport_2008.pdf

Davis, M. (2013). *Killing us with Hunger: Indigenous Perspectives on Nutrition, Food Aid and Food Sovereignty in Central Amazon of Peru*. London: Health Poverty Action.

Elliott, E., & Gunasekera, H. (2015). *The Health and Wellbeing of Children in Immigration Detention.* Report to the Australian Human Rights Commission. Retrieved from https://www.humanrights.gov.au/our-work/

asylum-seekers-and-refugees/publications/health-and-well-being-children-immigration

Iacono, T., & Bigby, C. (2019). The health of people with intellectual and developmental disabilities: strategies for change. In P. Liamputtong (Ed.), *Public Health: Local and Global Perspectives*, 2nd edn (Chapter 18). Melbourne: Cambridge University Press.

Ife, J. (2012). *Human Rights and Social Work: Towards a Rights-based Practice*. Melbourne: Cambridge University Press.

Kenna, P., & Fernández Evangelista, G. (2013). Applying a human rights-based approach to homelessness: from theory to practice. In S. Jones (Ed.), *Mean Streets: A Report on the Criminalisation of Homelessness in Europe* (pp. 31–52). Brussels: FEANTSA.

Kenyon, K.H., & Garcia, R. (2016). Exploring human rights-based activism as a social determinant of health: insights from Brazil and South Africa. *Journal of Human Rights Practice*, 8(2), 198–218. doi:10.1093/jhuman/huw008

Mariner, W. (2016). Beyond lifestyle: governing the social determinants of health. *American Journal of Law and Medicine*, 42, 284–309. doi:10.1177/0098858816658268

Mariner, W., & Annas, G. (2016). A culture of health and human rights. *Health Affairs*, 35(11), 1999–2004. doi:10.1377/hlthaff.2016.0700

McDonald, E., Bailie, R., & Morris, P. (2017). Participatory systems approach to health improvement in Australian Aboriginal children. *Health Promotion International*, 32(1), 62–72.

Mitrou, F., Cooke, M., Lawrence, D., Rovah, D., Mobilia, E., Guimond, E., & Zubrick, S. (2014). Gaps in indigenous disadvantage not closing: a census cohort study of social determinants of health in Australia, Canada and New Zealand from 1981–2006. *BMC Public Health*, 14, 201. doi:10.1186/1471-2458-14-201

NPBRC (National Pro Bono Resource Centre) (2011). *What is Social Justice?* Sydney: University of New South Wales. Retrieved from https://www.probonocentre.org.au/wp-content/uploads/2015/09/Occ_1_What-is-Social-Justice_FINAL.pdf

NRHA (National Rural Health Alliance) (2013). Improving the social determinants of rural and remote health. *Australian Journal of Rural Health*, 21(2), 135. doi:10.1111/ajr.12026

Panaretto, K., Lee, H., Mitchell, M., Larkins, S., Manessis, V., Buettner, P., & Watson, D. (2005). Impact of a collaborative shared antenatal care program for urban Indigenous women: a prospective cohort study. *Medical Journal of Australia*, 182(10), 514–519.

Ramos, A. (2018). A human rights-based approach to farmworker health: an overarching framework to address the social determinants of health. *Journal of Agromedicine*, 23(1), 25–31. doi:10.1080/1059924X.2017.1384419

Reisch, M. (2002). Defining social justice in a socially unjust world. *Families in Society*, 83(4), 343.

Robertshaw, L., Dhesi, S., & Jones, L. (2017). Challenges and facilitators for health professionals providing primary healthcare for refugees and asylum seekers in high-income countries: a systematic review and thematic synthesis of qualitative research. *BMJ Open, 7*(8) (e015981). doi:10.1136/bmjopen-2017-015981

Steen, A. (2018). The many costs of homelessness. *Medical Journal of Australia*, 208(4), 167–168. doi:10.5694/mja17.01197

Stephanie, R., & Thurston, W. (2015). Mapping the role of structural and interpersonal violence in the lives of women: implications for public health interventions and policy. *BMC Women's Health*, 15. Retrieved from https://search-proquest-com.elibrary.jcu.edu.au/docview/1779685795?accountid=16285

Stronks, K., Toebes, B., Hendriks, A., Ikram, U., & Venkatapuram, S. (2016). *Social Justice and Human Rights as a Framework for Addressing Social Determinants of Health.* Final Report of the Task Group on Equity, Equality and Human Rights. Review of the Social Determinants of Health and the Health Divide in the WHO European Region. Geneva: World Health Organization. Retrieved from http://www.euro.who.int/__data/assets/pdf_file/0006/334356/HR-task-report.pdf?ua=1

Sundram, S., & Ventevogel, P. (2017). The mental health of refugees and asylum seekers on Manus Island. *Lancet*, 390(10112), 2534–2536. doi:10.1016/S0140-6736(17)33051-9

Taket, A. (2012). *Health Equity, Social Justice and Human Rights.* London: Routledge.

Taket, A. (2019). Human rights, social justice and public health. In P. Liamputtong (Ed.), *Public Health: Local and Global Perspectives*, 2nd edn (Chapter 10). Melbourne: Cambridge University Press.

UN General Assembly (1948). *Universal Declaration of Human Rights*, 217 [III] A. Paris. Retrieved from http://www.un.org/en/universal-declaration-human-rights/

UN General Assembly (1966). *International Covenant on Civil and Political Rights.* Retrieved from http://www.ohchr.org/EN/ProfessionalInterest/Pages/CESCR.aspx

VicHealth (2012). Disability and Health Inequalities in Australia: Addressing the Social and Economic Determinants of Mental and Physical Health. Research summary. Melbourne: VicHealth. Retrieved from https://www.vichealth.vic.gov.au/media-and-resources/publications/disability-and-health-inequalities-in-australia

Voigt, K. (2010). Smoking and social justice. *Public Health Ethics*, 3(2), 91–106. doi:10.1093/phe/phq006

Walsh, T. (2006). A right to inclusion? Homelessness, human rights and social exclusion. *Australian Journal of Human Rights*, 12(1), 185–204.

Whelan, S., & Wright, D. (2013). Health services use and lifestyle choices of Indigenous and non-Indigenous Australians. *Social Science and Medicine*, 84, 1–12. doi.org/10.1016/j.socscimed.2013.02.013

WHO (World Health Organization) (2014). *Health in all Policies: Helsinki Statement. Framework for Country Action.* Geneva: World Health Organization. Retrieved from http://apps.who.int/iris/bitstream/handle/10665/112636/9789241506908_eng.pdf;jsessionid=16A756A7634B5BE720C24ABBCB5B5ABD?sequence=1

WHO (World Health Organization) (2017). *Violence against Women*. Fact Sheet. Retrieved from http://www.who.int/mediacentre/factsheets/fs239/en/

WHO (World Health Organization) (2018). *Tobacco*. Fact Sheet. Retrieved from http://www.who.int/mediacentre/factsheets/fs339/en/

WWDA (Women with Disabilities Australia) (2013). *Dehumanised: The Forced Sterilisation of Women and Girls with Disabilities in Australia.* WWDA Submission to the Senate Inquiry into the involuntary or coerced sterilisation of people with disabilities in Australia. Retrieved from http://wwda.org.au/wp-content/uploads/2013/12/WWDA_Sub_SenateInquiry_Sterilisation_March2013.pdf

Chapter 6

Health Promotion and Social Determinants of Health

Kate McBride, Freya MacMillan, Emma George and Genevieve Steiner

Topics covered

This chapter covers the following topics:

- principles of health promotion
- Ottawa Charter: priority action areas and principles in health promotion
- theoretical frameworks underpinning health promotion
- primary healthcare
- social marketing

Key terms

evaluation
community engagement
health promotion
logic model
needs analysis
primary healthcare
social determinants of health
social marketing

Introduction

As defined by the World Health Organization, health is 'a state of complete physical, mental and social well-being and not merely the absence of disease or infirmity' (WHO 2005). **Health promotion** is therefore 'the process of enabling people to increase control over, and to improve, their health, moving beyond a focus on individual behaviour towards a wide range of social and environmental interventions' (WHO 2005). When thinking about planning interventions to improve health and well-being, researchers and students commonly make the mistake of focusing on one particular life-style behaviour and/or education in a particular area of health need. However, there are a multitude of factors that can potentially impact an individual's health (WHO 2005). Life-style behaviours are just one piece of the complex health and well-being puzzle. **Social determinants of health**, such as factors affecting equity and equality, can also have substantial impacts on health and well-being (see Chapters 1, 13 & 14 in this volume). Health promotion interventions need to tackle these broad areas alongside life-style behaviours in order to have maximal impact on overall health.

Health promotion
The process of enabling people to increase control over and to improve their health.

Social determinants of health
A number of factors, including social, cultural, economic and political, which can impact on the health of individuals.

Having a low level of knowledge in one particular area of health may indeed hinder an individual's ability to follow a healthy life-style. However, viewing an issue through such a narrow lens misses the fact that limited knowledge levels may be accompanied by a number of other barriers to following a healthy life-style, for example poor literacy levels, lack of social support, limited access to healthy choices, cultural and equity factors, as well as gender. It is therefore imperative that health promotion education is delivered in conjunction with structural support, to enhance the likelihood of successful behaviour change. Looking at health promotion as an educational intervention that targets only life-style behaviour therefore limits the likeliness of interventional impact on overall health. For example, providing educational interventions only on following a healthy diet, to a target group from a low socio-economic background with limited access to healthy foods, is not likely to be efficacious. However, when paired with the introduction of community gardens to increase access to fresh fruit and vegetables, and practical sessions on how to grow and cook fruits and vegetables to increase community members' capacity in this skill, an educational intervention would be more likely to positively impact the target group.

We discuss the basic principles of health promotion and theoretical models underpinning health promotion approaches, before examining the five Ottawa Charter for Health priority action areas. We explore these five areas—developing personal skills, strengthening community action, creating supportive environments, re-orienting healthcare services towards prevention of illness and promotion of health, and building healthy public policy—using obesity as a focus.

Principles of health promotion

Health promotion can be conceptualised in a number of ways, as shown in the Ottawa Charter. The Ottawa Charter describes health promotion as 'the process of enabling people to increase control over, and to improve, their health' (WHO 1986). It provides a structure for the broad range of health promotion interventions aimed at different types of target groups (e.g. working with individuals, groups, communities, or settings such as the workplace), and encompassing different strategies or intervention tools (e.g. capacity-building, built environment development, group education). Given that the Ottawa Charter underpins almost all health promotion activities, this chapter is structured in the context of the Charter and provides examples of interventions that align with its action areas.

The first step in health promotion intervention development is the undertaking of a **needs analysis** to identify the target group (who) and area/s of health that require intervention (what). Deciding which health promotion intervention strategies or tools should be utilised (how), and the dose of the intervention (when), is next. This is followed by planning how to evaluate the intervention, which may involve exploring efficacy, reach and sustainability. Each of these stages can be guided by health promotion theories and logic modelling.

Needs analysis
A process to assess the health status and needs of individuals, populations and communities.

Theoretical models in health promotion can be mapped to intervention components. This is useful for explaining an area of health need, for the design of health promotion interventions, and to guide the strategies or tools that may be useful. Common theoretical models utilised in health promotion include the Health Belief Model, the Transtheoretical Model, and Stages of Change (Becker 1974; Prochaska & DiClemente 1984). These theories will be discussed in more detail in the 'Developing personal skills' section.

Logic models are the road map of a health promotion program. They incorporate the theory underpinning a program and how the program is expected to impact on outcomes. Logic models, like the RE-AIM framework or the PRECEDE-PROCEED model, are useful for the **evaluation** of interventions (Glasgow et al. 1999; Green & Kreuter 2005). Logic models should be created in the early planning stages of a health promotion program to ensure that the program 'makes sense' (e.g. the intervention strategies being applied are likely to impact on the identified outcomes of the target group). They are also important in the development stage of a health promotion program, when establishing a project's budget, to identify what resources are required for delivery and evaluation of the program, and when they are needed. During implementation, logic models ensure the intervention stays on track and can be modified with learnings made through the roll-out process. Following the program, logic models assist in evaluation to identify what impact has been made, how it was made, and what adjustments can be made to improve the program in the future. Depending on the area of need and resources, logic models can be very simple or very complicated. In their simplest form, they consider inputs, outputs and outcomes. More complex models, such as the PRECEDE-PROCEED model, may include greater detail (Green & Kreuter 2005).

Logic model
A graphical or narrative representation of the health promotion process and how it is supposed to work by identifying strategies and desired outcomes.

Evaluation
The structured process of assessing the success of a project in meeting its goals, and reflecting on lessons learned.

More often than not, health promotion interventions are not evaluated or do not have a rigorous evaluation approach (Lobo et al. 2014; Smith et al. 2016). This is often due to lack of resources or limited knowledge and skills in evaluation processes (Denford et al. 2018). Without a thorough evaluation, it can be challenging to financially sustain health promotion programs, as funders will seek evidence of efficacy and sustainability. Models are useful in planning appropriate evaluation and should be used from the design phase right through to the implementation and review/improvement of interventions.

Social marketing
An approach used to develop activities aimed at changing or maintaining people's behaviour to benefit both themselves and society as a whole.

Well-thought-out **social marketing** strategies may also need to be developed to increase the reach and retention of an intervention to a target group. Broadly speaking, social marketing occurs when marketing techniques are applied to social issues (Birkenshaw 1988). Without effective marketing and adherence strategies, regardless of the efficacy of an intervention, an intervention is unlikely to be cost-effective or sustainable—the target population needs to accept it and show willingness to adopt the intervention (Ward 1986). Social marketing is not just about recruitment and retention into interventions, but is geared towards encouraging behaviour change.

Ottawa Charter

In 1986, a call by the WHO for governments, organisations and local communities to strive for 'Health for All' through health promotion was made via the launch of the Ottawa Charter at the first international conference on Health Promotion (WHO 1986). The Ottawa Charter includes five priority action areas for health promotion (see Figure 6.1):

1. developing personal skills
2. strengthening community action
3. creating supportive environments
4. re-orienting healthcare services toward prevention of illness and promotion of health
5. building healthy public policy.

Figure 6.1 The Ottawa Charter

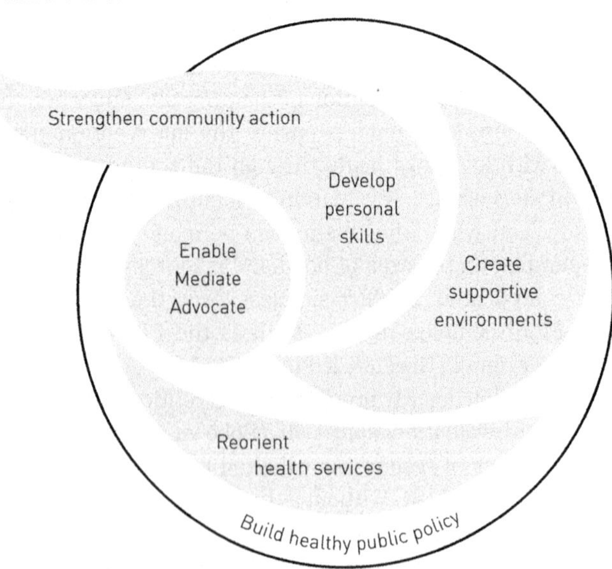

Advocating, enabling and mediating are key health promotion principles that can help achieve these action areas. These areas, and the incorporation of principles from the Ottawa Charter, are contextualised below in the obesity health issue example.

Obesity: a worldwide problem—needs analysis

Worldwide, approximately 13 per cent of adults and 7 per cent of children are obese, and around 39 per cent of adults and 18 per cent of children are overweight (WHO 2017). Both developed and developing countries show high rates of obesity and, since 1975, global obesity rates have almost tripled (WHO 2017). Obesity is associated with the most common non-communicable diseases: cardiovascular disease, type 2 diabetes and some forms of cancer (WHO 2013). Physical inactivity and dietary intake are key contributors to obesity and, traditionally, health promotion programs focused on obesity have targeted these specific risk factors. However, when examining the problem with a wider socio-economic lens, there are many social and economic factors that can increase risk for obesity. In Australia, for example, Aboriginal and Torres Strait Islander people are 1.6 times more likely to be obese than non-Indigenous Australians (ABS 2014), and those living in rural areas are more likely to be obese (69 per cent) compared to those living in metropolitan areas (61 per cent) (ABS 2015). Tackling obesity effectively therefore requires multi-sectoral and multi-strategy interventions targeting not only physical activity and diet, but wider contributing factors. Culturally sensitive and built environment interventions may also be important (see Chapters 3 and 11).

Stop and Think

Kiran, a Samoan woman in her late 50s, was told that she is pre-diabetic after a blood glucose reading at a pop-up health check stall in her local mall. She lives alone—she is divorced, and her son lives with his girlfriend. Kiran works part-time in a bakery, where she is one of the lead bakers. Despite her senior role, her salary is the minimum wage. Kiran has friends through her church network, but she does not see them much as she tends to work on weekends. Although she likes the idea of joining an exercise class, the local gym is the only place that runs classes and she cannot afford its fees. She would prefer a native dance-style class, but this does not exist. There are walking trails near where she lives (a rural town in Queensland, Australia) but these are not safe at night, when she is most likely to be available to exercise, and none of her friends are able to accompany her at night. Kiran enjoys eating foods popular in the Samoan culture, including turkey tails and mutton flaps. An ulcer has started to form on her right foot and is sore when she stands for too long. She does not attend a doctor regularly in Australia as she has not been able to find a GP who understands the Pacific way of life;

she believes that God is in charge of her health and will ultimately decide when her time is up. Think about the social determinants of health.

- What do you think are the potential facilitators and barriers to Kiran changing her life-style to prevent her from developing diabetes?
- Bearing in mind that health promotion involves not only life-style and behaviour change, but should also incorporate strategies targeting wider social determinants of health, what health promotion intervention strategies could help Kiran to lead a healthier life-style?

Stop and Think

Consider the case of Kiran presented above. Maslow's Hierarchy of Needs is a theory incorporating different levels of human need (Maslow 1943). The five layers of this theory (from highest importance to lowest) are:

1. physiological (food, shelter, warmth)
2. safety needs (basic needs)
3. belongingness and love needs
4. esteem needs (psychological needs)
5. self-actualisation (self-fulfilment).

- What do you think might be priority needs in Kiran's life? Think about how these needs would fit into Maslow's Hierarchy—which needs do you think could play a role in her risk of developing diabetes? Think about why considering the hierarchy of needs is important when developing a health promotion intervention.

Developing personal skills

Within the context of the Ottawa Charter, the action area focused on individual health behaviours that people can control encompasses the development of personal skills (Naidoo 2009). Empowering individuals to take control of their health and make healthy life-style choices is imperative to health behaviour change, and these skills often evolve and change as people enter different life-stages. Providing information and skills to give individuals control over their health is a key principle in health promotion, and this must be facilitated in a broad range of contexts. It is important to develop personal skills across the life-span and utilise a multi-sectoral approach, comprising the school, home, work and community settings.

As mentioned earlier, a number of factors can increase a person's risk of becoming overweight or obese. However, many of the risk factors associated with obesity are modifiable at an individual level. Physical inactivity and dietary intake, for example, are two of the leading causes of obesity and can lead to the development of other non-communicable diseases including cardiovascular disease and diabetes (WHO 2017). Developing personal skills to improve these individual life-style behaviours is therefore important for preventing obesity across all life-stages.

Theoretical models that are commonly used to inform interventions targeting personal skills and behaviour change include the Health Belief Model (Becker 1974), the Theory of Reasoned Action and Planned Behaviour (Ajzen & Fishbein 1980), and the Transtheoretical (or Stages of Change) Model (Prochaska & DiClemente 1984; Bidewell 2019).

The Health Belief Model (Becker 1974) is a framework that helps explain perceptions of health—specifically, why some individuals take action to avoid developing specific health conditions such as obesity. The model considers the likelihood of an individual taking action based on the:

- perceived seriousness and severity of the disease (e.g. the impact the disease might have on their quality of life or ability to earn a living)
- perceived likelihood of developing the disease (i.e. their susceptibility to the disease)
- perceived benefits associated with taking action (e.g. the benefits of cancer screening and early detection) (Talbot 2014)
- perceived barriers to taking action (e.g. time, cost or discomfort).

The Theory of Reasoned Action and Behaviour (Ajzen & Fishbein 1980) is underpinned by a belief that an individual's 'intention to act is the most immediate determinant of behaviour, and that all other factors influencing behaviour will be mediated through behavioural intention' (Nutbeam et al. 2010, p. 12). In this model, behavioural intentions are thought to be influenced by:

- an individual's attitude towards the specific behaviour
- subjective norms, that is, the beliefs that the individual thinks others hold (i.e. whether others think they should or should not engage in the behaviour)
- the perceived control an individual has over the specific behaviour.

The Transtheoretical (or Stages of Change) Model (Prochaska & DiClemente 1984) considers the different levels through which an individual may progress when attempting to change a behaviour (Talbot 2014). The model identifies five key stages of behavioural change:

1. precontemplation: includes individuals who are not considering behaviour change at all, or who are consciously intending not to change
2. contemplation: includes those who are thinking about changing a specific behaviour
3. preparation (or determination): includes those who have made a commitment to change behaviour and have taken steps to prepare for the change
4. action: the individual's behaviour has changed, but is not yet habitual
5. maintenance: the stage at which the behaviour is sustained and the individual is beginning to achieve health benefits.

Not all behaviour change attempts are successful, and some individuals may relapse and re-enter the cycle of change (Nutbeam et al. 2010; Bidewell 2019).

Case Example 6.1

The 'Healthy Dads, Healthy Kids' intervention

The 'Healthy Dads, Healthy Kids' (HDHK) intervention is an excellent example of a research study that developed participants' (n=53 fathers) personal skills (Morgan et al. 2011). The three-month program comprised educational sessions targeting weight loss, physical activity and healthy eating, which encouraged men to focus on setting specific, individualised behaviour change goals. Men identified individual barriers to weight loss and learnt practical strategies to overcome these barriers, developing personal skills to encourage health behaviour change. Three of the eight sessions involved practical activities designed for fathers and children to participate in together, and the importance of being a good role model for health behaviours was consistently reinforced.

The study resulted in significant between-group differences for weight loss, with intervention fathers losing more weight (7.6 kg) than control group fathers (0.0 kg). Fathers in the intervention also reduced their waist circumference and BMI, and increased physical activity; children also increased their physical activity levels (Morgan et al. 2011).

Stop and Think

- Case 1: Ahmed is a 23-year-old man, originally from Afghanistan. Ahmed is studying Law at university and works two jobs to support his family. He has been struggling to stay on top of his studies, but is the first in his family to attend university and does not want to let his parents down. Due to work, study and family commitments, Ahmed has little time to himself and any spare time is usually spent watching sport and playing computer games. Ahmed has recently noticed that his clothes are not fitting as well as they used to, and he is starting to put on weight. He snacks a lot in between lectures and shifts at work and usually purchases takeaway food for dinner as he has no time to prepare his own meals. Ahmed used to spend a lot of time playing football and going to the gym with his friends, but he no longer has time for these activities and does not see them as a priority.
- Case 2: Alison is a 45-year-old single mother of two teenage boys. After separating from her long-term partner and dedicating much of her life to raising her sons, Alison decided that she needed to spend some time focusing on herself. She joined a local gym, cut out all processed foods from her diet and signed up to a public speaking course at a local community college. She gained confidence and was the healthiest she had ever been. Six months ago, Alison fractured her wrist in an accident at work. She could not participate in any of her favourite fitness classes for eight weeks, while she was in a cast. She tried a few new activities including aqua aerobics and running but did not enjoy them, and soon found she was not engaging in any physical activity. When her cast was removed, Alison was excited to get back into the gym

but felt like she was starting from scratch. She was too out of shape to feel like she could resume her fitness classes—although she wants to get back into exercise, the thought of going to the gym is causing her to feel anxious and overwhelmed.

Consider the cases of Ahmed and Alison in relation to the Transtheoretical Model. Which stage of change are Ahmed and Alison currently in? As a health professional, how would you encourage behaviour change based on their current stage within the model? Why is it important to consider an individual's stage of change when encouraging behaviour change?

Strengthening community action

Empowerment is about assisting communities in taking ownership of their health. Community development processes provide communities with support to be able to make decisions based on the community's priorities, and to plan and implement their own health promotion actions. This increases the likeliness of adoption by the community, and the effectiveness and long-term sustainability of the actions on health (Labonte & Laverack 2008; Heritage & Dooris 2009). The more involved community members are in making decisions and taking action, the more empowered they become. Community involvement can be at various levels, and draws upon the resources already within the community. Communities can include individuals who live within the same geographical area or those with a shared social identity. Partnerships and collaboration across sectors are important in strengthening the community action.

Four main components in relation to strengthening community actions are (Laverack & Mohammadi 2011):

- identifying shared priorities through engagement with communities
- developing community capacity (increasing competency and capacity of individuals)
- clear processes for funding, which are flexible
- creativity to up-scale and translate health promotion programs to wider areas.

A challenge is identifying enough community members, with a genuine interest in the health of the wider community, to ensure that all issues within the community are captured. It is also important to ensure that **community engagement** is not tokenistic, and that community values, preferences and concerns are incorporated into any decision-making.

Community engagement
A process where community values, concerns and aspirations are actively sought out and incorporated into decision-making processes.

Creating supportive environments

Developing personal skills and building healthy public policy can encourage healthy life-style behaviours. But, in order to sustain positive health behaviours, it is important to create environments that support behaviour change. These environments include the settings in which people live, work, learn and play, such as workplaces, schools, healthcare facilities and local neighbourhoods. The settings-based approach to health promotion is grounded in the understanding that health is created in these specific settings (Sebar et al. 2019). There are many examples of health promotion interventions and policies that have created supportive environments that are conducive to good health. The NSW Healthy School Canteen Strategy (discussed below) is one such example (NSW DoE 2017). The Strategy encourages schools to limit discretionary (or occasional) foods, making healthy choices the norm for school students. Combined with education on healthy eating and physical activity, and compulsory physical education lessons, schools can create an environment that encourages healthy life-style behaviours.

Case Example 6.2

Healthy stadiums

Across the world, attending sporting events is a common leisure activity. However, sports stadiums are not the most supportive environments for healthy life-style behaviours. Most sport fans tend to be inactive for the majority of their time, and many complain about the cost and nutritional quality of food at sporting stadiums (Parry et al. 2018). Most food options at stadiums are high in carbohydrates, sugar and fat; if healthy food options are available, they tend to be higher in price and less appealing than the unhealthy options, which are prepared fresh, and are quick and easy to eat. In recent years, sports stadiums have come under pressure from governments, fans and other stakeholders to provide a setting that improves and supports public health outcomes (Parnell et al. 2017). Sporting organisations are beginning to harness the power of sport to promote health (Hunt et al. 2014). The European Healthy Stadia Network has been established to showcase and promote examples of good public health practice across sporting clubs and governing bodies, research institutions and public health organisations. Healthy Stadia encourages sporting organisations and stadiums to prohibit or limit smoking, encourage active transport to and from the venue (e.g. by providing free public transport for fans), and provide healthy catering guidance through online menus so fans can look at available food and associated nutritional value before arriving at the stadium. By encouraging these healthy behaviours, sports stadiums can play a role in creating supportive environments that encourage healthy behaviours.

Reorienting health services

Another of the Ottawa Charter's five priority action domains is the reorienting of health services (WHO 1986). Health service reorientation includes investment in primary and prevention services in order to focus holistically on individuals' health needs (Ziglio et al. 2011). Such investment can provide long-term, sustainable preventative health and health promotion services at a population level. The reorientation of health services acknowledges the important contribution of health systems to health promotion. However, progress is often slow as a result of:

- increasing pressures of health services to demonstrate cost-effectiveness (Ziglio et al. 2011)
- preference for investment in tertiary services that develop or provide clinical interventions (Wise & Nutbeam 2007)
- a focus on the social determinants of health (Wise & Nutbeam 2007)
- practitioners' perceptions that health promotion and preventative health is 'dull' and not within their remit (Stuckler et al. 2011).

Health systems become unsustainable and unaffordable when they are primarily focused on providing clinical interventions via tertiary services (Wanless 2002; Lim et al. 2014; see also Chapter 13 in this volume). The reorientation of health service investment to focus on health promotion and prevention is not only in line with the WHO's definition of health systems 'whose primary purpose is to promote, restore, or maintain health' (Reinhardt & Cheng 2000), but is essential for the global sustainability of health systems, particularly with the rising pressures of non-communicable diseases and risk factors, such as obesity.

Case Example 6.3

Obesity and people with intellectual disabilities

The obesity epidemic is a global health concern, particularly in first-world countries. As noted above, obesity is associated with, and a risk factor for, many other health conditions including cancer, cardiovascular disease and diabetes (AIHW 2015, 2018; WHO 2017). It is also incredibly complex, as it is associated with a range of factors including societal, vocational and technological trends (e.g. agriculture, transportation), physical activity, food and health systems (Lang & Rayner 2007). This complexity means that obesity poses a significant challenge and opportunity for health promotion and its potential to reorient health services for obesity.

Some populations, including people with intellectual disabilities, have a higher prevalence of obesity than non-disabled people (van Schrojenstein Lantman-De Valk et al. 2000), with some studies estimating prevalence rates of overweight and obesity of over 70 per cent (Ranjan et al. 2018; Russell et al. 2018). It has also been noted that people with intellectual disabilities experience difficulties accessing health services (Kerr et al. 1996; Robertson et al. 2011; Iacono & Bigby 2019).

A study aimed at reorienting health services for obese and overweight intellectually disabled people ran a health promotion program delivered by disability nurses in a community health clinic (Marshall et al. 2003). The program was focused on health literacy, promoting the importance and benefits of physical activity and diet in an enjoyable and engaging way. Over a six-week period, participants' (n=20) weight dropped by an average of 3.4 kg (*SD*=17. kg).

This reorienting of health services to focus on health promotion, rather than being reactive and crisis-driven, demonstrates the important role that intellectual disability services and primary care can take in the promotion of weight loss (Marshall et al. 2003).

Building healthy public policy

Prevention of chronic disease is by far a better option than the social and economic cost of treatment, yet most risk factors for chronic disease lie beyond the direct control of the health sector (Krech 2011; Pinto et al. 2015). Creation of healthy public policy is therefore required to address environmental and structural determinants of health, such as development of green spaces, reshaping of food chains or the establishment of laws and funding policies. Essentially, healthy public policy should provide the structures necessary to make healthy choices easier (or even the easiest) in order to support health promotion education (Sebar et al. 2019). A number of reductions in disease incidence can be attributed to healthy public policy, including a reduction in deaths from road traffic accidents thanks to legislation of seatbelt usage, and regulation of workplace health and safety. In future, however, multi-level approaches will be increasingly important, especially where both the issue and solutions are systemic and complex, for conditions like obesity (Krech 2011). There are downsides to the creation of healthy public policy—this approach can be seen as 'top-down' and overly directive, with resistance from the population if policy is unpopular. Certain stakeholders may also lobby heavily against changes in legislation; for example, tobacco companies and soft drink manufacturers if they stand to lose from the new policy. However, there is evidence that initially unpopular policy can later become popular; for example, anti-smoking legislation in Australia, where cigarette smoking is now considered unacceptable by a large majority of the population (Sebar et al. 2019).

Nonetheless, there are challenges around the creation of healthy public policy. A number of social, economic and political forces can exert influence on those forming healthy public policy, such as different levels of government (Brownson et al. 2009). For example, despite the massive costs of chronic diseases and the fact that many are largely preventable through adoption of healthy life-style choices, governments worldwide place little value on prevention and health promotion. Instead, they make large investments in healthcare for management once the disease has developed. Generally, there is also insufficient evidence on the efficacy of policy interventions, which has resulted in a lack of evidence-based policy development (Sebar et al. 2019).

Case Example 6.4

Healthy School Canteen Strategy

The Australian Healthy School Canteen Strategy is a good example of how policy is being used. It is part of a multi-strategy campaign targeted at reducing childhood overweight and obesity by 5 per cent by 2025. The policy, which is based on lengthy consultation with stakeholders such as school canteen managers and parents, has been designed to benchmark what can be sold in school canteens. The aim is to provide students with a taste for healthy foods as well as making healthy food the easiest choice. All government schools in New South Wales were required to transition to the strategy over a three-year period (2017–2019) and independent and Catholic schools were strongly encouraged to participate (NSW DoE 2017). As the program is in its infancy, there is no evidence yet that it is effective in achieving the goal of reducing overweight and obesity among children in New South Wales. However, it is a good example of building healthy public policy as part of an overall health promotion strategy.

Primary healthcare

Another essential element of health promotion is **primary healthcare**. Primary healthcare is the first contact with care that most people have as they access the health system, and encompasses the principle of universal access to basic healthcare (Blackberry 2019).

Primary healthcare
Essential healthcare that is accessible to all.

As stated in the Declaration of Alma-Ata, primary healthcare is integral in the provision of 'healthcare for all' (WHO 1978). It forms the core of accessible, affordable and equitable healthcare for the whole community (Guzys & Petrie 2014), and should involve partnerships between government, community and individuals to address issues from different social, cultural, economic or political contexts. Core components of primary healthcare should include (Blackberry 2019):

- immunisation
- provision of essential drugs
- maternal and child healthcare
- prevention and control of local endemic diseases
- education on health literacy
- promotion of the food supply and correct nutrition.

In Australia, primary healthcare is informed by the First National Primary Healthcare Strategy (2009), which refers to the comprehensive first level of care in the health system. It comprises a wide range of services in both the public and private sectors. Health professionals in this first level of care work together as multi-disciplinary teams to provide comprehensive, person-centred care. Although general practitioners (GPs) provide much of the primary healthcare to Australians, others with an important role in the delivery of primary care include Aboriginal health services, pharmacists, community nurses, dentists and allied health professionals (Willis et al. 2016). These providers deliver a range of services including prevention and screening, treatment and health promotion, which may be targeted at specific population groups (e.g. youth health or Aboriginal people) or at specific conditions (e.g. cancer or maternal health). Primary healthcare is therefore an essential element of effective health promotion as it not only provides a setting from which to deliver health promotion, but also the services to facilitate universal access to health for all.

Social marketing

Social marketing 'aims to persuade or motivate people to adopt specific courses of action or behaviour which are generally accepted as being beneficial' (Luca & Suggs 2013; Smith et al. 2018; see also Chapter 12). Thus, social marketing is important for raising awareness and encouraging healthy behaviours, but it does not create the behaviour itself. The key concepts—the '4 Ps' of Product, Place, Price and Promotion—of commercial marketing can be applied to the development of social marketing campaigns. Social marketing differs from that of general marketing, as the ultimate aim in social marketing is to promote health.

Product

The area of health that is being targeted must be of interest and importance to the individuals that are the audience of the marketing campaign. Conducting a needs analysis that includes consultation with the target group will assist in this process. Additionally, it is important to ensure that the target audience feels the product (i.e. the health promotion intervention that might be a service or material) is usable and appropriate for them.

Place

The social marketing campaign needs to be accessible to the target audience. That is, it needs to reach the end-users via a location where the individuals are likely to be.

Price

The financial cost and the perceived value of the behaviour change being promoted will impact on whether an individual decides to make that particular change. If value is perceived as high, then individuals are more likely to be prepared to pay a high financial cost (if they have the income to do so). If value is perceived as low, then even a relatively cheap intervention is unlikely to be adopted. Price can cover other areas such as the time burden, reduced pay (if time off work has to be taken) and response costs (e.g. fear of reactions from others).

Promotion

Timing needs to be pitched appropriately to assist in encouraging the behaviour change; for example, January is often a good time to target diet and physical activity messages when individuals are setting New Year's resolutions. The message needs to be visible (in a place where the individual would expect to see the message) and it must be easy to understand. The method of message delivery should therefore be carefully planned to match the characteristics of the target group. Examples of delivery methods include social media (Facebook, Twitter, Instagram etc.), television, billboards, radio, newsletters and newspapers, community organisations and community meetings, schools and workplaces, and word of mouth. The methods selected are often dictated by the financial resources of the social marketing intervention. Flyers and posters may be cheaper than films or newspaper advertisements, but distribution costs may be high depending on where the target audience is located. Social media has the potential to reach a large audience very quickly if tailored appropriately to the target group. Messages that are surprising to the audience, often through humour, shock or novelty, are more likely to gain attention. Concise, repeated messages are more likely to reach the target group. When working with particular cultural groups, it is essential to ensure the message is correctly interpreted. Literacy level is also important to consider.

Reflection Exercise

Health promotion programs need to consider health issues in their widest context. That is, targeting not just life-style behaviours, but also the associated socio-ecological factors that impact on health and well-being. The 'best' interventions (most effective and sustainable) are those incorporating intervention strategies that focus on all layers of the Ottawa Charter, and relate to the areas of health need that are important to the target population.

Evaluation is not just for researchers. Health promotion practitioners also need to carefully plan ways of evaluating their programs. Evaluation is essential for the sustainability of a program, and to argue the case for funding to support its continuation. Without evidence that a program is efficacious and has a reasonable reach into the target group, funders are unlikely to continue to support it.

A health promotion program may be efficacious at improving an area of health but, in order to be effective overall, it must also be sustainable and reach the target group. Social marketing is a tool used to reach a target group to raise awareness and encourage their consideration and participation in behaviour change. Inclusion of a target group in the development and implementation process of a health promotion program can assist in long-term participation by a particular community group and the sustainability of a program.

- Think about a health promotion program that you have heard of or taken part in. How do you think this program could be evaluated? As a health promotion professional, what do you think might affect (hinder or facilitate) the outcomes that you decide to evaluate?
- Think about a priority health issue in the country where you live. Search the internet to find if there are any current health promotion programs or campaigns underway to target this issue in your country. Are there current interventions at all levels of the Ottawa Charter? If so, who are the collaborators and partners delivering those interventions? If not, where are the gaps? What would you recommend to fill the gaps or to strengthen existing strategies?
- Select a theory used in health promotion to develop interventions, then think about a health issue. Can the theory explain all aspects of this issue? What is missing? Is there another theory/theories that might be useful in addition to the original theory?
- Think about a health issue that affects people of any age. Would it be possible to create a health promotion campaign to target this health issue across the life-span? How might a campaign differ if targeted at a teenager compared to an elderly individual, to increase its chances of having impact?
- Integrated health promotion programs that involve all areas of the Ottawa Charter require strong collaborations and partnerships. Think about the different organisations and entities that might be involved in an intervention. What do you think would assist in ensuring collaborative working? What might hinder and cause tension between those involved?

Summary

Historically, there has been a focus on treating the sick instead of addressing the causes of illness. Health promotion disrupts this perspective by focusing on the promotion of health and the prevention of disease through carefully planned and implemented initiatives. We have provided an overview of the principles of health promotion within the context of the Ottawa Charter framework, using obesity to show how ill health is multi-faceted and can be viewed from a number of perspectives. Multi-faceted problems require multi-pronged approaches. We also highlighted theoretical frameworks underpinning health promotion, the important role played by primary healthcare, and the required elements for successful social marketing campaigns. All these play important parts in developing and rolling out health promotion interventions.

Given the increasingly complex nature of health, and the multiple social and environmental determinants that can affect well-being, it is important that health promotion is guided by the Ottawa Charter to emphasise social and personal resources as well as physical capacities when addressing health. Health promotion strives to use a multi-level approach, involving collaboration between governments, communities, individuals and health services. This is essential, given that health promotion can and should occur population-wide, to the community level and at individual or clinical level. Importantly, we outlined that health promotion is not just the responsibility of the health sector, but goes beyond to society as a whole. Integrating multiple health promotion strategies via collaboration and partnerships for health, through to community-based approaches, provides opportunities for holistic interventions to prevent the complex health issues that our society faces.

Tutorial exercises

1. Identify a current area of health promotion need in the geographical area where you live. Search for sources of information to support the case for an intervention. Now write a needs analysis arguing the case for a health promotion intervention. In your argument, include the different sources of information that support your case, and your suggestions for gathering additional evidence that could support your case for an intervention.
2. Find a health promotion intervention research article that reports an intervention's design (e.g. a protocol paper) or the outcomes of an intervention. Draw a logic model incorporating the inputs, outputs and outcomes of the intervention. Write a brief summary on whether the evaluation plan was appropriate for the planned aims of the intervention. What would you suggest could be added/adjusted to strengthen the evaluation plan? What project restrictions or challenges do you think might have impacted on the evaluation plan?
3. For the article identified above, read about the recruitment strategies that were utilised to promote the intervention. Thinking about the target audience, plan a social marketing campaign to support this intervention, considering the 4 Ps. Remember to consider how you would encourage the audience to actually consider the behaviour change, rather than just inform it that an issue exists.

Further reading

Bayer, R. (2008). Stigma and the ethics of public health: not can we but should we. *Social Science and Medicine*, 67, 463–472.

Bidewell, J. (2019). Individual models of behaviour change. In P. Liamputtong (Ed.), *Public Health: Local and Global Perspectives*, 2nd edn (Chapter 8). Melbourne: Cambridge University Press.

Blackberry, I. (2019). Primary health care and community health. In P. Liamputtong (Ed.), *Public Health: Local and Global Perspectives*, 2nd edn (Chapter 4). Melbourne: Cambridge University Press.

Glasgow, R.E., Vogt, T.M., & Boles, S.M. (1999). Evaluating the public health impact of health promotion interventions: the RE-AIM framework. *American Journal of Public Health*, 89(9), 1322–1327.

Green, L., & Kreuter, M.W. (2005). *Health Program Planning: An Educational and Ecological Approach*, 4th edn. New York: McGraw-Hill.

Guzys, D., & Petrie, E. (2014). *An Introduction to Community and Primary Health Care*. Melbourne: Cambridge University Press.

Nutbeam, D., Harris, E., & Wise, M. (2010). *Theory in a Nutshell: A Practical Guide to Health Promotion Theories*, 3rd edn. Sydney: McGraw-Hill.

Talbot, L. (2014). *Promoting Health: The Primary Health Care Approach*, 5th edn. Sydney: Elsevier Australia.

World Health Organization (1986). *The Ottawa Charter for Health Promotion*. Available from http://www.who.int/healthpromotion/conferences/previous/ottawa/en/

Websites

http://www.who.int/en/news-room/fact-sheets/detail/obesity-and-overweight

This website has useful information on the worldwide obesity crisis.

http://www.who.int/en/news-room/fact-sheets/detail/obesity-and-overweight

This website is the World Health Organization page for health promotion and contains links to WHO programs and activities.

https://www.bttop.org/sites/default/files/public/W.K.%20Kellogg%20LogicModel.pdf

Developed by the Kellogg Foundation, this is a valuable online resource to assist with logic model development.

https://www.cdc.gov/eval/resources/

Hosted by the Centers for Disease Control, this website hosts a number of useful evaluation resources.

http://lgreen.net/

This website contains resources to guide use of the PRECEDE-PROCEED model for health program planning.

https://ctb.ku.edu/en/developing-intervention

The Community Toolbox is a service of the Center for Community Health and Development at the University of Kansas, and provides support for developing community interventions.

https://health.gov/

This US government website is hosted by the Office of Disease Prevention and Health Promotion and provides links to a number of healthy life-style resources.

https://www.australia.gov.au/information-and-services/health/health-promotion

This Australian government website provides information about health promotions and initiatives to help with a healthy life-style

References

ABS (Australian Bureau of Statistics) (2014). *Australian Aboriginal and Torres Strait Islander Health Survey: Updated Results, 2012–13.* ABS Cat. No. 4727.0.55.006. Retrieved from Canberra: http://www.abs.gov.au/ausstats/abs@.nsf/mf/4727.0.55.001

ABS (Australian Bureau of Statistics) (2015). *National Health Survey: First Results Australia 2014–15.* Cat. No. 4364.0.55.001. Retrieved from http://www.ausstats.abs.gov.au/ausstats/subscriber.nsf/0/CDA852A349B4CEE6CA257F150009FC53/$File/national health survey first results, 2014–15.pdf

AIHW (Australian Institute of Health and Welfare) (2015). *Risk Factors, Disease and Death.* Canberra: Australian Institute of Health and Welfare.

AIHW (Australian Institute of Health and Welfare) (2018). *Australia's Health 2018.* Canberra: Australian Institute of Health and Welfare. Accessed 20 June 2018 from https://www.aihw.gov.au/getmedia/7c42913d-295f-4bc9-9c24-4e44eff4a04a/aihw-aus-221.pdf.aspx?inline=true

Ajzen, I., & Fishbein, M. (1980). *Understanding Attitudes and Predicting Social Behavior.* New Jersey: Prentice-Hall.

Becker, M.H. (1974). *The Health Belief Model and Personal Health Behavior.* Thorofare, NJ: C.B. Slack.

Bidewell, J. (2019). Individual models of behaviour change. In P. Liamputtong (Ed.), *Public Health: Local and Global Perspectives*, 2nd edn (Chapter 8). Melbourne: Cambridge University Press.

Birkenshaw, M. (1988). *Social Marketing for Health.* Retrieved from http://apps.who.int/iris/bitstream/handle/10665/62146/HMD_89.2.pdf

Blackberry, I. (2019). Primary health care and community health. In P. Liamputtong (Ed.), *Public Health: Local and Global Perspectives*, 2nd edn (Chapter 4). Melbourne: Cambridge University Press.

Brownson, R.C., Chriqui, J.F., & Stamatakis, K.A. (2009). Understanding evidence-based public health policy. *American Journal of Public Health*, 99(9), 1576–1583. doi:10.2105/AJPH.2008.156224

Denford, S., Lakshman, R., Callaghan, M., & Abraham, C. (2018). Improving public health evaluation: a qualitative investigation of practitioners' needs. *BMC Public Health*, 18. doi:10.1186/s12889-018-5075-8

Glasgow, R.E., Vogt, T.M., & Boles, S.M. (1999). Evaluating the public health impact of health promotion interventions: the RE-AIM framework. *American Journal of Public Health*, 89(9), 1322–1327.

Green, L., & Kreuter, M.W. (2005). *Health Program Planning: An Educational and Ecological Approach*, 4th edn. New York: McGraw-Hill.

Guzys, D., & Petrie, E. (2014). *An Introduction to Community and Primary Health Care*. Melbourn: Cambridge University Press.

Heritage, Z., & Dooris, M. (2009). Community participation and empowerment in Healthy Cities. *Health Promotion International*, 24, 45–55. doi:10.1093/heapro/dap054

Hunt, K., Wyke, S., Gray, C.M., Anderson, A.S., Brady, A., Bunn, C. ... & Leishman, J. (2014). A gender-sensitised weight loss and healthy living programme for overweight and obese men delivered by Scottish Premier League football clubs (FFIT): a pragmatic randomised controlled trial. *Lancet*, 383(9924), 1211–1221.

Iacono, T., & Bigby, C. (2019). The health inequalities of people with intellectual and developmental disabilities: strategies for change. In P. Liamputtong (Ed.), *Public Health: Local and Global Perspectives*, 2nd edn (Chapter 18). Melbourne: Cambridge University Press.

Kerr, M., Fraser, W.I., & Felce, D. (1996). Primary health care for people with learning disabilities. *British Journal of Learning Disabilities*, 24, 2–8. doi:10.1111/j.1468-3156.1996.tb00192.x

Krech, R. (2011). Healthy public policies: looking ahead. *Health Promotion International*, 26 (Suppl 2), II268–272. doi:10.1093/heapro/dar066

Labonte, R., & Laverack, G. (2008). *Health Promotion in Action: From Local to Global Empowerment*. London: Palgrave Macmillan.

Lang, T., & Rayner, G. (2007). Overcoming policy cacophony on obesity: an ecological public health framework for policymakers. *Obesity Reviews*, 8 (Suppl.1), 165–181. doi:10.1111/j.1467-789X.2007.00338.x

Laverack, G., & Mohammadi, N.K. (2011). What remains for the future: strengthening community actions to become an integral part of health promotion practice. *Health Promotion International*, 26, II258–262. doi:10.1093/heapro/dar068

Lim, J., Chan, M.M.H., Alsagoff, F.Z., & Ha, D. (2014). Innovations in non-communicable diseases management in ASEAN: a case series. *Global Health Action*, 7, 13–22. doi:10.3402/gha.v7.25110

Lobo, R., Petrich, M., & Burns, S.K. (2014). Supporting health promotion practitioners to undertake evaluation for program development. *BMC Public Health*, 14, 1315. doi:10.1186/1471-2458-14-1315

Luca, N.R., & Suggs, L.S. (2013). Theory and model use in social marketing health interventions. *Journal of Health Communication*, 18(1), 20–40. doi:10.1080/10810730.2012.688243

Marshall, D., McConkey, R., & Moore, G. (2003). Obesity in people with intellectual disabilities: the impact of nurse-led health screenings and health promotion activities. *Journal of Advanced Nursing*, 41(2), 147–153. doi:10.1046/j.1365-2648.2003.02522.x

Maslow, A.H. (1943). A theory of human motivation. *Psychological Review*, 50(4), 370–396. doi:http://dx.doi.org/10.1037/h0054346

Morgan, P.J., Lubans, D.R., Callister, R., Okely, A.D., Burrows, T.L., Fletcher, R., & Collins, C.E. (2011). The 'Healthy Dads, Healthy Kids' randomized controlled trial: efficacy of a healthy lifestyle program for overweight fathers and their children. *International Journal of Obesity*, 35(3), 436.

Naidoo, J. (2009). *Foundations for Health Promotion*, 3rd edn. New York: Baillière Tindall/Elsevier.

NSW DoE (Department of Education) (2017). *The Revised Healthy School Canteen Strategy.* Retrieved from https://www.healthykids.nsw.gov.au/campaigns-programs/nsw-healthy-school-canteen-strategy

Nutbeam, D., Harris, E., & Wise, M. (2010). *Theory in a Nutshell: A Practical Guide to Health Promotion Theories*, 3rd edn. Sydney: McGraw-Hill.

Parnell, D., Curran, K., & Philpott, M. (2017). Healthy stadia: an insight from policy to practice. *Sport in Society*, 181–186. doi:https://doi.org/10.1080/17430437.2016.1173914

Parry, K., Rowe, D., George, E., & Hall, T. (2018). Healthy sport consumption: moving away from pies and beers. In D. Parnell & P. Krustrup (Eds), *Sport and Health: Exploring the Current State of Play.* London: Routledge.

Pinto, A.D., Molnar, A., Shankardass, K., O'Campo, P.J., & Bayoumi, A.M. (2015). Economic considerations and 'Health in All Policies' initiatives: evidence from interviews with key informants in Sweden, Quebec and South Australia. *BMC Public Health*, 15, 9. doi:10.1186/s12889-015-1350-0

Prochaska, J.O., & DiClemente, C.C. (1984). *The Transtheoretical Approach: Crossing Traditional Boundaries of Therapy*. Homeward, Ill: Dow-Jones Irwin.

Ranjan, S., Nasser, J.A., & Fisher, K. (2018). Prevalence and potential factors associated with overweight and obesity status in adults with intellectual developmental disorders. *Journal of Applied Research in Intellectual Disabilities*, 31, 29–38. doi:10.1111/jar.12370

Reinhardt, U., & Cheng, T. (2000). The world health report 2000: health systems—improving performance. *Bulletin of the World Health Organization*, 78(8), 1064–1064.

Robertson, J., Roberts, H., Emerson, E., Turner, S., & Greig, R. (2011). The impact of health checks for people with intellectual disabilities: a systematic review of evidence. *Journal of Intellectual Disability Research*, 55, 1009–1019. doi:10.1111/j.1365-2788.2011.01436.x

Russell, R., Chester, V., Watson, J., Nyakunuwa, C., Child, L., McDermott, M. … & Alexander, R.T. (2018). The prevalence of overweight and obesity levels among forensic inpatients with learning disability. *British Journal of Learning Disabilities*, 46(2), 101–108. doi:10.1111/bld.12220

Sebar, B., Morgan, K., & Lee, J. (2019). Health promotion principles and practice: addressing complex public health issues using the Ottawa Charter. In P. Liamputtong (Ed.), *Public Health: Local and Global Perspectives*, 2nd edn (Chapter 3). Melbourne: Cambridge University Press.

Smith, B.J., Rissel, C., Shilton, T., & Bauman, A. (2016). Advancing evaluation practice in health promotion. *Health Promotion Journal of Australia*, 27(3), 184–186. doi:10.1071/HEv27n3_ED2

Smith, J., Zheng, X., Lafreniere, K., & Pike, I. (2018). Social marketing to address attitudes and behaviours related to preventable injuries in British Columbia, Canada. *Injury Prevention*, 24, I52–I59. doi:10.1136/injuryprev-2017-042651

Stuckler, D., Basu, S., & McKee, M. (2011). Commentary: UN high level meeting on non-communicable diseases— an opportunity for whom? *British Medical Journal*, 343, d5336. doi:10.1136/bmj.d5336

Talbot, L. (2014). *Promoting Health: The Primary Health Care Approach*, 5th edn. Sydney: Elsevier Australia.

van Schrojenstein Lantman-De Valk, H.M., Metsemakers, J.F., Haveman, M.J., & Crebolder, H.F. (2000). Health problems in people with intellectual disability in general practice: a comparative study. *Family Practice*, 17(5), 405–407.

Wanless, D. (2002). *Securing our Future Health: Taking a Long-term View*. Retrieved from https://www.yearofcare.co.uk/sites/default/files/images/Wanless.pdf

Ward, G.W. (1986). How to sell health. *World Health Forum*, 7, 169–177.

WHO (World Health Organization) (1978). *Declaration of Alma-Ata*. Paper presented at the International Conference on Primary Health Care, Alma-Ata, USSR.

WHO (World Health Organization) (1986). *Ottawa Charter for Health Promotion*. Retrieved from http://www.who.int/hpr/NPH/docs/ottawa_charter_hp.pdf

WHO (World Health Organization) (2005). *Constitution of the World Health Organization*. Geneva: World Health Organization.

WHO (World Health Organization) (2013). *Global Action Plan for the Prevention and Control of Non-communicable Diseases 2013–2020*. Geneva: World Health Organization.

WHO (World Health Organization) (2017). *Obesity and Overweight*. Retrieved from http://www.who.int/en/news-room/fact-sheets/detail/obesity-and-overweight

Willis, E., Keleher, H., & Reynolds, L. (2016). Introduction to understanding the Australian health care system. In E. Willis, L. Reynolds & H. Keleher (Eds), *Understanding the Australian Health Care System*, 3rd edn (pp. 3–15). Sydney: Elsevier.

Wise, M., & Nutbeam, D. (2007). Enabling health systems transformation: what progress has been made in re-orienting health services? *Promotion and Education*, 14(2 suppl.), 23–27. doi:10.1177/10253823070140020801x

Ziglio, E., Simpson, S., & Tsouros, A. (2011). Health promotion and health systems: some unfinished business. *Health Promotion International*, 26(Suppl.2), ii216–225. doi:10.1093/heapro/dar079

Chapter 7

Economic Determinants of Health and Disease

Elizabeth Martin and David Brain

Topics covered

This chapter covers the following topics:

- role of health economics
- impact of economics on health and disease
- initiatives to address economic determinants of health
- gender differences in health outcomes and the role of economics

Key terms

demand
economic welfare
economics
gender-based health inequality
health insurance
scarcity
supply

Introduction

The term 'economic determinants of health and disease' is often assumed to mean the association between increasing wealth and better health. However, examining the concept in detail provides opportunities to understand how economics can inform decisions that address inequities. Decisions need to be made about how to spend resources to address all types of inequities, not only access to healthcare, and thus maximise the welfare of society. Economics seeks to understand the choices made by people, governments and other organisations, and uses this information to predict the effect of an intervention. As the focus of economics is on the welfare of society, there is an inextricable link between the social and economic determinants of health.

In this chapter we will define economics and challenge the idea that economic growth is the solution to addressing the social determinants of health. We will then examine how economists have contributed to identifying the economic determinants of health, and where changes should be made in society to improve health outcomes. We provide examples of how governments and other organisations have adopted the knowledge generated by economics to address the economic determinants of health. We finish by focusing on the economic determinants of gender-based health inequality, and reinforcing the close relationship of social and economic factors in shaping the health outcomes of women.

Economics

Economics
The study of the choices made in relation to the production, consumption and distribution of goods and services in a scenario of scarcity.

Scarcity
Limited availability of goods and services.

At its most basic level, **economics** can be described as the science of choice. As humans with a natural instinct for unlimited wants, we are met with a dilemma—our unlimited wants outstrip what we can have. The inability to satisfy all of our wants is described by economists as the concept of **scarcity**.

Scarcity exists at many levels. On a societal level, we face scarcity because as a nation we want to have access to high-quality healthcare, great schools and universities, a successful Olympic team, well-maintained roads and a reliable public transport system, all the while ensuring our borders are kept safe and secure by a well-resourced and fully functioning defence force. There are not enough resources to ensure that everything we want can be provided. At an individual level, the concept of scarcity is easily understood—we have all been faced with the problem of wanting to purchase more goods than we have the means to pay for. Scarcity forces us to make a decision that involves trading-off one outcome with another.

At an individual level, we make decisions by comparing the cost to our perception of benefit—does the benefit of buying some new clothes outweigh the benefits of ensuring we have paid our car registration and can legally use our vehicle? Economics studies the choices of multiple players in society—individuals, businesses and governments—as they respond to scarcity.

Measuring economic welfare

Several common indicators are used to measure **economic welfare**, particularly on a societal or national level. Economic indicators such as gross domestic product (GDP), unemployment rate, wage growth, inflation rate and import/export data are often used to describe the prosperity of a nation on an overall level. Generally, we would expect there to be a direct link between higher GDP and improved standards of living, but increased wealth does not prevent healthcare-related inequities, nor does it automatically improve health outcomes. Case Example 7.1 describes how economic growth can be a problem for healthcare.

Economic welfare
The capacity to make choices due to economic stability at both an individual and societal level—the better your economic welfare, the more choices available to you.

There are numerous examples of a country that has a large total GDP but its citizens do not enjoy the health benefits that should be associated with that large GDP. For example, China, Brazil and Russia have large total GDP but poorer life expectancy than nations that have a smaller GDP, such as Spain, Ireland and Sweden (OECD 2017). This is because an individual's economic welfare is impacted by many elements, including, but not limited to, personal political freedom, environmental quality and hours spent at work. For example, according to the World Bank (2018), India's total GDP is nearly double that of Australia's (US$2 597 491 million vs US$1 323 421 million), yet there are stark differences in life expectancy, pollution levels and equity in service access between the two countries. The majority of Australians enjoy a higher quality of life than their Indian counterparts, despite the lower total GDP (WHO 2018).

It is important to understand the difference between societal-level indicators of economic welfare, particularly for understanding the impact of economic factors on health and healthcare. The performance of a nation's economy on a broad scale gives a useful view of the overall prospects of a country, but these measures can be limited in value for individuals, or for specific populations within a society.

Case Example 7.1

When economic growth turns into a healthcare problem

There is strong evidence from both developed and developing nations of a link between economic growth and increased diet-related healthcare problems. In earlier times, access to a nourishing and fulfilling diet was almost impossible for the common person. Diets were dictated by what could be grown or caught, and any available excess was traded for different types of food or other goods. This meant that a diet typically consisted of a small amount of meat and grain-based products, and a larger quantity of fruits and vegetables. However, since the 1970s there has been a significant shift in nutritional intake, particularly in countries that have experienced economic growth. There is increased access to supermarkets, a significant reduction in prices for certain food items, and a large rise in the availability of highly processed 'convenience' foods. Pre-packaged, frozen meals are abundant and sugar-sweetened drinks are widely sold. Additionally, as a result of economic growth, a larger proportion of people choose to spend a higher percentage of their income on food items that were not available a few decades ago. Due to this increased availability of food and change in behaviour, there is increased reliance on and desire for 'fast' food, which is typically energy-dense, with reduced nutritional value. Coupled with the trend towards a much more sedentary life-style due to mechanisation and technological advances, there has been a dramatic increase in obesity and diet-related diseases, such as diabetes, hypertension, stroke and heart disease. Figure 7.1 offers a visual explanation of the change in obesity levels in Australia between 1983 and 2012.

Figure 7.1 Change in obesity levels in Australia by state and territory, 1983–2012

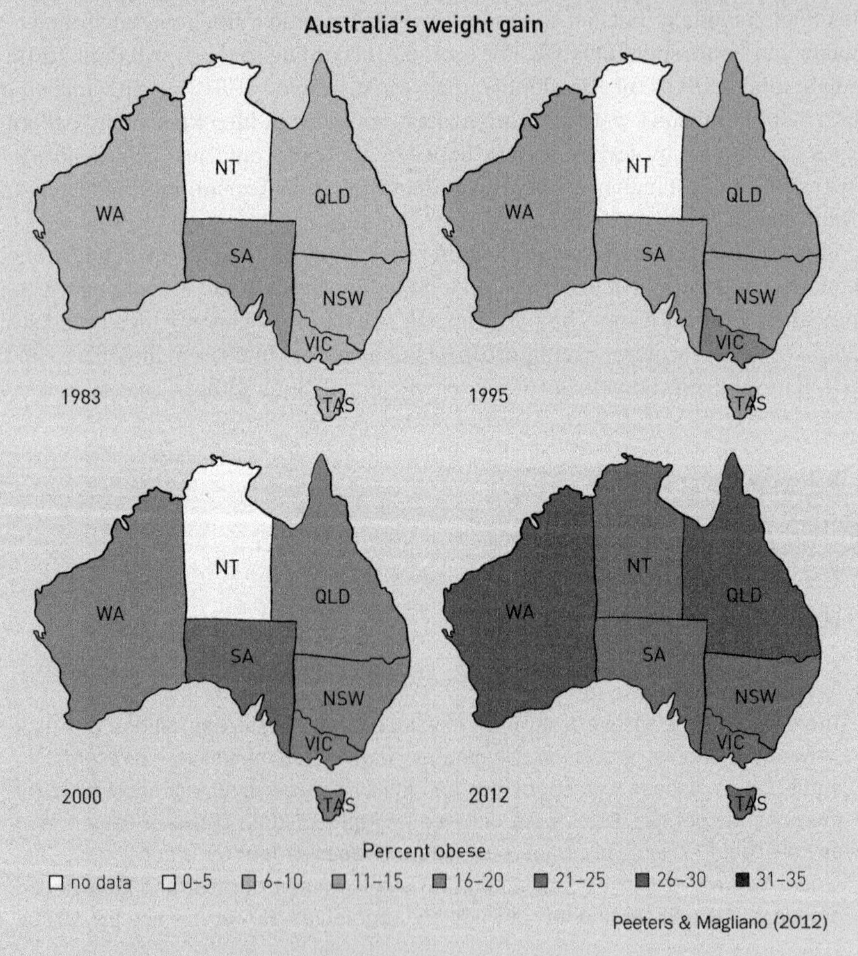

Peeters & Magliano (2012)

Impact of economics on health and disease

There is a well-established connection between wealth and health (see Chapters 1, 2, 13 and 14 in this volume), and the detrimental effects of national wealth (discussed in Case Example 7.2). However, understanding the role of economics in healthcare is not as simple as thinking that nations with greater wealth will inevitably have greater individual health outcomes and better access to healthcare. The distribution of a nation's wealth and the way that a country utilises its overall budget for healthcare has a significant impact on the health outcomes of its citizens. Economics contributes to healthcare because it helps inform decisions about how a scarce healthcare budget should be spent, how we decide which healthcare services should be provided and to whom these services should be made available. Economic evaluation in healthcare is primarily concerned with understanding how much health gain we can expect from our investment in health services—answering a simple question about value for money in order to inform our response to the issue of scarcity. Case Example 7.2 gives an example of how economics was used to impact the Australian healthcare setting. Deeble and Scotton used economic theory to address reasons for the inequity in access to healthcare, as a key determinant of health is inequity between people and between countries (Marmot 2015). This inequity occurred prior to the introduction of Medicare in the 1970s, because of the failure of the free market in healthcare. We will now examine the characteristics of healthcare markets that drive inequities in access to health and healthcare.

Case Example 7.2

Economics and universal healthcare

Before the mid to late 1970s, Australians were not covered by a universal healthcare system. The system was user-pays, with services provided to citizens who could pay for the healthcare they needed. This was similar to the way that services are still provided in some countries, most notoriously, the US. A user-pays system unfairly favours those who have a greater capacity to pay for services, and tends to allow healthcare costs to increase substantially. To address what was deemed to be an unfair and inappropriate system, health economists John Deeble and Dick Scotton devised a plan for a universal healthcare system in Australia. Using economics as their building block, they designed a funding system that provided a wide coverage of health services for a wide range of patients. The system, known as Medicare, is funded through taxation, with those who are deemed to have more capacity to pay contributing a slightly higher amount of their income than others. There is some top-up funding from the federal government. The key benefit of the Medicare system is that it offers a large range of services via public hospitals for no cost, and subsidised services from privately owned and managed healthcare providers, such as dental care, optometry services and some diagnostic imaging and pathology. It can be argued that Deeble and Scotton's plan for universal healthcare was driven by a desire to address issues relating to scarcity and capacity to pay for something that we all need—healthcare services. Their approach was underpinned by basic principles of economics. It is an excellent example of how economics can make a contribution to health and healthcare policy—the implementation of Medicare involved a fundamental shift in the provision of healthcare in Australia (see also Chapter 13).

A market is any arrangement or mechanism that facilitates trading. It is not solely about the trade of goods and services; within any economy there are also markets for items that assist production such as land, labour and capital, which are the equipment, tools and buildings that can be used in production. The market coordinates the individual decisions of buyers and sellers through the constant adjustment of prices. Price can be used as a device to allocate scarce resources by guiding them into the production of goods and services most desired by society. According to economic theory, under certain conditions, a perfectly competitive market can result in the maximisation of society's welfare (McPake 2013).

Demand
Relationship between the price of a good or service and the amount of that good or service people are willing to buy at that price.

Supply
The relationship between price of a good or service and the quantity the suppliers are willing to supply.

By examining the concepts of **demand** and **supply**, we are able to see how price can be used to guide the production of goods and services. Individuals choose the goods and services they wish to consume, and express those demands in the market. Demand is a relationship between the price of a good or service and the amount of that good or service people are willing to buy at that price (McPake 2013). The solid demand curve in Figure 7.2 shows this relationship: at a price of $4 per packet, people only seek (demand) one packet of paracetamol. At a price of 50c per packet, people seek 22 packets. Supply is the relationship between price of a good or service and the quantity the suppliers are willing to supply (McPake 2013). This relationship is represented by the dashed supply curve in Figure 7.2, whereby at a price of 50c per packet, suppliers are willing to supply only one packet of paracetamol per person per day. The market is in equilibrium where the demand and supply curves cross. This point is marked by the grey circle in Figure 7.2, indicating that both suppliers and consumers reach maximum satisfaction in terms of the price and quantity of paracetamol. Maximum satisfaction is where society's welfare is also maximised due to the right allocation of scarce resources (McPake 2013).

However, many conditions of a perfectly competitive market are not met in healthcare. This is called market failure. Key characteristics of healthcare that cause market failure are information asymmetry, externalities, public goods and market power (McPake 2013).

Information asymmetry is a situation where the consumer and/or the supplier does not have enough knowledge to make informed decisions in the market

Figure 7.2 Demand and supply: a relationship between price and quantity

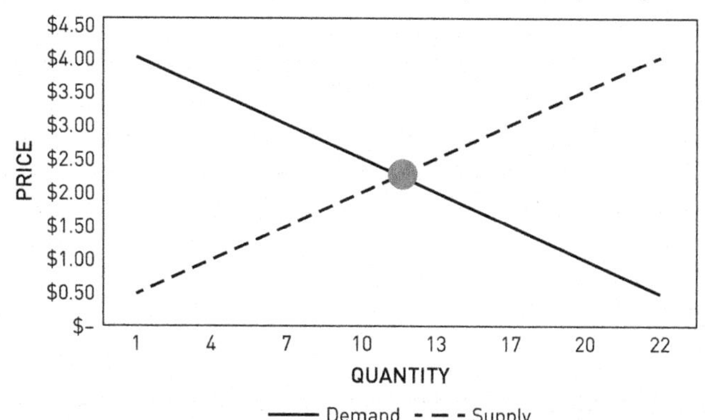

(McPake 2013). Having perfect information is a condition of a perfectly competitive market; however, consumers are unlikely to have as much knowledge as the health carers, who train for years to practise in their specialty. Nor will consumers have full access to or understanding of the research related to their health condition, despite the internet being widely used. The demand for healthcare is affected because it may be too high or low, depending on consumers' access to information. Consumers may also withhold information, resulting in too much or too little healthcare being supplied.

Externalities are side effects of the consumption or production of goods or services which are not traded on the market or taken into account in setting a price (McPake 2013). For example, negative externalities exist in the case of cigarette smoking. The detrimental effect of passive smoking is a cost to healthcare systems, but is not costed into the price of a packet of cigarettes. An example of a positive externality is vaccination. If a case of measles is prevented, other people are not infected. If 95 per cent of the population receive vaccinations, the unvaccinated minority are likely to be protected. The costs of treatment averted through vaccination would not be taken into account in setting its price in a perfectly competitive market.

Public goods are those that may be consumed by one person without preventing simultaneous consumption by another (a non-rival good), and that nobody can be excluded from consuming (a non-excludable good) (McPake 2013). Public health initiatives such as health promotion campaigns and air quality surveillance programs are examples of public goods (see Chapters 6 & 11). A non-rival good creates market failure because the cost of the health promotion campaign drops to zero for each additional person provided with it, after person 1. The supply curve becomes meaningless and the point of equilibrium uncertain. Non-excludability results in the total cost of supply usually exceeding consumers' willingness to pay. There may not be anyone who values good air quality enough to fund a whole program. Under these circumstances, public goods are rarely provided in a perfectly competitive market.

When there is a small number of suppliers within a healthcare system, they exert considerable market power. A small number of suppliers may exist because there are many barriers to entering the market, such as the high fixed costs of establishing a hospital or developing a new piece of technology, or legal barriers such as pharmaceutical patents and workforce accreditation. Monopolies and oligopolies may form when a single or a small number of suppliers control the market, resulting in higher prices for the quantity of goods or services supplied (McPake 2013).

The conditions of a perfectly competitive market are not met in healthcare. The market fails, and some form of intervention is required to correct the point of equilibrium and to enhance society's welfare and equity.

Stop and Think

In May 2014, the Australian government proposed the introduction of a $7 co-payment for a General Practitioner (GP) consultation, out-of-hospital pathology and imaging services. The co-payment was to be applied to services that were then bulk-billed and those that charged additional fees above the standard bulk-billing. The aim was to reduce demand for the affected services, especially bulk-billed services, by encouraging consumers to value them more through the $7 price signal. The co-payment was also intended to contribute to the Medical Research Future Fund, which funds health and medical research. Health professionals and politicians objected to the proposed co-payment and, in March 2015, the plan was abandoned.

- In what ways could a $7 co-payment reduce the demand for GP services? Have you or a family member experienced an under-supply of GP services? How did this affect health outcomes?
- How might a shift in the demand for GP services impact the demand for emergency services or acute services in hospital?

Addressing economic determinants of health and disease

Governments and non-government organisations have a role in addressing healthcare market failure and the ensuing inequities in access and health outcomes (see Chapters 13 & 14). This occurs because the purpose of government in particular is to maximise the welfare of its people, often expressed through a constitution and legislation (Parliament of Australia 2018). These sets of rules for governing lay out how the country will provide for public goods and adjust for undesired market results. Democratic governments mostly represent the will of the people. If an undesired market results, such as poor air quality results in respiratory problems and high healthcare costs, the public usually expects a response from government. This section provides contemporary examples of government and non-government intervention in both the health and non-health sectors. They will demonstrate how market failure and the social determinants of health can be addressed through public policy.

Health sector interventions

Health insurance
A publicly or privately organised risk management scheme that provides protection from financial loss associated with purchasing healthcare.

Private **health insurance** in Australia is regulated through the *Private Health Insurance Act 2007* (Australian Government 2016). The Act is the Australian government's response to information asymmetry problems faced in the private health insurance market. A key element of health insurance is the pooling of risk. This means that people with high needs for healthcare and those who currently have low needs both contribute to the pool of funds used for 'purchasing' healthcare from the provider on behalf of the consumers. However, private insurers may want to decline insurance or charge higher premiums to high-risk people. A phenomenon called 'adverse selection' may also occur, where healthy people do not purchase private health insurance and therefore do not subsidise the sick (McPake 2013). In accordance with the Act, private health insurance in Australia is community-rated and not risk-rated. As a result, everyone is entitled to buy any insurance product and private insurers cannot refuse insurance to consumers on the basis of health status or expected frequency of claims. This results in equitable access to private health insurance and the maintenance of a large risk pool. Universal healthcare is also better supported through this policy because a high enrolment in private health insurance results in less demand for public hospital beds, outpatient appointments and other goods and services. These resources can then be redirected to supply more healthcare goods and services focusing on those most in need.

In contrast, private health insurers in the US can charge higher premiums to people with certain medical conditions, people of a certain age or living in a particular geographical area, or people who work in industries that have higher healthcare costs (*Patient Protection and Affordable Care Act 2010*). There are few incentives to provide equitable insurance access for high-risk consumers. The *Patient Protection and Affordable Care Act*, commonly known as Obamacare, mandates that most individuals purchase health insurance, which increases the risk pool and partly addresses adverse selection. As part of the Act, a regulation regarding the cost of insurance was introduced in 2014: small insurers are compensated for high-risk consumers purchasing their insurance policies. This is called a 'risk adjustment program'. While the introduction of the Affordable Care Act improved issues associated with access, affordability and quality of care in the US (Obama 2016; Courtemanche et al. 2017), the private health insurance market remains unstable, with insurers leaving the market, and small risk pools in some states (Gostin & Connors 2010; Khazan 2017; Soffen & Uhrmacher 2017; The Economist 2017).

Non-health sector interventions

It is not only the healthcare market that produces goods or services that affect health. Interventions in the non-health sector can occur when public health professionals seek to address the upstream determinants of health (see Chapters 1 & 13).

Aboriginal and Torres Strait Islander people in remote Australian communities experience challenges in access to, and affordability of, quality nutritious foods. This affects their overall nutritional status, risk of nutrition-related chronic disease and quality of life (Davy 2016; see also Chapter 8). Privately owned local food stores are established in the communities if there is both a commercial real estate market and a food market that they can participate in freely. These stores supply the quantity and type of food that consumers demand, at a price they are willing to pay. However, a community's geographical isolation and/or tropical weather may make it expensive to transport food there, and the quality of fresh produce may be compromised because of long transport times. Consequently, Aboriginal and Torres Strait Islander community members are more likely to purchase cheaper food products that do not deteriorate during transport, such as sugar-sweetened beverages and snack foods (Davy 2016). This failure of the food market affects health outcomes—there may be a monopoly of food providers, and the cost of the negative health externalities associated with poor nutrition are not incorporated into the price of the cheaper food products.

The challenges in supplying nutritious food to remote Aboriginal and Torres Strait Islander communities has been well-acknowledged by governments. In 2006, the Australian government intervened in the food supply market in remote Aboriginal and Torres Strait Islander communities by establishing 27 stores through the Outback Stores initiative (Davy 2016; Outback Stores 2018). The aim of Outback Stores was to improve the price and quality of nutritious food, and introduce better store management practices such as implementing health and safety standards. To do this, the government managed local food stores, subsidising the cost of nutritious food and returning profits to the community. Outback Stores has reported a reduction in sugar-sweetened beverage sales and an increase in fruit and vegetable sales, and a 5 per cent reduction in costs since the initiative commenced (Lee et al. 2009; Outback Stores 2018). However, Outback Stores has been criticised because the communities do not have decision-making powers over store operations, and the interference in both the commercial real estate and food supply markets inhibits other suppliers from entering the market in communities with more than 1000 residents (Hudson 2010).

Internationally, northern European countries and parts of the US have excelled at providing public goods such as infrastructure that promotes healthy living and addresses environmental determinants of health. In particular, active transport infrastructure that promotes incidental cycling and walking, is an example of how the non-health sector funds interventions that are a public good. The positive externalities of active transport are valued by the government and private investors. Copenhagen is often considered the cycling capital of the world (Sallis et al. 2016), a reputation that has been assisted by dense urban environments, short distances and flat terrain. The demand for cycling has been met with the supply of an extensive and well-designed system of cycling tracks, resulting in an estimated US$91 million saving for the Danish healthcare system per year from reduced morbidity and mortality (Baykal 2011). In Norway, the benefits of investment in walking and cycling tracks were estimated to be five times the cost of such investment (Sælensminde 2004). The health benefits of active transport investments are not only related to physical activity but also relate to reduced carbon dioxide emissions, less noise and lower traffic congestion (Sælensminde 2004; Sallis et al. 2016).

Stop and Think

The health impacts of climate change in terms of more heat waves, natural disasters, food-borne disease and displaced climate refugees are well recognised. Climate change is influenced by the emission of greenhouse gases, including carbon dioxide, through the human-driven production of good and services such as coal-fired electricity (Garnaut 2008; also see Chapter 11). The Australian government has attempted to support the implementation of initiatives that reduce carbon emissions, for example through the carbon pricing scheme of 2011–2014, and the Emissions Reduction Fund that commenced in 2014 (DoEE 2018). These schemes use government funds to pay organisations which store or avoid the production of carbon.

- Why might some people argue that the energy market in Australia fails, requiring government intervention such as an Emissions Reduction Fund?
- Investigate how a carbon market could be created with the introduction of government carbon-reduction incentives. How might a carbon market help address the climate-change determinants of health?

This section examined the role of governments and the non-government sector in addressing economic market failures that impact the social determinants of health. Interventions can occur in both the healthcare and non-health markets to improve inequities and health outcomes.

Gender, economics and health outcomes

As indicated in Chapter 1, gender is one of the social determinants of health that can have an influence on health and well-being. This section explores how an individual's economic welfare is impacted by their gender, and how this may influence their health outcomes.

Differences in health outcomes between genders

Health is not only impacted by genetic and biological differences between genders but by other variables such as societal structure, economic inequality, educational attainment and employment status (see Chapters 1 & 9). Numerous studies have shown that inequality between men and women has contributed to disproportionately negative health outcomes for women (Krieger 2000; Cooper 2002).

The difference in health status between men and women has been studied and reported upon frequently in Australia and in other countries. The Australian

Gender-based health inequality
The difference in health outcomes between genders.

Longitudinal Study on Women's Health (ALSWH) is an example of a large, long-term cohort study, with data collected from more than 50 000 women across Australia to gain a better understanding of women's health outcomes, service usage and factors that impact women's health (ALSWH 2018). However, **gender-based health inequality** may not always be revealed in commonly reported summary statistics, such as life expectancy. For example, based on global life expectancy averages, women can expect to live longer lives than men—this trend is maintained even when countries are grouped into low-, middle- and high-income brackets (WHO 2014). The issue is that average scores for a broad summary outcome, such as life expectancy, mask variation within and across countries. They also exclude other important outcome measures such as access to and use of services, discrimination associated with service provision or capacity to pay for healthcare. The reasons for inequality are not entirely clear, or easy to understand in isolation, and there is a link between social and economic determinants of health which is difficult to disentangle.

Difference in economic welfare between genders

Gender can influence an individual's economic welfare in a number of ways. For example, factors associated with the labour market disadvantage women in a disproportionate way compared to men (WGEA 2018). On average, Australian men are paid $253 per week more than women and some studies suggest that women are less likely to rise to higher-paid roles, remaining at the lower end of their chosen field (WGEA 2018). One explanation for this is that women remain largely responsible for child-rearing. Child-rearing consistently impacts on career building like no other life event, and there is no comparative life event that consistently impacts men in the way that childbirth does for women. In many societies there is less expectation that men will interrupt their careers when a child is born, and there is a strong social expectation that women will put paid work and a career aside to care for children (Rahim 2014). When women do re-enter the workforce after childbirth, they are more likely to balance paid and unpaid work—compared to men, a higher proportion of women will work in casual or part-time roles, negatively impacting on their earning capacity and limiting their career progression (ABS 2018).

Other societal factors also impact women more negatively than men. Studies have shown that a larger range of social barriers exist for women, impeding their capacity to independently build economic welfare (Austen 2014). For example, there is strong evidence that age discrimination is more prevalent against women, meaning that it can be more difficult for women to re-enter the workforce after a period of absence (Neumark 2015). Other studies also show that, remarkably, men are less likely to have their job credentials questioned, increasing their scope of employment as they are likely to have greater access to jobs they may not be qualified for (Murray 2014). Indeed, there are many countries where women are prohibited from certain roles or where a husband can legally prevent his wife from working (The Economist 2018). In traditional relationship settings, men are more frequently in charge of dividing the household budget, regardless of who earned the majority of the income. This leaves women vulnerable to economic abuse. Examples of economic abuse against women could include the male withholding money from their partner, spending a larger proportion of the household income on his own interests rather than on shared goods, or controlling financial transactions in some other way.

As a result of these factors, it is more common for women to depend on men, from an economic perspective (Jacobsen 2007). Economic reliance is an important issue when it comes to capacity to pay for goods or services, and there is evidence to suggest that capacity to pay for healthcare is a decisive factor in overall quality of life and health-related outcomes. An individual's capacity to pay for healthcare services can be diminished if they have reduced individual capacity, or lack economic support from a partner. Likewise, if their capacity to pay for services is overstretched because they are responsible for paying for more than just their own healthcare needs, then it is likely that they will suffer worse health outcomes than others who have a stronger economic framework.

Economic welfare is undoubtedly influential when it comes to health-related quality of life, but it is difficult to disentangle other societal factors that can negatively impact upon health. It is prudent to view gender-based differences in health outcome with a broad lens, and important to include as many influential factors as possible in understanding the inequalities that exist.

Case Example 7.3

Maternal mortality in the US

Of the 4 million women who give birth in the US each year, more than 50 000 experience severe life-threatening complications and 740 die. In 2015, the US had a higher maternal mortality rate than Kazakhstan, a country that is perceived to experience more challenging determinants of health than the US. While the maternal mortality rate in many sub-Saharan countries is decreasing, the rate has been increasing in the US for 20 years (Mapping Health 2018). There does not appear to be any sense of urgency in the federal or state governments, or philanthropic organisations, to fund healthy public policy for maternity services. For example, one venture capital fund raised $146 million over four years for pregnancy, fertility and women's health initiatives. In contrast, in only one year $220 million was raised for male-pattern baldness (RockHealth 2018). The funding available for maternity services does not supply a sufficient quantity or quality of care. Why does the funding shortfall exist?

The maternal mortality rate for African American women is four times higher than for all American women (Mapping Health 2018). The reasons for this are not clear, and assumptions involving African American women's economic welfare and access to healthcare should be challenged. Often, it is assumed that these women are not insured or are under-insured for antenatal and birthing care. However,

African American women from all socio-economic quintiles experience higher rates of adverse events and mortality during birth. It has been proposed that the root cause of this inequity is not only economic factors, but also racism and bias in medical practice. The care African American women receive cannot be separated from historical ideas about African American women's bodies, biased cultural norms, and stereotypes and moral judgment about African American women as mothers. African American women's judgment about the care they need and how they should be treated is said to be not always respected, and relationships between pregnant African American women and their caregivers are often a source of stress, anger and distress (Martin & Montagne 2017; Allers 2018; New York Times Magazine 2019). It is therefore not only economic welfare that determines maternal health outcomes for African American women in the US, but also social well-being and respect.

Stop and Think

Economic freedom is not experienced in the same way for both genders, due to a multitude of reasons. Economic freedom and capacity to pay for healthcare services are linked and there is evidence to suggest that capacity to pay for healthcare is crucial in experiencing good health outcomes. The universal basic income (UBI) is an economic strategy that has become the feature of much debate across the globe in recent years. The UBI could replace all government-based welfare payments, such as the age pension, carer's payments and unemployment benefits. All the funds involved with current welfare payments, including the large administration costs associated with managing the welfare system, would be channelled into the UBI. All citizens over a specified age would receive an income that would cover basic needs such as food, clothing and shelter, regardless of whether they were earning money through other means. The UBI would be paid equally to people who work full-time and those not currently in paid work. The current welfare system involves numerous checks and tests before people can receive payments—the UBI would be provided to all citizens, without stringent criteria for eligibility. This radical change in welfare policy is being trialled in socially progressive countries such as the Netherlands and Finland, to see how well it works and how best to administer the new system.

Think about this radical change, and use the following questions to generate discussion about the merits and pitfalls associated with a change in approach to welfare.

- How could a radical change to welfare policy reduce the difference in gender-related health outcomes?
- Would UBI be a fairer system for both genders in Australian society, or would it unfairly advantage one gender group?
- How could UBI be seen as an important investment?
- What problems might politicians face with introducing the UBI? Would there be strong political support for a changed approach to welfare in Australia?

Reflection Exercise

- Imagine you are a state Minister for Health. In a cabinet meeting, you hear that a business consortium would like your capital city to host the Olympic Games. Your concern is that health funding may be reduced to pay for investments in transport and infrastructure associated with hosting the Olympic Games. How could you use the economic concepts discussed in this chapter to realise health benefits for your department and health consumers in your state?
- Think about how economics aims to maximise the welfare of all society by informing choices made in a scenario of scarcity. How could you influence other ministers in your state to invest in non-health areas that could improve health outcomes? Do you think you could convince other ministers that the existence of public goods and externalities may result in market failure and poor health outcomes in your state? What is the reasoning behind your thoughts?
- Investigate the impact of hosting major events, such as the Olympic Games, on the economic welfare of the host state. Do you think this is a sensible use of scarce resources for an Australian capital city? What might be the legacy of hosting an Olympic Games?

Summary

Economics seeks to understand the choices made by people, governments and other organisations in a scenario of scarcity. This information can be used to predict whether an initiative to address the social determinants of health will be successful. The economic determinants of health are the ways society is funded and organised and these societal systems are often informed by key economic concepts. We have examined the economic concept of market failure, and how knowledge about it can inform the way society is funded and organised. We discussed how governments and organisations can intervene in the free market through changing societal systems to reduce inequities and improve social welfare. When examining gender-based health inequity, we emphasised that factors other than economics are involved in the poorer quality of life experienced by women. Social and historical factors also play a large part in gender-based health inequity. There is an inextricable link between the social and economic determinants of health, but economics cannot provide all the answers despite its focus on the welfare of society.

Tutorial exercises

Watch the Four Corners program *Mind the Gap* which is about out-of-pocket costs for surgical patients in Australia: http://www.abc.net.au/4corners/mind-the-gap/9809314

1. Identify aspects of market failure that drive the out-of-pocket costs described in the program.
2. What could all stakeholders do to rectify the variation in out-of-pocket costs?

Read the latest Australian Institute of Health and Welfare *Mothers and Babies* report (AIHW 2018).

3. Which groups are vulnerable to higher morbidity and mortality? Why this is so?
4. In small groups, discuss the impact of a UBI on your family and friends. Can you think of a situation where the current welfare system let you, or someone you know, down? Would that situation have been different if the UBI were implemented?

Further reading

Hotchkiss, J.L., Pitts, M.M., & Walker, M.B. (2017). Impact of first birth career interruption on earnings: evidence from administrative data. *Applied Economics*, 49(35), 3509–3522. doi:10.1080/00036846.2016.1262523

Jacobsen, J.P. (1994). *The Economics of Gender*. Cambridge, MA: Blackwell.

Popkin, B.M., Kim, S., Rusev, E.R., Du, S., & Zizza, C. (2006). Measuring the full economic costs of diet, physical activity and obesity-related chronic diseases. *Obesity Reviews*, 7, 271–293. doi:10.1111/j.1467-789X.2006.00230.x

Websites

http://www.heatwalkingcycling.org

The Health Economic Assessment Tool (HEAT) was developed by the World Health Organization to examine infrastructure and transport investments in walking and cycling.

https://www.everymothercounts.org/

Every Mother Counts is a non-profit organisation dedicated to making pregnancy and childbirth safe for every mother.

https://www.wgea.gov.au

The Workplace Gender Equality Agency website is a resource for understanding the gender pay gap in Australia.

https://www.youtube.com/watch?v=aIL_Y9g7Tg0

In this TEDx talk, Rutger Bregman explains the potential benefit of the Universal Basic Income and the economic theory underpinning it.

References

ABS (Australian Bureau of Statistics) (2018). *Labour Force, Australia.* Cat. No. 6291.0.55.001. Retrieved from http://www.abs.gov.au/ausstats/abs@.nsf/mf/6291.0.55.001

AIHW (Australian Institute of Health and Welfare) (2018). *Australia's Mothers and Babies 2016: In Brief.* Retrieved from https://www.aihw.gov.au/reports/mothers-babies/australias-mothers-babies-2016-in-brief/contents/table-of-contents

Allers, K.S. (2018). *Ending the Doom and Gloom: Shifting the Narrative about Black Maternal Health*. Retrieved from https://womensenews.org/2018/04/ending-the-doom-gloom-shifting-the-narrative-about-black-maternal-health/

ALSWH (Australian Longitudinal Study on Women's Health) (2018). *Australian Longitudinal Study on Women's Health.* Retrieved from https://www.alswh.org.au/publications-and-reports/published-papers

Austen, S., Jefferson, T., & Ong, R. (2014). The gender gap in financial security: what we know and don't know about Australian households. *Feminist Economics*, 20(3), 25–52. doi:10.1080/13545701.2014.911413

Australian Government (2016). *Private Health Insurance Act 2007.* Retrieved from https://www.legislation.gov.au/Details/C2016C00911

Baykal, A. (2011). *Copenhagen City of Cyclists: Bicycle Account 2010.* Retrieved from https://web.archive.org/web/20120929230131/http://www.kk.dk/sitecore/content/Subsites/CityOfCopenhagen/SubsiteFrontpage/LivingInCopenhagen/CityAndTraffic/~/media/439FAEB2B21F40D3A0C4B174941E72D3.ashx

Cooper, H. (2002). Investigating socio-economic explanations for gender and ethnic inequalities in health. *Social Science and Medicine*, 54(5), 693–706.

Courtemanche, C., Marton, J., Ukert, B., Yelowitz, A., & Zapata, D. (2017). Early impacts of the *Affordable Care Act* on health insurance coverage in Medicaid expansion and non-expansion states. *Journal of Policy Analysis and Management*, 36(1), 178–210. doi:10.1002/pam.21961

Davy, D. (2016). Australia's efforts to improve food security for Aboriginal and Torres Strait Islander peoples. *Health and Human Rights*, 18(2), 209–218.

DoEE (Department of the Environment and Energy) (2018). *Emissions Reduction Fund.* Retrieved from http://www.environment.gov.au/climate-change/government/emissions-reduction-fund

Garnaut, R. (2008). *The Garnaut Climate Change Review.* Melbourne: Cambridge University Press.

Gostin, L., & Connors, E. (2010). Health care reform in transition: incremental insurance reform without an individual mandate. *Journal of the American Medical Association*, 303(12), 1188–1189. doi:10.1001/jama/2010.375

Hudson, S. (2010). *Healthy Stores, Healthy Communities: The Impact of Outback Stores on Remote Indigenous Australians.* Retrieved from http://www.cis.org.au/app/uploads/2015/07/ia122.pdf

Jacobsen, J.P. (2007). *The Economics of Gender*, 3rd edn. Malden, MA: Blackwell Publishing.

Khazan, O. (2017). *Why so many Insurers are Leaving Obamacare*. Retrieved from https://www.theatlantic.com/health/archive/2017/05/why-so-many-insurers-are-leaving-obamacare/526137/

Krieger, N. (2000). *Discrimination and Health*. Oxford: Oxford University Press.

Lee, A.J., Leonard, D., Moloney, A.A., & Minniecon, D.L. (2009). Improving Aboriginal and Torres Strait Islander nutrition and health. *Medical Journal of Australia*, 190(10), 547.

Mapping Health (2018). *Mapping Maternity Care and Birth Outcomes*. Retrieved from http://www.mappinghealth.com/maternitycare

Marmot, M. (2015). *The Health Gap: The Challenge of an Unequal World*. New York: Bloomsbury.

Martin, N., & Montagne, R. (2017). *Nothing Protects Black Women from Dying in Pregnancy and Childbirth*. Retrieved from https://www.propublica.org/article/nothing-protects-black-women-from-dying-in-pregnancy-and-childbirth

McPake, B. (2013). *Health Economics: An International Perspective*, 3rd edn. Abingdon: Routledge.

Murray, R. (2014). Quotas for men: reframing gender quotas as a means of improving representation for all. American Political Science Review, 108(3), 520-532. doi.org/10.1017/S0003055414000239

Neumark, D., Burn, I., & Button, P. (2015). *Is it Harder for Older Workers to Find Jobs? New and Improved Evidence from a Field Experiment*. Working Paper No. 21669. Cambridge, MA: National Bureau of Economic Research. doi.org/10.3386/w21669

New York Times Magazine (2019). *Black Mothers Respond to Our Cover Story on Maternal Mortality*. Retrieved from https://www.nytimes.com/2018/04/19/magazine/black-mothers-respond-to-our-cover-story-on-maternal-mortality.html

Obama, B. (2016). United States health care reform: progress to date and next steps. *Journal of the American Medical Association*, 316(5), 525–532. doi:10.1001/jama.2016.9797

OECD (Organization for Economic Cooperation and Development) (2017). *Health at a Glance 2017*. Retrieved from http://dx.doi.org/10.1787/health_glance-2017-en

Outback Stores (2018). *Outback Stores: Working with Communities*. Retrieved from https://outbackstores.com.au/about/

Parliament of Australia (2018). *The Constitution*. InfoSheet 13. Retrieved from https://www.aph.gov.au/About_Parliament/House_of_Representatives/Powers_practice_and_procedure/00_-_Infosheets/Infosheet_13_-_The_Constitution

Patient Protection and Affordable Care Act, 42 U.S.C. § 18001 et seq. (2010).

Peeters, A., & Magliano, D. (2012). *Mapping Australia's Collective Weight Gain*. Retrieved from https://theconversation.com/mapping-australias-collective-weight-gain-7816

Rahim, F. (2014). Work–family attitudes and career interruptions due to childbirth. *Review of Economics of the Household*, 12, 177–205. doi.org/10.1007/s11150-013-9180-2

RockHealth (2018). *RockHealth*. Retrieved from https://rockhealth.com/

Sælensminde, K. (2004). Cost–benefit analyses of walking and cycling track networks, taking into account insecurity, health effects and external costs of motorized traffic. *Transportation Research Part A: Policy and Practice*, 38(8), 593–606. doi:10.1016/j.tra.2004.04.003

Sallis, J.F., Bull, F., Burdett, R., Frank, L.D., Griffiths, P., Giles-Corti, B., & Stevenson, M. (2016). Use of science to guide city planning policy and practice: how to achieve healthy and sustainable future cities. *Lancet*, 388(10062), 2936–2947. doi:10.1016/S0140-6736(16)30068-X

Soffen, K., & Uhrmacher, K. (2017). *Where the Obamacare Exchanges Lost Insurers for 2018*. Retrieved from https://www.washingtonpost.com/graphics/2017/national/obamacare-marketplace-insurers/?noredirect=on&utm_term=.e720f82cf243

The Economist (2017). *States Hurry to Fix Health-insurance Markets*. Retrieved from https://www.economist.com/united-states/2017/08/31/states-hurry-to-fix-health-insurance-markets

The Economist (2018). *Labour Laws in 104 Countries Reserve Some Jobs for Men Only*. Retrieved from https://www.economist.com/finance-and-economics/2018/05/26/labour-laws-in-104-countries-reserve-some-jobs-for-men-only

WGEA (Workplace Gender Equality Agency) (2018). *Australia's Gender Pay Gap Statistics*. Retrieved from https://www.wgea.gov.au/sites/default/files/gender-pay-gap-statistics.pdf

WHO (World Health Organization) (2014). *Large Gains in Life Expectancy*. Retrieved from http://www.who.int/mediacentre/news/releases/2014/world-health-statistics-2014/en/

WHO (World Health Organization) (2018). *Global Health Observatory: Summary Statistics*. Retrieved from Geneva: http://www.who.int/gho/data/node.country

World Bank (2018). *GDP (Current US$)*. Retrieved from https://data.worldbank.org/indicator/NY.GDP.MKTP.CD?name_desc=false

Part II

Social Determinants of Health and Applications

Chapter 8

Social Determinants of Australia's First Peoples' Health: A Multi-level Empowerment Perspective

Lisa Jackson Pulver, Megan Williams and Sally Fitzpatrick

Topics covered

This chapter covers the following topics:

- First Peoples' holistic health and well-being
- social and emotional well-being
- 'social' in social determinants from First Peoples' perspectives
- cultural, historical and political determinants of First Peoples' health
- structural determinants and racism
- multi-level empowerment and self-determination
- relationships, partnerships and accountability
- role of the reflective practitioner

Key terms

Australia's First Peoples
community engagement
critical reflection
multi-level empowerment
self-determination
social support
socio-ecological model
strengths-based approach

Introduction

We acknowledge the Traditional Owners on whose Lands, Waters and Skies the writing of this chapter took place, and we pay respects to Ancestors and Spirits of Nungeen-tya Mother Earth (in the language of the Wiradjuri peoples, from who the authors Jackson Pulver and Williams are descended). We think of future generations and those who came before us; it is upon their shoulders we stand today.

There is no doubt that the work by Wilkinson and Marmot in the late 1990s drew attention to the role of social determinants in explaining inequities in life experience between different groups of people (Wilkinson & Marmot 1998). These social determinants include the social gradient, stress, early life, social exclusion, work, unemployment, social support, addiction, food and transport (see also Chapters 1 and 2 in this volume). This has had a profound influence on western notions of health and health promotion, and is the basis of much progressive health policy.

However, we argue that contemporary western understandings of social determinants of health need to be expanded and extended to more fully reflect the experiences of Aboriginal and Torres Strait Islander people, **Australia's First Peoples**. Australia's First Peoples is the preferred term for referring to Aboriginal peoples. It is the collective term for the sovereign peoples of mainland Australia and Tasmania, as well as Torres Strait Islander peoples, the sovereign peoples of the islands between Cape York and Papua New Guinea. There are approximately 500 Aboriginal nations and 17 inhabited islands in the Torres Straits. The term 'Indigenous' can mean any person born in, or flora or fauna originating from, a particular country, but is often used to refer to Aboriginal and Torres Strait Islander peoples. Many of Australia's First Peoples dislike the term Indigenous, and we use it here only in the international context.

Australia's First Peoples
The preferred term for referring to Aboriginal peoples. It is the collective term for the sovereign peoples of mainland Australia and Tasmania, as well as Torres Strait Islander peoples, the sovereign peoples of the islands between Cape York and Papua New Guinea.

Australia's First Peoples are leading world citizens in the struggle for health equity and justice. They are leaders in culturally responsive, safe and respectful social support services, social and emotional well-being promotion and comprehensive primary healthcare practice. Despite their wisdom and innovation, these services and practices are severely constrained by external, socially determined factors. Assumptions are too often made when applying a western framework to non-western cultures. We must question 'Who is the social in social determinants?' and 'What is the contemporary compared to the historical, social context?' Importantly, these questions must be asked from First Peoples' perspectives.

In this chapter we will explore three different yet interrelated sets of factors implicated in the health and well-being of Australia's First Peoples: cultural, historical and structural determinants. We explore First Peoples' experience of determinants, and present examples of strengths-based, community-led services, programs and research. We then extend our understanding of determinants using a socio-ecological model of health that incorporates multi-level empowerment, with a particular focus on social support and the centrality of the value of relatedness. This provides a scaffold for our discussion about how all healthcare and social care providers can develop confidence in engaging with and providing support to First Peoples' families and communities, and be a good partners within and through their practice.

Laying claim to a future that embraces health for all

> Australians are truly one of the world's great human populations and a very ancient one at that, with deep connections to the Australian continent and broader Asian region. About this now there can be no dispute (Curnoe, cited by AGS & AAP 2011; Rasmussen et al. 2011, pp. 96–98).

Evolving out of more than 65 000 years of intergenerational sharing of knowledges and practice, and a profound sense of belonging to this land, the First Peoples of Australia are the world's oldest continuing cultures. Their definition of health involves both social and emotional well-being and their determinants:

> '**Aboriginal health**' means not just the physical wellbeing of an individual but refers to the social, emotional and cultural wellbeing of the whole Community in which each individual is able to achieve their full potential as a human being, thereby bringing about the total wellbeing of their Community. It is a whole of life view and includes the cyclical concept of life–death–life (NACCHO 2011, pp. 5–6, emphasis in original; cf NAHSWP 1989, p. ix).

This understanding of health, in which the well-being of the individual is inextricably linked to that of the community, society and environment, and vice versa, is the basis of the comprehensive primary healthcare model that emerged early in the 1970s, led and still used today by Aboriginal Community Controlled Health Services (ACCHSs) (Grant et al. 2008). This model preceded (Mazel 2016) yet has similarities to the Declaration of Alma-Ata (ICPHC 1978) and Ottawa Charter (WHO 1986), although those documents were developed largely from a western perspective and without the strategic inclusion of Indigenous peoples (McPhail-Bell et al. 2013). Our conscious use of the Aboriginal definition of health acknowledges the pre-eminence of its relational model as cultural, as well as the importance of working to decolonise mainstream models by centring Aboriginal ways of being, doing and knowing (Smylie et al. 2006; Mazel 2016), minimising the ongoing influence of colonisation and westernisation (Vickery et al. 2004). The effect, over time, is 'to establish more equitable Indigenous–non-Indigenous relationships based on principles of **self-determination**, empowerment and coexistence' (Mazel 2016, pp. 325–326).

For Australia's First Peoples to experience their holistic conceptualisation of health, several challenges must be addressed. These largely relate to 'the 97 per cent'—the general Australian population who, because of their overwhelming majority in numbers and as voting citizens (Mohamed & Sweet 2017), control how governments plan for and respond to First Peoples, as well as how First Peoples are conceptualised and treated, and the extent to which human rights abuses are allowed to occur. That is, Australia's First Peoples are a minority population, comprising 3 per cent of all Australians, without formal political power through collective representation. Almost half are not of voting age. Poor determinants of health have been, and continue to be, reinforced by the choices and ubiquity of the dominant Anglo cultures that have shaped contemporary Australia.

Self-determination

Self-determination became a legal right for all peoples in 1960. Decades later the collective rights of Indigenous peoples to self-determination were articulated in Article 3 of the UN Declaration on the Rights of Indigenous Peoples, which stated 'Indigenous peoples have the right to self-determination. By virtue of that right they freely determine their political status and freely pursue their economic, social and cultural development' (UN 2008, p. 4).

British colonisers were quick to judge Aboriginal people as uncivilised (Reynolds 1999) and closer to apes than humans (Wilkins 2009), and to deny citizenship rights (Chesterman & Galligan 1997). These assumptions persist in various forms, with an 'historical emotionality … strongly tied to meanings of the past still existent within Australian society … [reinforcing] assimilative intent and subjugations' (Arbon 2008, p. 145). These politically and socially position First Peoples at the lowest rung on Australia's social ladder (Tripcony 2000; Danalis 2009). They also place all Australians as witness to and complicit in the poor social determinants of health experienced by First Peoples, including social inequality and institutional and interpersonal racism. Contemporary Australia is a place of great wealth yet profound disparities. Opportunity is not equally shared and many First Peoples experience health and social lives similar to people in developing countries.

We agree with Arabana scholar, Veronica Arbon (2008, p. 145), that many in the wider Australian population also feel disempowered:

> All, including the invaded, are now expected to struggle to find their individual place along this road even if they are to be forced to transform, to exist within this created philosophical, scientific and ideological pathway. Individuality, subjugation and development for economic gains are all existent and central here.

The individuality and economic gains of Australians come at great cost to First Peoples' families and communities. The forced removal of First Peoples from their homelands by colonisers, and the social policies and economic development strategies that involve unequal power relations, perpetuate disadvantage among First Peoples. The dominant power of Anglo culture is now institutionalised through imported forms of governance, education systems and the narrative about the character of Australia and its citizens.

British colonisers have been described as unimaginative in their failure to recognise First Peoples' highly developed legal, health, science, kinship, agriculture and land care systems (Pascoe 2014). The subjugation of First Peoples' knowledges from colonisation to now (Arbon 2008) is seen in persistent disregard for models of holistic health and social and environmental practices that First Peoples offer, based on their cultural ways of knowing, being and doing. These ways could enrich the lives of many. We are fortunate today that out-of-date methods of disempowerment are being superseded by examples of positive and progressive strategies with the potential to stabilise negative trajectories and promote First Peoples' health and well-being.

It is with a spirit of humility and respect for the strengths of First Peoples that we write this chapter, moving away from merely describing the problems, deficits, risks and gaps, and governments' imposed and ill-thought-out 'solutions' to health inequity. It is with utmost regard that we engage with First Peoples' ways of knowing, being and doing, including the intergenerational, relational and place-based values central to the Aboriginal definition of health. These have inherent value for everyone.

Shape of Australia: the 'social' in social determinants

Australia is 'one of the most ethnically diverse societies in the world' (Australian Government, 2018, para 1). Of the estimated population of almost 25 million Australians (ABS 2018) 28 per cent were born overseas, with 5.1 per cent born in the UK, followed by New Zealand (2.6 per cent), China (2 per cent), India (1.8 per cent) and the Philippines and Vietnam (both 1 per cent) (ABS 2017a). This is a profoundly different society from that of 1901, when the colonies became a federation of states and territories. The population census then counted 3 773 801 people, with 18 per cent born in the UK (ABS 2006). The vast majority of citizens were Caucasian and Christian immigrants or descendants of immigrants from Britain, Ireland and central Europe. Chinese people made up the third-largest immigrant group (DIBP 2017, p. 4). Australia's First Peoples were not reported in the counts (Madden & Jackson Pulver 2009). Soon after federation, the Australian parliament legislated to prevent further Chinese people and labourers from the Pacific Islands arriving, in what became known as the White Australia Policy (DIBP 2017).

By 1950, Australia had welcomed over a million post-war immigrants, particularly from central and western Europe. By 1961, 9 per cent of the 10.5 million Australians were from countries other than Britain, predominantly Italy, Germany, Netherlands, Greece and Poland (DIBP 2017, p. 36). Many brought cultural practices from their homelands, including Indigenous peoples' cultures and practices. Further changes in migration policies that welcomed people from all over the world have created a potent, multi-dimensional 'intercultural space' (Yunkaporta & McGinty 2009). If nurtured, this rich mixing of cultures and insights could provide a dynamic position from which to develop solutions to the exclusion and disadvantage of Australia's First Peoples, particularly if led by younger Australians who have grown up among multiple cultures, with their unique intergenerational weaving together of historical narratives and value systems.

Australia's First Peoples on average are young, too. There are 500-plus clans with an estimated 649 171 people, making up approximately 3 per cent of the Australian population (ABS 2017b), of whom one in three are under the age of 25. A third (34 per cent) are under 15 (ABS 2017b), and the fertility rate is higher than that of the whole Australian community (ABS 2017c). There is an opportunity for major social change by developing the strengths of young people early, preventing ill health before it begins, and investing in support to maintain well-being and its determinants.

The broader reality, however, is that Australia has an ageing population. The average age is 37.2, and the birth rate is declining (ABS 2017d). Very different health and social policies are required to serve this majority, ageing population, rather than the young population of First Peoples. It is this demographic profile of Australians overall—the overwhelming dominance of the 97 per cent—that very much shapes the 'social' in social determinants of health, including those of First Peoples. That is, current social policies, health systems and societal expectations are geared towards mainstream population needs, which at times are very different from the needs of the country's First Peoples.

There is well-publicised worsening in well-being and determinants of health for many First Peoples (Markham & Biddle 2018; Seccombe 2018). Efforts over the past decade at 'closing the gap' in health inequality are 'not on track' (DPMC 2018, p. 9). Targeted strategies self-determined by First Peoples have not been invested in and government directives for First Peoples' access to mainstream services have not worked. Neither have they been given ample time or resources to work.

On almost every indicator of health and well-being, Australia's First Peoples fare worse than other Australians. The overall burden of disease is 2.3 times greater (AIHW 2016), and First Peoples born between 2010 and 2012 can expect to live approximately 10–11 years less than other Australians (AIHW 2018, p. 29).

This gap has often been blamed on First Peoples, with assertions such as they are genetically predisposed to illness, are negligent or apathetic (Saggers & Gray 1991, p. 6). The continuing focus on 'deficits' in the planning and delivery of services positions First Peoples as 'too sick' and 'the problem', rather than as developing solutions (Anderson 1988, pp. 134–139; Fogarty et al. 2018). Despite better education among the millennial generation and abundant contemporary evidence to the contrary, these prevailing beliefs remain entrenched in the mainstream health and policy environment.

Social determinants: expanding to understand First Peoples' views

Holistic, multi-level view

Peter Moodie was among the first researchers of the health gap between First Peoples and other Australians. He aimed to set a baseline from which to observe future progress (Moodie 1973, p. 2), and rejected common theories about the gap. He questioned the assumption that Aboriginal people 'have—or should have—the same "health values" as white Australians' (Moodie 1973, p. 18). Moodie took what is akin to a social-ecological approach to health, identifying five categories of factors determining Aboriginal health status: demographics, environment, diet, economy and contact with health and medical services (Saggers & Gray 1991, p. 6). Moodie stated that Aboriginal health status was not due to failings of Aboriginal people in those five categories, and he located causes of ill-health in socio-economic factors. He called for strategies that solved economic and social problems in concert with medical improvements, and pointed out that participation by Aboriginal people was 'essential to any efforts to improve their health status' (1973, p. 8).

Almost 50 years later, First Peoples and their allies continue to advocate for change, including for a paradigm shift to understand and address the particular social determinants of First Peoples' health. This means highlighting the impact of past and current processes and effects of colonisation and racism, and the importance of a human rights framework, strengths-based approaches and cultural understandings of health (Fisher et al. 2018).

These more nuanced social determinants are best understood as 'multiple, interconnected [factors that] develop and act across the life course from conception to late life' (Zubrick et al. 2014, p. 93). Importantly, these factors may differ between population groups, given the diversity of Aboriginal and Torres Strait Islander communities across Australia (Moodie 1973, p. 22; Carson et al. 2007).

Diversity of Australia's First Peoples

How different are determinants from First Peoples' perspectives from those described by Wilkinson and Marmot? Let's consider the value of work as an organising principle, which features in the famous Whitehall Studies renowned for demonstrating the impact on well-being of power and control (Marmot et al. 1991). The relevance of work status, across different First Peoples' communities, was questioned by Palawa academic Ian Anderson (2007, p. 26). Anderson noted that an individual's sense of purpose is constituted by a variety of roles, only one of which is work.

What if we were to consider culture instead of work? For example, in remote areas of Australia, positive impacts on social emotional well-being have been shown to accrue from a strong cultural identity (Dockery 2011, p. 14). Aboriginal people living in remote areas have higher self-rated senses of social and emotional well-being than Aboriginal people in urban areas, despite often having extremely limited healthcare access, relatively high unemployment and poorer living conditions (ABS 2011). Those whose cultural identity is less strong or who experience the cultural dissonance of 'living between two worlds' face the potential for higher levels of psychological stress and anxiety, possibly associated with a sense of doubt over the persistence or survival of valued aspects of their culture, or asking themselves 'what their role would be should their connection with that culture be severed' (Dockery 2011, pp. 13–14).

More favourable socio-economic outcomes have been shown among those with stronger attachment to or engagement with their traditional culture. Higher educational attainment and probability of being employed are also associated with stronger cultural identity (Dockery 2011, p. 10). Responsibilities and obligations between some Aboriginal families can mean that family members are required to relocate in order to fulfil intergenerational caring roles, maintain connections and obligations to family, and access seasonal work, healthcare and educational opportunities (Memmott et al. 2006). Burbank (2011, p. 136), in her study of stress, conveys the tensions experienced by her participants when their relationships, needs and emotions 'about getting on with life' in the intercultural setting of Numbulwar in the Northern Territory were at odds with the different value hierarchies of westerners who lived there. Anderson (2007, p. 26) writes:

> In this light, it is not unreasonable to hypothesise that Indigenous extended families continue to have a relatively more significant influence on Indigenous sociality (compared with the social world of work) as people continue to negotiate social relationships within a system of reciprocity.

Anderson is referring to values inherent in the holistic worldview suggested by the Aboriginal definition of health and well-being. These values of relatedness and locatedness (Arbon 2008) are shared by Indigenous peoples around the world. For Australia's First Peoples, identity is fundamentally tied to Country and the obligations within the web of relationships associated with that connection to Country. An individual's fulfilment of these obligations is through reciprocity, the purpose to which Anderson alludes. As Arbon (2008, p. 34) reflects, 'becoming who you are is accomplished by knowing your reciprocal relationships'. This is the same whether or not an individual is living on Country—for the many people living in the city, away from Country and kin, 'strong cultural determinants of health can still be enabled and maintained through languages, relationships, customs and community networks' (DoH 2017, p. 7). Embedding these values into mainstream health systems is the challenge with which 'the social' is currently grappling.

Community engagement
The sustained process of creating meaningful relationships and developing empowering strategies with community members to participate in decision-making, developmental actions and services that affect their lives, in order to create positive change. It includes the monitoring and evaluation of outcomes.

Strengths-based approach
A commitment to actively identifying strengths of an individual, family, community and/or service, as well as assets and available resources to build and invest in these, respecting and taking into account but choosing not to focus on or reinforce deficits, gaps, negatives or needs.

A particular area of difficulty is achieving the human rights principle of effective participation (see also Chapter 5). We often hear about this in terms of **community engagement** and the struggle by Aboriginal and Torres Strait Islander peak organisations to have their voices heard (Thorpe et al. 2016).

It is of 'deep concern' that 'Federal Government policies continue to be made for and to, rather than with, Aboriginal and Torres Strait Islander people', and opportunities for reform, reconciliation and renewal are ignored (NCAFP 2016, p. 2).

Case Example 8.1 highlights strong engagement and leadership by First Peoples, and their community and cultural strengths, in the urban community of Inala in the city of Brisbane, Queensland. 'Strong in the City' was among the first Aboriginal and Torres Strait Islander health promotion projects to document a **strengths-based** health promotion framework, which ensured that community members were adequately involved in decisions that affected their well-being (Vignette 1), helping inform the successful development of a government health service (Vignette 2).

Case Example 8.1

An urban Aboriginal community showcasing its strengths

Vignette 1: Strong in the City

The aim of Inala's Strong in the City was to identify participating community strengths through the eyes of community members themselves. Using participatory action research led by First Peoples, five key strengths were identified (Brough et al. 2004, pp. 217–218):

- Strength 1: extended family
- Strength 2: commitment to community
- Strength 3: neighbourhood networks
- Strength 4: community organisations
- Strength 5: community events.

In order to establish and provide a basis for supporting community-initiated ideas and problem-solving strategies, the Strong in the City team developed working partnerships with a range of Aboriginal and Torres Strait Islander agencies. More than 50 ideas and strategies were put forward over a period of two years, and were considered on the basis of how they engaged with the five strength themes.

The Strong in the City collaboration identified the important enabling resources as:

- professional support and development
- networking resources
- management support
- specialist support
- financial support (pp. 218–219).

The research identified that instead of 'a passive community "waiting" for top-down public health interventions', it found 'a community already working hard towards health improvement goals' (p. 219). However, people were usually working with limited resources and in unsupported roles. The constraints were not only financial but in the 'connections and commitments made by mainstream structures to support the efforts of Indigenous communities to create their own mix of strategies and solutions' (p. 219).

Vignette 2: Connectedness and cultural richness

Also in Inala, local non-Indigenous general practitioner Dr Geoff Spurling's research found that the Aboriginal and Torres Strait Islander community had a keen awareness of and sought active engagement in breaking the cycle of 'complex, interrelated, intergenerational' social, cultural and environmental determinants of health such as 'poverty, racism, housing, mental health, grief, loss, education, and employment' (2017, p. 102).

Spurling's interviewees described how they were able to negotiate the social, cultural and environmental challenges of their youth with the support of parents, family members and positive peer groups. The local community-based health service was seen as a trusted part of participants' lives. Overwhelmingly, collective strength 'owing to its connectedness and cultural richness' sustained the Inala community (Spurling 2017, p. 110).

In a presentation to the Research Translation Conference co-hosted by Australia's National Health and Medical Research Council and the Lowitja Institute (2017), Spurling acknowledged how hard it is for practitioners trained in western models of healthcare, research and support to transform their practices to support the design and delivery of First Peoples' collective, family and community-based models of healthcare. He highlighted the need for non-Indigenous people to be honest about what they do not know, to commit to developing relationships with First Peoples, to be a resource rather than to lead, and to commit to ongoing learning about First Peoples' historical and contemporary experiences, needs and aspirations (McInerney 2017).

Cultural determinants of health

First Peoples' cultural determinants connect sense of identity with purpose and practices. The *My Life My Lead* report (DoH 2017, p. 7) states that cultural determinants:

> encompass the cultural factors that promote resilience, foster a sense of identity and support good mental and physical health and wellbeing for individuals, families and communities … [They] are enabled, supported and protected through traditional cultural practice, kinship, connection to land and Country, art, song and ceremony, dance, healing, spirituality, empowerment, ancestry, belonging and self-determination.

Cultural determinants also connect individuals to their environment:

> Cultural determinants originate from and promote a strength-based perspective, acknowledging that stronger connections to culture and Country build stronger individual and collective identities, a sense of self-esteem, resilience and improved outcomes across the other determinants of health including education, economic stability and community safety (Brown, cited in DoH 2017, p. 7).

Further to the connection between the individual and environment, cultural determinants reinforce a way of being, knowing and doing:

> The accepted and traditionally patterned ways of behaving and a set of common understandings shared by members of a group or community. Includes land, language, ways of living and working artistic expression, relationships and identity (Australian Museum 2017).

These perspectives on culture and cultural determinants and their relationship to health and well-being must be contrasted with behaviours that are manifestations of poor health, intergenerational trauma, social marginalisation and poverty. Trans- and intergenerational trauma and poverty have accumulated among Australia's First Peoples as a result of decades of systemic oppression and disempowerment.

My Life My Lead affirms overwhelmingly that for First Peoples:

> strong connections to culture and family are vital for good health and wellbeing … The best results are achieved through genuine partnerships with

> communities ... The impacts of trauma on poor health outcomes cannot be ignored ... [and that] systemic racism and a lack of cultural capability, cultural safety and cultural security remain barriers to health system access (DoH 2017, pp. 7–8).

These points highlight determinants that have a particular influence on the lives of First Peoples, including historical factors, policy and related structural issues. These are explored further below (see also 'Culture as a social determinant of health' in Chapter 3).

Historical and political determinants of health

Prior to colonisation, people 'were able to determine their "very-being", the nature of which ensured their psychological fulfilment and incorporated the cultural, social and spiritual sense' (NAHSWP 1989, p. ix). This was permanently disrupted by British colonial forces in 1788 and the subsequent resistance and warfare (Gapps 2018), which continued well into the 20th century (Stanner 1969; Jackson Pulver 2003). The trauma of 1788 and colonisation did not disappear—the late Australian ethnographer and anthropologist, Patrick Wolfe (2006), argued that invasion is a structure and not merely an event, and the same can be said for settler colonisation.

The roots of colonial society were steeped in disrespect born of the invaders' sense of entitlement and desire to profit, which rested on the settler-colonial 'logic of elimination' (Wolfe 2006). This is 'premised on the securing—the obtaining and the maintaining—of territory. This logic certainly requires the elimination of the owners of that territory, but not in any particular way' (2006, p. 402). It includes disempowering First Peoples through oppressive government regulation, disparaging their cultures, social exclusion, not bringing to account perpetrators of frontier violence, and Stolen Generations. Wolfe (2006, p. 403) describes their collective impact as 'structural genocide', which continues into the present.

The creation of a free market was paramount (Havemann 2001). In this new economy, Aboriginal families actively participated despite the disruption. They worked as shepherds, labourers and farmers, at the same time maintaining fundamentals of their social behaviours and belief (Elkin 1951). Massacres, introduced diseases and the introduction and abuse of alcohol contributed to high death rates and lower birth rates (Jackson Pulver 2003). As early as the 1860s commentators were expecting Aboriginal people to become extinct (Reynolds 2001).

Segregationist government policies from the 1890 to the 1950s forced Aboriginal people to live on small government reserves of land and church missions. Biological and social factors were set in motion that profoundly influence health today, including oppression and disempowerment, profound grief and loss, the premature death of loved ones, sedentary and institutionalised life-styles, malnourishment and trauma (Saggers & Gray 1991; Jackson Pulver 2003).

The assimilationist policy era of the 1950s–1960s reinforced the devaluing of First Peoples' cultures and humanity. Wolfe (2006, p. 402) argues that:

> depending on the historical conjuncture, assimilation can be a more effective mode of elimination than conventional forms of killing, since it does not involve such a disruptive affront to the rule of law that is ideologically central to the cohesion of society.

The high rates of government-enforced child removals that characterised this period and were enforced by policy and practice into the 1970s resulted in multiple 'Stolen Generations'. It is suggested that no Aboriginal family has been unaffected by the forcible removal of children. Trauma, grief and loss arising from these policies impacts communities today (HREOC 1997).

The overarching intent was assimilation, and restrictions remained; for example, on access to social security until 1966. A successful referendum in 1967 meant the Commonwealth could make laws for Aboriginal people and include them when enumerating the Australian population (Madden & Jackson Pulver 2009). The short-lived policy era of integration (1967–1972) lifted hope, but threw up other challenges arising from Australia's federated political system. Aboriginal people led a growing civil rights movement that advocated for land rights, self-determination and an end to racism, particularly in the health system, yet little attention was paid to the poor health and social conditions produced by generations of oppression (Eckermann et al. 2010).

Community frustration with inaction by the Commonwealth led to the development of Aboriginal community-controlled housing, legal and health services, such as the Redfern Aboriginal Medical Service in 1971. Community-controlled health organisations were organised locally, regionally and nationally as a response to racism and exclusion within the mainstream health system (NAHSWP 1989; Foley 1991; Mazel 2016). They embodied a social health model that sought to address factors such as cultural connections and access to housing (NAHSWP 1989; Gillor 2012).

However, with the dismissal of the Whitlam Labor government, a short-lived policy period of self-determination (1972–1975) was wound back to a more conservative policy of self-management (Sullivan 2011). Nevertheless, the phase ushered in a period (1989–2005) of political participation through the Aboriginal and Torres Strait Islander Commission, a statutory authority that was directly elected by First Peoples. The Commission was important because it not only recognised First Peoples' unique place in 'the Australian social and political system … it also legitimized an approach that acknowledged difference on the basis of equality' (Mazel 2016, pp. 341–342). Self-management lasted into the 1990s and was overlapped by a formal decade of attempts at reconciliation (1991–2000) (ANTR 2010). The current policy period of normalisation involves a shift toward mainstreaming, and interventions designed to enforce western cultural norms (Sullivan 2011). The elimination of First Peoples continues in the fact that the property right of native title has rarely been experienced; their rights to land are presumed to have been swept aside by the tide of history (Olney, cited in Wolfe 2006, p. 393). Top-down, disempowering policies derived from the 2007 Northern Territory Emergency Response have resulted in deepening poverty, particularly in very remote communities (Altman 2017; Markham & Biddle 2018); overpolicing; 50 per cent of pensions and other welfare payments being quarantined, able to be spent only in government-prescribed ways; forced participation in work for the dole schemes; and the perpetuation of stigma (NCAFP 2018).

It is important to note that all these policies towards First Peoples are produced by people and thus are socially produced. Hence, whether historical, political or structural, they are social determinants.

Structural determinants of health: 'institutional racism'

As well as at times being in conflict with each other (Sanders 2013), the overwhelming influence of the policies described above has been the manifestation of forms of institutional racism that, for example, restrict First Peoples from 'receiving better healthcare outcomes, securing long-term employment or gaining meaningful and appropriate education' (Holland 2018, p. 12). Effectively, such inequality of opportunity breaches human rights principles, and the Australian government is obligated to quantify and remedy such inequalities progressively over a reasonable period of time (see Chapter 5 for more information about human rights and social justice).

The wide range of material discussed earlier demonstrates deeply entrenched 'othering' of Australia's First Peoples as separate from the general population (Smith 2012; Quayle et al. 2016). One of the most important questions to ask here is 'What is the link between racism and First Peoples not achieving their self-determined strategies to improve social determinants of health?'

First, racism occurs at the interrelated levels of 'interpersonal racism, internalised racism and systemic or institutional racism' (Kelaher et al. 2014, p. 44).

At the interpersonal level, First Peoples frequently experience racism in healthcare, education, employment and the criminal justice system (AHRC 2015). This is associated with psychological distress, depression, poor quality of life, and substance misuse, all of which contribute significantly to the overall ill-health experienced by Aboriginal and Torres Strait Islander people. Prolonged experience of stress can have physical health effects, such as on the immune, endocrine and cardiovascular systems (Anderson 2013, p. 7).

Stop and Think

- Have you experienced racism? Why or why not?
- Have you experienced stigma? Why or why not?
- Have you been disempowered by institutions? If so, how?

Think about the different ways that racism might impact on your willingness to access health and other welfare services.

Poor health, depression, disempowerment and victimhood are visible manifestations of internalised racism and oppression (Fanon 1967; Paradies 2007) that in turn disempower communities to exert their local norms and caregiving mechanisms (Gooda 2014). This is made even more complicated when First Peoples are blamed for their situation, and discourses of fairness and human rights struggle to find traction or be addressed (AHRC 2015). Jiman-Bundjalung scholar, Judy Atkinson (2002), has shown how the impact of such trauma is cumulative and compounding and has impacts across the life course. First Peoples are not alone here. For example, the breakdown of Canadian Aboriginal families and loss of traditions, custom and culture has had a cumulative effect on generations of residential school survivors, with many turning to 'alcohol and other drugs ... as a means to cope with the complex effects of poverty, despair, discrimination, loss of language and traditional territories and the erosion of culture' (Craib et al., cited in Treloar et al. 2016, pp. 19–20).

Such manifestations of trauma fuel inappropriate assumptions and lack of empathy for First Peoples, which become 'embedded' into healthcare and social care, policy and planning mechanisms and governance systems (Anderson 2013, p. 7).

Historically, there have been poor strategies to engage First Peoples in government policy and programming, and lack of trust to allow First Peoples' solutions to flourish. Quayle et al. (2016) discuss a perceived social distance between First Peoples and the broader population. Paradoxically, while there is absence or disregard for First Peoples' interests in so many spheres of influence, at the same time they are hypervisible, either as Australia's cultural icons or as social problems perpetuated through racial profiling in mainstream media (Quayle et al. 2016, p. 81; see also Paradies 2007; Sweet et al. 2017). Stereotypes abound, intensifying the lack of trust between both groups. First Peoples quickly become disenchanted with the consultation and program planning process. Lack of good processes around participation contribute to service inaccessibility, to the extent that First Peoples:

> may be reluctant to seek much-needed health, housing, welfare or other services from providers whom they perceive to be unwelcoming or who they feel may hold negative stereotypes about them (Anderson 2013, p. 7).

Stop and Think

- Describe Aboriginal and Torres Strait Islander peoples—Australia's First Peoples—in your own words (even things you would not tell other people).
- What is your experience engaging with Aboriginal and Torres Strait Islander peoples?
- How did you learn about Aboriginal and Torres Strait Islander peoples?
- Of that information, what did you seek out for yourself?

While it is one step to identify racism at individual and interpersonal levels, many Australians find it difficult to identify structural racism, let alone identify strategies to dismantle it (Dwyer et al. 2016; Soutphommasane 2017). Alyawarre Elder Pat Anderson AO (Anderson 2013, p. 7) has stated this is not necessarily the result of individual ill-will by health practitioners, for example, but a reflection of how systems for healthcare are designed and implemented.

Three implications for care providers arise from this dynamic:

1. the dominance of the western biomedical paradigm, and its neoliberal emphasis on the individual, limits holistic care that could ameliorate the impact of negative determinants (Baum et al. 2013); for example, through family-centred care and by strengthening First Peoples' cultures
2. social inequality reinforces inequality in the relationships between the professional support providers and service users (Sheaff 2005) that are so essential to breaking the trauma cycle
3. we are 'unlikely to accommodate the provision of programs designed to assist Aboriginal groups pass on their culture to the next generation' (Spurling 2017, p. 180).

These statements highlight how institutional and interpersonal racism are linked. In practical terms, assumptions influence the design of whole programs of health interventions, as well as decisions about resource allocation, staffing, delivery and evaluation. They are based on the worldview, power and values of the 97 per cent of Australians who are not First Peoples, and thus rarely reflect First Peoples' perspectives and practices, and are rarely self-determined by ACCHSs (Blignault & Williams 2017).

This is despite Australia being party to the UN Declaration of the Rights of Indigenous Peoples, which recognises self-determination as a special and collective right of First Peoples (Mazel 2016). First Peoples have remained vulnerable, highly politicised and without collective representation in governments. A recent example of the denial of the right to self-determination is the Australian government's rejection of First Peoples' recommendations for future directions outlined in the Uluru Statement from the Heart (FNNCC 2017).

Once again, this is the interface between social and structural determinants. It is political will that shapes determination to reform entrenched structural barriers to change (Mazel 2016). Often, development and assimilative intentions take precedence over First Peoples' aspirations, contributing to a 'status quo that is not of an Indigenous definition' (Arbon 2008, p. 86).

The powerful forces of oppression and history cannot be overlooked (Fanon 1967), including the 'depth at which colonialism can submerse itself in a society' (Hilton 2011, p. 51), whether this is intentional, hidden or unintentional. Lasting change at interpersonal and structural levels and relatively peaceful coexistence between First Peoples and others will ideally come about by recasting relationships through a peace-building process (Fitzpatrick 2003). Strategies include the ongoing promotion of anti-racist values and beliefs within government leadership (Paradies 2007), a national truth-telling process, a voice in the Australian parliament, and treaty frameworks (NCAFP 2016; FNNCC 2017). Also vital is workforce development and strategies to enable parity in workforce participation by First Peoples (DoH 2015; AIDA 2016).

These important proposals are being discussed and nationally debated, and there are excellent exemplars of leadership based on the experiences of healthcare and social care professionals. These professionals, who are grappling with their own position, privilege, confusion and strategies for inspiring change in others, suggest that a shift in the 'social' is happening.

Multi-level empowerment

Importance of relationships and collective healing for all

There is an axiom that there can be no self-determination without healing. Healing for First Peoples 'is a holistic process which addresses mental, physical, emotional and spiritual needs and involves connections to culture, family, community and land' (Muru Marri with Blignault & Arkles 2015, p. 4). Collective healing is of particular relevance to First Peoples as a culturally informed, strengths-based process that encompasses how issues, responsibilities and opportunities for change exist within and between personal, cultural and structural domains. In this way, collective healing reflects a socio-ecological model of health, incorporating the processes of **multi-level empowerment**.

Multi-level empowerment
Empowerment is commonly understood as an enhanced sense of 'control of destiny' with respect to forces that affect an individual's daily life (Syme 2004). Multi-level empowerment is the potential for and process of positive change at individual, family, community, services, system and environmental levels. Changes occur at these separate levels, and are interconnected and interactive.

Research into multi-level empowerment among First Peoples affirms an enhanced sense of personal empowerment that flows from participation in and having influence over activities at the community or organisational level, for example through volunteering or political action (Tsey et al. 2010). This can be through either a sense of direct control or influence or a sense of perceived control, for example through participating in organisations (Shulz et al. 1995, p. 312).

Another way of thinking about multi-level empowerment is to consider how it can be promoted and nurtured. Research among First Peoples shows how the dynamic interaction between collective and personal empowerment 'encompasses the extent that a person can live a life that honours their identity, values and abilities in harmony with others' (Haswell et al. 2010, p. 798).

An empowered community of First Peoples in Australia cannot grow or flourish unless awareness, understanding, engagement and respect by all Australians also grow, and the value of First Peoples' cultures are embraced. For example, studies of social capital and Indigenous people from around the world have found that their health and well-being depend on connections with communities (Richmond et al. 2007). Connection is important not only within First Peoples' communities but also with the general community. This was affirmed by Sir Michael Marmot (2011, p. 21), who pointed out that in addition to addressing social disadvantage, attention was needed with respect to 'the particular relationship with Indigenous Australians to mainstream society'.

A multi-level empowerment perspective therefore requires us to understand that Australian society as a whole has an important role in bringing about improved health equity, making it 'everyone's business' (Virdun et al. 2013). Relationship—our basic need to be connected socially and to belong—along with the need for freedom to live autonomously and the need for competence to be effective in life, are theorised as essential to the well-being of everyone (Deci & Ryan 2000, 2008).

Figure 8.1 Socio-ecological empowerment model for First Peoples' health and well-being

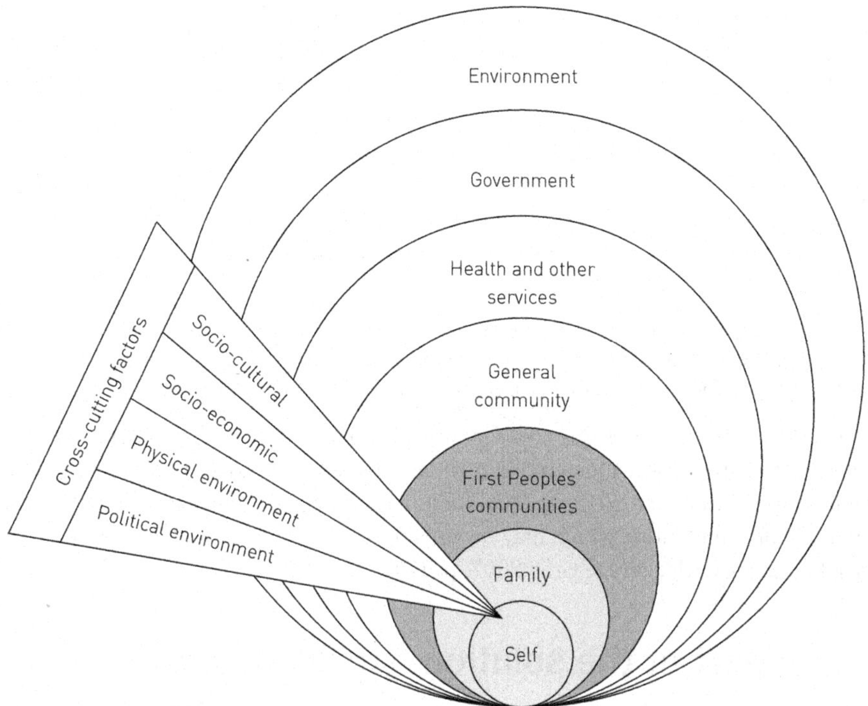

Figure 8.1 illustrates the multiple levels of relationships significant to the well-being of First Peoples, from self to family, Aboriginal community, general community, health and other services, government (policy, bureaucracy, politics) and environment (Country, world, biosphere, universe and time) and back again: a dynamic ripple effect. There are also cross-cutting factors (adapted from Anderson 1988, pp. 127–139):

- socio-cultural (identity, inclusivity, intercultural space, colonisation)
- socio-economic (access to employment, income, health and education, goods and services)
- physical environment (place, demographics, climate and living conditions, food sovereignty)
- political environment (control, self-determination, participation, coexistence and economy).

Each factor includes the potential for positive empowerment and negative stressors; they exist on a continuum and within a context of constant change.

Multi-level empowerment is the social action process that occurs within and between the levels and domains of a **socio-ecological model** (Wallerstein 1992). A socio-ecological model is often depicted as a nested Venn diagram, onion rings or ripples in a pond. The centre depicts the individual, moving out to the 'microsystem' of family, peers, schools and community groups, extending to the 'exosystem' of social

Socio-ecological model
A perspective that respects the multiple interconnected relationships between a person and their social and environmental contexts.

services and systems, to the 'macrosystem' of cultural, societal, economic, geographic and political factors. The socio-ecological model respects cumulative influences over the life-span, as the underlying 'chronosystem' (Bronfenbrenner 1977; Santrock 2007).

Positive collective identity, social support and enhanced confidence are all possible, particularly when 'individuals and organizations participate in processes which enable the community to meet the needs of its constituents' (Schulz et al. 1995, p. 311).

Collective healing is an example of this process, in that it 'broadens the scope for *who* does healing and *who* healing is for' (Muru Marri with Blignault et al. 2014, p. 14, emphasis in original).

> It means moving from a model where expert professionals work with individuals to a model where individuals develop their own skills and capacities to empower healing in themselves and their families and communities.

Collective healing engages participants 'as workers for healing so that working together we grow the wider circles of relationships necessary to develop healing communities' (Sheehan 2012, p. 108). Included here are psychosocial determinants such as cultural identity, which may be considered a mediator, such as in relation to social inequality (Saggers & Gray 2007, p. 15).

Being part of the solution: social support

As discussed above, Aboriginal social structures are based on kinship systems (Anderson 1988). The collecti-vist or communi-vist worldview held by First Peoples allows people to know who they are in terms of their affiliations, kin relations, social standing, roles, responsibilities and obligations to each other and to society as a whole (SNAICC 2011). Relationships and reciprocal responsibilities and obligations that flow from these are highly valued. This network of relationships sustained Aboriginal society since time immemorial, by locating people in a collective network of cultures where reciprocity and mutuality are the norm, and reinforcing the role and purpose of the individual as well as their health and well-being. Relationships between individuals are the logical site of caregiving and **social support**, which in turn influence multiple other levels.

Social support
Social support is widely acknowledged as a determinant of health, and as having direct health-giving effects. It is an individual's sense that their needs may be met with assistance and reinforcement from others, whether in practical, instrumental or emotional ways.

Social support is widely acknowledged as a determinant of health, and as having direct health-giving effects. It is an individual's sense that their needs may be met with assistance and reinforcement from others, whether in practical, instrumental or emotional ways. There are many types of cultural and social influences on how needs and assistance are defined, including by whom, the timing of assistance and the evaluation of its effectiveness. Social support is a multi-level construct, required and experienced by individuals, families and communities. It involves interplay between these domains.

Individual-level social support is well identified as a significant independent determinant of health (Bloom 1990; Schwarzer & Leppin 1991; Uchino et al. 1999; Schwarzer & Knoll 2007; Taylor et al. 2007). It includes several 'entwined dimensions' of interpersonal relationship mechanisms, which protect people from stress (Cohen et al. 2000; Ball & Elliot 2005); and resources that people can give or receive to reduce stress (Stansfeld 2006). Social support can be tangible, such as provision of financial resources, or intangible such as reassurance (Weber 1998). It can also be experienced as an individual's belief that they are loved, valued and cared for because their relationships with others provide this (Cobb 1976, cited in Stansfeld 2006, p. 148). The main effect of social support on health is that an individual's sense of well-being increases as a result of being part of a supportive network (Cohen & Syme 1985; Cohen 1988). That is, the health-giving effects of social support arise from interactions and transactions with others (Stansfeld 2006, p. 150).

What is the healthcare and social care practitioner's role? Clarifying this is essential for psychosocial empowerment, as it provides insights into relevant steps for action and for self-care. To paraphrase Quayle et al. (2016, p. 81), for practitioners to work in solidarity means centring and listening to First Peoples' voices, to critically discern power relations, to revise meanings attributed to experience, and to affirm identities and communities. Understanding history and context is key as this stimulates critical reflection (discussed below). Once we begin to reflect, critically heightened self-awareness becomes possible, providing a clarity that reduces fear of saying or doing the 'wrong thing' or being overwhelmed at the complexity of issues. It also serves to prevent resentment when positive change does not occur at a broader level—and helps to appreciate the small shifts that may have occurred in an individual's immediate sphere of influence.

Relating well and being critically reflective

> Social justice is what faces you in the morning ... a life of choices and opportunity, free from discrimination. (Dodson, cited by NCAFP 2016, para 1).

When 'realities' in one culture are out of sight from another, there develops a gulf in understanding. This can easily be racialised and characteristics of difference can be magnified (see Chapter 3). Commitment to health equity and addressing social determinants of First Peoples' health means being confident to challenge racialisation, and instead develop and participate in meaningful relationships with each other at the 'cultural interface' (Nakata 2007). This means stepping into a relational domain in which an individual has a strong sense of the influence of their own culture, privilege and bias, and where a reflexive sense of their role can be developed and provide a solid basis for learning.

Developing a relational domain is not just about, for example, meeting the needs of First Peoples. As mentioned, it is also about truth-telling, recognising the history of Australia, and embracing First Peoples' cultures towards forging a new national identity. This can stimulate re/connection with deeper ways of being often overlooked by western society, including, for example Europeans' tendency in recent generations to see themselves as separate from nature (Anderson 2011). It is also important for moving beyond learning about, to *learning with* and *learning from* First Peoples. There is much to learn, particularly because of the great diversity among First Peoples that existed both pre- and post-colonisation. Each community has its own and multiple protocols for engaging, relating and working together. And as stated earlier, the holistic conceptualisation of health, intergenerational care and relational and place-based values have inherent value for everyone.

To know what and how we can contribute and meet the needs and aspirations of First Peoples' communities requires ongoing **critical reflection**. The purpose of critical reflection is to learn from and make meaning of an individual's position, to stimulate decision-making and steps for self-improvement in personal and professional relationships with others, committed to the empowerment of others. This offers a means by which to identify 'inconsistencies between formal theories and practice theories' (Bennett et al. 2016, p. 2). Critical reflection values 'practical wisdom'—by reflecting on an incident or text, we may gain new insights that are potentially generalisable. Critical reflection opens the potential to question actions, strategies and assumptions that render healthcare professionals complicit in maintaining an established order. Critical reflection is a key tool in self-care as well. It helps in knowing our role and setting our boundaries. It helps us to be discerning and not dominating as advocates.

Critical reflection
The practice and process of developing awareness about oneself, examining experiences, ideologies, identity, social location, biases, motivations, contradictions and assumptions that might overtly or unconsciously influence behaviours, actions and ways of relating to and engaging with others.

The final Stop and Think includes some useful critical reflection questions, adapted from social work scholar Jan Fook (2009) and Fitzpatrick (2011).

Stop and Think

- How do I influence what I see?
- How does what I look for influence what I find?
- How could I learn directly from Aboriginal and Torres Strait Islander peoples?
- What holds me back?
- What steps can I take to overcome these factors, and make connections?

Community-empowered approaches

The model of multi-level empowerment is embodied in Aboriginal community-controlled health organisations (Mazel 2016). As well as delivering a world-leading comprehensive primary healthcare model, these organisations are the largest employer of Aboriginal people. They provide a benchmark for culturally safe care and self-determination through locally elected boards of management (NACCHO 2013; Mazel 2016). Their sector peak bodies advocate and mobilise other service providers, parliamentarians and community members to demand structural change

(NCFP 2016), and extend the example of multi-level empowerment. An indicator of the success of the sector and its constituents is the successful embedding of social and cultural determinants at the centre of the national implementation plan for Aboriginal and Torres Strait Islander health (Fisher et al. 2018).

From an intervention perspective, we can understand multi-level empowerment through the factors and conditions required for a program to enable participants to achieve their full potential, as proposed in the Aboriginal definition of health. Case Example 8.2 summarises four sets of critical success factors that were found to influence the ability of a program or service to do so at service provider, organisational and system levels. These factors were elicited from case studies of social and emotional well-being programs for Aboriginal and Torres Strait Islander young people (Haswell et al. 2013) and women leaving prison (Haswell et al. 2014, pp. 89–92).

Case Example 8.2

Critical success factors in First Peoples' programs

Effectiveness factors

To be 'effective', programs must work from strengths; be relational; model reliability and consistency; facilitate connection to culture; be non-judgmental; have rules and boundaries; model openness, honesty and trust; enable choice; and celebrate achievement.

Sustainability factors

To be 'sustainable' program establishment processes must be inclusive; embed Aboriginal ways of being and doing; engage with the community and strengthen the local knowledge base; reflect a shared vision between participants and workers; foster innovation and collaboration; have accountability and monitoring processes; demonstrate value through achievements; have emotionally safe working environments; manage change respectfully; and put time into relationships with stakeholders.

Resourcing factors

Critical 'resourcing' factors involve flexible funding attuned to local circumstances; connections with other services; pre-program grassroots consultation; culturally informed evaluation processes and tools; realistic funder and community expectations; support by continuous funding strategies that facilitate growth, strengthen the workforce and accommodate flexible and internally relevant accountability.

Landscape factors

Within the wider landscape, critical factors include cross-sectoral alliances; avoiding competitive funding processes; the capacity to demonstrate meaningful accountability; systematic mechanisms to share information among stakeholders; clearly articulated roles, responsibilities and expectations across sectors; leadership and management by experienced, skilled and empowered Aboriginal people and recognised professional and community allies; extensive Aboriginal and Torres Strait Islander community networks and mechanisms that support the collection of culturally informed data on program performance.

Haswell et al. (2014, pp. 89–92); Haswell et al. (2013)

Engaging in multi-level empowerment and holistic health perspectives requires relating with a wide range of stakeholders at individual, service, community and policy levels. For decades, there have been calls for governments to break down silos in policy development and program delivery. For example, in 2008 the Close the Gap Statement of Intent, instigated by a First Peoples'-led coalition of national health sector peak bodies and social justice organisations, was described as a compact between Australian governments and Australia's First Peoples (Holland 2018, p. 3). Its aims included 'working collectively to systematically address the social determinants that impact on achieving health equality for Aboriginal and Torres Strait Islander peoples' (Indigenous Health Equality Summit, cited in Holland 2018, p. 13). This must be achieved in tandem with financial and other resource inputs that address issues such as infant and maternal health, chronic and communicable diseases, social and emotional well-being, along with strategies that reduce health system discrimination and racism (Mazel 2016; Holland 2018).

Kungarakan Elder Tom Calma AO (Calma 2008) provides the crucial elements for interaction and partnership across the multiple domains:

> To me, these principles reflect what social workers are striving for and of course, [what] many social workers are actually practicing already:
>
> 1. People are recognised as key actors in their own development, rather than passive recipients of commodities and services.
> 2. Participation is both a means and a goal.
> 3. Strategies are empowering, not disempowering.
> 4. Both outcomes and processes are monitored and evaluated.
> 5. Analysis includes all stakeholders.
> 6. Programmes focus on marginalized, disadvantaged, and excluded groups.
> 7. The development process is locally owned.
> 8. Programmes aim to reduce disparity.
> 9. Both top-down and bottom-up approaches are used in synergy.
> 10. Situation analysis is used to identify immediate, underlying, and basic causes of development problems.
> 11. Measurable goals and targets are important in programming.
> 12. Strategic partnerships are developed and sustained.
> 13. Programmes support accountability to all stakeholders.

These elements represent ways of working together that protect trust, respect and integrity while moving towards common goals. In essence—how to be a good partner. Marmot (2005, p. 1102) has suggested 'that both material or physical needs and capability, spiritual, or psychosocial needs are important to the gradient in health'.

One important example aligned with this approach is First 1000 Days, based on a global initiative to reduce undernutrition in low- and middle-income countries (Arabena et al. 2016). First 1000 Days Australia is an early childhood development intervention led by First Peoples working with a multi-disciplinary team of experts. In introducing the concept, the First Peoples-led Australian team conducted a year-long engagement process:

> linking early-life researchers, research institutions, policy makers, professional associations and human rights activists with Australian Indigenous organisations and families. The resultant model, First 1000 Days Australia, broadened the international concept beyond improving nutrition (Ritte et al. 2016, p. 1).

First 1000 Days Australia focuses on 'bringing together disparate programs—home nursing, child protection and fathering support—with evidence-based very early learning programs' (Arabena 2014, p. 442). The partners are committed to developing an enabling environment, by building on strengths and reinforcing resilience.

This approach, while not yet fully evaluated, is critical to respecting community needs and values, overcoming service fragmentation and building practice-based evidence of programs that address the 'complex effects of social and community environments on children's development' (Arabena 2014, p. 442). Drawing from this program, Case Example 8.3 talks about the role and aspirations of family, and therefore the types of supports, healing and development required.

Case Example 8.3

First 1000 Days Australia

The focus on the First 1000 Days is important because while the family life of Aboriginal and Torres Strait Islander people is predominantly centred around complex kinship systems and clan structures, with clear lines of rights and obligations to others, an increasing number of our children are vulnerable and at risk. We recognise that, until recently, the education and socialisation of young children took place within the rhythms of family life, the extended family and their Country. We also recognise the intrinsic value of children within our communities.

However, we also acknowledge that these ideals have been radically disrupted for some families, particularly those who have suffered the separation of their children, the destruction of extended family networks, and decades of living in oppressive circumstances—as evidenced by poor health and early deaths, substandard housing, poor educational outcomes, high unemployment and large numbers of Aboriginal and Torres Strait Islander people in custody.

Despite these hardships, family remains the primary and preferred site for developing and protecting culture and identity in our children. We also acknowledge, then, the importance of family-strengthening initiatives, the crucial role played by men in raising children and the importance of the First 1000 Days to the future prosperity of Aboriginal and Torres Strait Islander societies. By initiating an early and continued investment in the next generation, we can mitigate connections between adverse early experiences and a wide range of costly problems, such as lower educational achievement and higher rates of criminal behaviour and chronic disease. The First 1000 Days focuses on reducing the burdens of significant adversity on families with young children (Arabena et al. 2015, p. 1).

The family-strengthening, transgenerational care and complex issues identified in Case Example 8.3 require efforts across multiple domains of the community, including government departments, community organisations, community members and families and individuals. The diverse, transdisciplinary teams call for much care to be taken by individuals and the organisations and interest groups they represent, given the potential for professional differences, cultural differences and inevitable power differentials (Whiteside et al. 2011, p. 228).

Whiteside et al.'s writing (2011) is valuable further reading—it provides an example of a theoretical, multi-level empowerment framework, which can be applied to a range of contexts. This type of framework is valuable as an evaluative and critical reflection tool:

> When used in a critically reflective way [a multi-level empowerment framework can help make sense of complexity and allow] the practitioner to place values at the forefront of any engagement and assist people to envision how things could be different (Whiteside et al. 2011, pp. 228–229).

A multi-level empowerment framework is also useful in monitoring and evaluation of processes and programs. The critical success factors identified in Case Example 8.2 include factors at the individual, family, community, service and policy levels of a multi-level empowerment framework. To genuinely understand processes, outcomes and impacts of projects and programs with, by or for First Peoples, evaluations and research must adhere to ethical guidelines (NHMRC 2003) and be led by or, at the very least, involve First Peoples, ideally from the decision to do the evaluation or research, through to the translation of the results (Williams 2018). Evaluation and research require critical engagement with socially and culturally relevant questions, and agreement by local First Peoples about data and indicators of success to be used. The misuse of simple demographics, such as nationally aggregated data rather than local data, can have major implications in research, particularly when making recommendations for the design and delivery of health and social support programs, addressing social determinants and prevention, and training of future generations of support providers. It is imperative to ask who is doing the measurement, and why (Walter & Andersen 2013). These questions are not culturally neutral.

There are also ethical concerns and implications of research. Too often, evaluations are executed to satisfy grant conditions, yet programs shown to be successful are not supported or do not survive changes in government (Blignault & Williams 2017). It is vital to engage the end-users of evaluation and research, to ensure that outputs and recommendations are translated, as practically and realistically as possible, to meet the needs of all stakeholders and confidently address the complexities of multi-level empowerment frameworks.

Wisdom, particularly practical wisdom grounded in a sound moral and ethical framework, is at the core of effective Aboriginal and Torres Strait Islander social work. Emergent wisdom is when we recognise that the whole is greater than the sum of its parts—a shift from independence and individualism to interdependence (Bassett 2005). It involves a shift in standpoint from 'I am a good person' to 'I am complicit'. This means that a person recognises themselves as part of the larger whole, whether their participation is willing or not. Thus, even those who are not working directly with Aboriginal and Torres Strait Islander people can still work to effect change in prevailing structures and systems of oppression. We can call out racism wherever we see it. We can respect all life forms and contribute to the common good of this planet.

There is great potential for a mutually beneficial future; where one culture's aspirations and needs are not in competition with another's, where 'others' are seen not as a threat but as an opportunity for enrichment and improvement.

The key step in achieving health equity is to learn to relate well with Aboriginal and Torres Strait Islander people, based on knowing oneself, one's position and bias, one's strengths and what one has to offer in supporting the Aboriginal and Torres Strait Islander leaders to meet their self-determined aspirations and needs. Learning to be reflective, in order to become more critically self-aware and able to understand one's own biases, is the crucial first step.

Without such a shift in mainstream Australia, there is the potential for ever-widening health and social inequality. Unless people can self-determine responses to their own issues, at individual and community levels, growth and empowerment is slow or impossible. Given the minority population and relative powerlessness of Australia's First Peoples, this requires everyone to work with, rather than for or against, First Peoples, supporting rather than rescuing, affirming rather than vilifying. Not only problem-focused, but also strengths-based. Learning about empowerment in ourselves first, in order to be empowering of others.

If there is no critically informed, inclusive action at all levels, there is no doubt that health inequity will widen.

It is an ethical decision for mainstream Australia—will we watch health inequity widen, or challenge ourselves critically on how we work with and respect First Peoples' knowledges and experiences for the good of the whole?

Reflection Exercise

Given that 3 per cent of the population is of Aboriginal and Torres Strait Islander heritage, 97 per cent is not. If you are one of the 97 per cent majority, your norms, practices, expectations, biases and judgments affect the 3 per cent. The social determinants of health described by Wilkinson and Marmot (1998) relate to food, transport, education and more, all mediated through and controlled by the dominant culture.

Accessing support as a determinant of health is also socially mediated. Australia's First Peoples have a clear vision of what good support strategies are, and how to ensure they are accessible. This is through mainstream services such as hospitals that are respectful, culturally safe and meet the needs of all Australians, as well as through locally oriented Aboriginal and Torres Strait Islander community-controlled services.

- How will you advocate for, respect and enact Aboriginal and Torres Strait Islander peoples' solutions?
- Will you make the effort to better understand your own culture, critically reflecting on what motivates your own actions, inactions and assumptions? Will you view the world through your cultural lens or open up to the lenses of others?
- Will you consciously and deliberately take up opportunities to establish good relationships with Aboriginal and Torres Strait Islander services?
- Will you learn from, not only about, Aboriginal and Torres Strait Islander peoples and share what you learn with others?

Summary

We have sought to extend and expand our understanding of the social determinants of First Peoples' health and well-being. We outlined the following propositions.

- The social is dominated by the 97 per cent who determine, and who should and could move to embrace First Peoples' cultures, including holistic approaches to health.
- This social is made up of multiple cultures and values to be embraced with respect for all.
- Racism is a grave legal, health and well-being concern.
- Solutions involve partnerships, with strategies for multi-level empowerment and self-determination to occur.
- Accountability is paramount, and must include community.
- Critical reflection will enable progress in providing social support.

Tutorial exercises

Watch the Australian feature film *Mad Bastards*, which is accessible in most university libraries or streaming services. The film has multiple narratives to help makes sense of concepts in this chapter, and has been described as a rare resource reflecting the lives of Aboriginal families.

1. What intergenerational transmission of the social determinants of First Peoples' health do you see in the film?
2. What factors are at play in TJ's life?
3. What factors work positively or negatively on TJ's sense of being able to parent?
4. What is the influence of cultural determinants of health?
5. What strengths do you see for Bullet to build on?
6. What could health and social support services do to help improve Bullet's options in the future?

The model shown in Figure 8.2 is informed by interviews with 13 Indigenous and 16 non-Indigenous people with extensive experience supporting Aboriginal groups in education, community development, health promotion, counselling, community management and health across remote, regional and metropolitan communities in Western Australia (Waterworth et al. 2015).

Figure 8.2 Factors influencing the health behaviour of Indigenous Australians from the perspective of people who support Indigenous groups

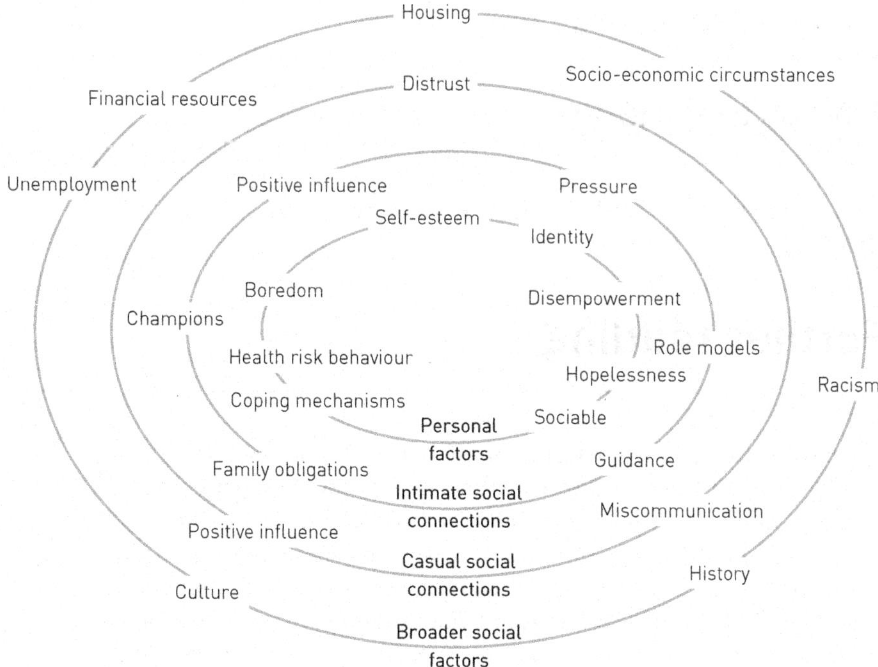

Waterworth et al. (2015, p. 6)

7. Describe the diagram in your own words—what is going on?

Accessing First Peoples' media.

8. How would you characterise mainstream media discourse regarding Aboriginal and Torres Strait Islander peoples?
9. Reflect on how many times you have accessed material from social media platform @IndigenousX. How often do you watch NITV?
10. What main themes do you hear and see?
11. What have you learned that is applicable to other parts of your life?

Access the Indigenous Allied Health Association, *Cultural Responsiveness in Action: An IAHA Framework* through http://iaha.com.au/policy/cultural-responsiveness/

12. What does Indigenous Allied Health Australia seek to do?
13. What is culturally responsive healthcare?
14. As a small group activity, discuss one of the six key capability statements in the Framework. Share your thoughts about these leadership statements.

In June 2016, all First Peoples' peak bodies and their supporters met and released the Redfern Statement. It calls on all Australian governments to genuinely engage with Aboriginal and Torres Strait Islander peoples to meaningfully address generations of disadvantage. Access the Redfern Statement at https://nationalcongress.com.au/redfern-statement/

15. What commitments does the Redfern Statement ask for, to ensure First Peoples' self-determined solutions to health and social issues?
16. What does it say is the role of partnerships in achieving this?
17. What would be your role, if you worked in mainstream health or social support?
18. Identify what holds you back from supporting and enacting the commitments asked for by leaders of Australia's First Peoples.

Acknowledgments

We are grateful for valued feedback from Rachelle Arkles, Melissa Haswell and Mark Ragg.

Further reading

Arabena, K., Ritte, R., Panozzo, S., Johnston, L., & Rowley, K. (2016). First 1000 days Australia: an Aboriginal and Torres Strait Islander-led early life intervention. *Aboriginal and Islander Health Worker Journal*, 40, 21–22.

Bassett, C. (2005). Wisdom in three acts: using transformative learning to teach for wisdom. In D. Vlosak, G. Kielbaso & J. Radford (Eds), *Appreciating the Best of What Is: Envisioning What Could Be. Proceedings of the Sixth International Conference on Transformative Learning*. East Lansing: Michigan State University & Grand Rapids Community College.

Calma, T. (2008). *The Role of Social Workers as Human Rights Workers with Indigenous People and Communities*. Sydney: Australian Human

Rights Commission. Retrieved from https://www.humanrights.gov.au/news/speeches/role-social-workers-human-rights-workers-indigenous-people-and-communities

DoH (Department of Health) (2017). *My Life My Lead: Opportunities for Strengthening Approaches to the Social Determinants and Cultural Determinants of Indigenous Health. Report on the National Consultations*. Retrieved from http://www.Health.Gov.Au/Internet/Main/Publishing.Nsf/Content/D2F6B905F3F667DACA2580D400014BF1/$File/My%20Life%20My%20Lead%20Consultation%20Report.Pdf

Pascoe, B. (2014). *Dark Emu: Black Seeds: Agriculture or Accident?* Broome: Magabala Books.

Schultz, C., Walker, R., Bessarab, D., McMillan, F., MacLeod, J., & Marriott, R. (2014). Interdisciplinary care to enhance mental health and social and emotional wellbeing. In P. Dudgeon, H. Milroy & R. Walker (Eds), *Working Together: Aboriginal and Torres Strait Islander Mental Health and Wellbeing Principles and Practice*, 2nd edn (pp. 221–242). Canberra: Commonwealth of Australia.

Whiteside, M., Tsey, K., & Cadet-James, Y. (2011). A theoretical empowerment framework for transdisciplinary team building, *Australian Social Work*, 64(2), 228–232.

Williams, M. (2018). Ngaa-bi-nya evaluation framework. *Evaluation Journal of Australasia*, 18(1), 6–20. doi:*10.1177/1035719X18760141*

Zubrick, S., Shepherd, C., Dudgeon, P., Gee, G., Paradies, Y., Scrine, C., & Walker, R. (2014). Social determinants of social and emotional wellbeing. In P. Dudgeon, H. Milroy & R. Walker (Eds), *Working Together: Aboriginal and Torres Strait Islander Mental Health and Wellbeing Principles and Practice*, 2nd edn (pp. 93–112). Canberra: Commonwealth of Australia.

Websites

Australian Indigenous Health*InfoNet*

http://www.healthinfonet.ecu.edu.au/

Fair Australia: Social Justice and the Health Gap. The 2016 Boyer Lectures by Professor Sir Michael Marmot

http://www.abc.net.au/radionational/programs/boyerlectures/series/2016-boyer-lectures/7802472

First 1000 Days Australia

http://www.first1000daysaustralia.org.au/

Healing Foundation

www.healingfoundation.org.au

Indigenous Allied Health Australia

http://iaha.com.au/

Lowitja Institute

https://www.lowitja.org.au/

National Aboriginal Community Controlled Health Organisation

www.naccho.org.au/

SNAICC – National Voice for Our Children

http://www.snaicc.org.au

Stronger safer together: A reflective practice resource and toolkit for services providing intensive and targeted support for Aboriginal and Torres Strait Islander families

https://aifs.gov.au/cfca/2017/07/27/stronger-safer-together

Western Australian Aboriginal Child Health Study

https://www.telethonkids.org.au/our-research/aboriginal-health/waachs/

Working Together

https://www.telethonkids.org.au/our-research/early-environment/developmental-origins-of-child-health/aboriginal-maternal-health-and-child-development/working-together-second-edition/.

There are many other useful chapters in this resource in addition to the one we suggest, as well as maps of Aboriginal Australia and helpful glossaries.

References

ABS (Australian Bureau of Statistics) (2006). *A Snapshot of Australia, 1901.* Retrieved from http://www.abs.gov.au/websitedbs/D3110124.NSF/24e5997b9bf2ef35ca2567fb00299c59/c4abd1fac53e3df5ca256bd8001883ec!OpenDocument

ABS (Australian Bureau of Statistics) (2011). *Social and Emotional Wellbeing: Positive Wellbeing*. Cat. No. 4704.0. Retrieved from http://www.abs.gov.au/AUSSTATS/abs@.nsf/lookup/4704.0Chapter400Oct+2010

ABS (Australian Bureau of Statistics) (2017a). *Migration, Australia, 2014–2015: Australia's Population by Country of Birth.* Cat. No. 3412.0. Retrieved from http://www.abs.gov.au/ausstats/abs@.nsf/Previousproducts/3412.0Main per cent20Features32014-15?opendocument&tabname=Summary&prodno=3412.0&issue=2014-15&num=&view=]

ABS (Australian Bureau of Statistics) (2017b). *Aboriginal and Torres Strait Islander Population.* Cat. No. 2071.0. Retrieved from http://www.abs.gov.au/ausstats/abs@.nsf/Lookup/2071.0main+features102016

ABS (Australian Bureau of Statistics) (2017c). *Aboriginal and Torres Strait Islander Births and Fertility.* Cat. No. 3301.0. Retrieved from http://www.abs.gov.au/ausstats/abs@.nsf/Latestproducts/3301.0Main per cent20Features62016?opendocument&tabname=Summary&prodno=3301.0&issue=2016&num=&view=

ABS (Australian Bureau of Statistics) (2017d). *Main Features: Population by Age and Sex, Regions of Australia.* Cat. No. 3235.0. Retrieved from http://www.abs.gov.au/AUSSTATS/abs@.nsf/mf/3235.0

ABS (Australian Bureau of Statistics) (2018). *Population Clock.* Retrieved from http://www.abs.gov.au/ausstats/abs per cent40.nsf/94713ad445ff1425ca25682000192af2/1647509ef7e25faaca2568a900154b63?OpenDocument

AGS & AAP (Australian Geographic Staff & Australian Associated Press) (2011). DNA confirms Aboriginal culture one of Earth's oldest. *Australian Geographic.* Retrieved from http://www.australiangeographic.com.au/news/2011/09/dna-confirms-aboriginal-culture-one-of-earths-oldest

AHRC (Australian Human Rights Commission) (2015). *Freedom from Discrimination: Report on the 40th Anniversary of the Racial Discrimination Act National Consultation Report.* Sydney. Retrieved from https://www.humanrights.gov.au/sites/default/files/document/publication/RDA40_report_2015_AHRC.pdf

AIDA (Australian Indigenous Doctors Association) (2016). *Racism in Australia's Health System.* Policy Statement. Canberra: Australian Indigenous Doctors Association. https://www.aida.org.au/wp-content/uploads/2017/08/Racism-in-Australias-health-system-AIDA-policy-statement_v1.pdf

AIHW (Australian Institute of Health and Welfare) (2016). *Australian Burden of Disease Study: Impact and Causes of Illness and Death in Aboriginal and Torres Strait Islander People 2011.* Canberra: Australian Institute of Health and Welfare. Retrieved from https://www.aihw.gov.au/reports/burden-of-disease/australian-burden-of-disease-study-impact-and-causes-of-illness-and-death-in-aboriginal-and-torres-3/contents/summary

AIHW (Australian Institute of Health and Welfare) (2018). *Australia's Health 2018: In Brief.* Cat. No. AUS 222). Canberra: Australian Institute of Health and Welfare. Retrieved from https://www.aihw.gov.au/getmedia/fe037cf1-0cd0-4663-a8c0-67cd09b1f30c/aihw-aus-222.pdf.aspx?inline=true

Altman, J. (2017). The debilitating aftermath of 10 years of the NT Intervention. *Land Rights News Northern Edition,* July, 20–21. Retrieved from https://www.nlc.org.au/media-publications/land-rights-news-northern-edition-july-2017-edition

Anderson, I. (1988). *Koorie Health in Koorie Hands: An Orientation Manual in Aboriginal Health for Health-care Providers.* Melbourne: Koorie Health Unit, Health Department Victoria.

Anderson, I. (2007). Understanding the processes. In B. Carson, T. Dunbar, R.D. Chenhall & R. Bailie (Eds), *Social Determinants of Indigenous Health* (pp. 21–40). Sydney: Allen & Unwin.

Anderson, K. (2011). Rethinking 'the human': in memory of Fay Gayle (AO). *Dialogue*, 31–70(2), 61.

Anderson, P. (2013). *Racism as a Public Health Issue*. Paper presented at the Dreaming Up the Future of Aboriginal and Torres Strait Islander Public Health Conference, University of New South Wales, Sydney. Retrieved from https://www.lowitja.org.au/sites/default/files/docs/Chairperson-unsw-public-health-symposium-oct2013_0.pdf

ANTR (Australians for Native Title and Reconciliation) (2010). *Are We There Yet? Ten Years on from the Decade of Reconciliation: A Reconciliation Progress Report*. Sydney: Australians for Native Title and Reconciliation.

Arabena, K. (2014). The First 1000 Days: catalysing equity outcomes for Aboriginal and Torres Strait Islander children. *Medical Journal of Australia*, 200(8), 442. doi:10.5694/mja14.00343

Arabena, K., Panozzo, S., & Ritte, R. (2015). *The First 1000 Days Researchers' Forum Report.* Melbourne: Onemda VicHealth Group, University of Melbourne.

Arabena, K., Ritte, R., Panozzo, S., Johnston, L., & Rowley, K. (2016). First 1000 Days Australia: an Aboriginal and Torres Strait Islander-led early life intervention. *Aboriginal and Islander Health Worker Journal*, 40, 21–22.

Arbon, V. (2008). *Arlathirnda Ngurkarnda Ityirnda: Being-Knowing-Doing. De-colonising Indigenous Tertiary Education*. Teneriffe, Qld: Post Pressed.

Atkinson, J. (2002). *Trauma Trails, Recreating Songlines: The Transgenerational Effects of Trauma in Indigenous Australia*. Melbourne: Spinifex Press.

Australian Government (2018). *Our People.* Paragraph 1. Retrieved from https://www.australia.gov.au/about-australia/our-country/our-people

Australian Museum (2017). *Glossary of Indigenous Australia Terms.* Retrieved from https://australianmuseum.net.au/glossary-indigenous-australia-terms

Ball, J., & Elliot, E. (2005). Measuring social support in Aboriginal early childhood programs. In J. Whitehead (Ed.), *Research Connections Canada: Supporting Children and Families*, 12, 41–58. Ottawa: Canadian Child Care Federation.

Bassett, C. (2005). Wisdom in three acts: using transformative learning to teach for wisdom. In D. Vlosak, G. Kielbaso & J. Radford (Eds), *Appreciating the Best of What Is: Envisioning What Could be. Proceedings of the Sixth International Conference on Transformative Learning*. East Lansing: Michigan State University & Grand Rapids Community College.

Baum, F.E., Laris, P., Fisher, M., Newman, L., & MacDougall, C. (2013) 'Never mind the logic, give me the numbers': former Australian health ministers' perspectives on the social determinants of health. *Social Science and Medicine*, 87, 138–146. doi:10.1016/j.socscimed.2013.03.033

Bennett, D., Power, A., Thomson, C., Mason, B., & Bartlett, B. (2016). Reflection for learning, learning for reflection: developing Indigenous competencies in higher education. *Journal of University Teaching and Learning Practice*, 13(2), 1–19. Retrieved from http://ro.uow.edu.au/jutlp/vol13/iss2/7

Blignault, I., & Williams, M. (2017). Challenges in evaluating Aboriginal healing programs: definitions, diversity and data. *Evaluation Journal of Australasia*, 17(2), 4–10. doi:10.1177/1035719X1701700202

Bloom, J. (1990). The relationship of social support and health. *Social Science and Medicine*, 30(5), 635–637. doi:10.1016/0277-9536(90)90162-L

Brofenbrenner, U. (1977). Toward an experimental ecology of human development. *American Psychologist*, 32, 513–531.

Brough, M., Bond, C., & Hunt, J. (2004). Strong in the city: towards a strength-based approach in Indigenous health promotion. *Health Promotion Journal of Australia*, 15(3), 215–220. doi:10.1071/HE04215

Burbank, V.K. (2011). *An Ethnography of Stress: The Social Determinants of Health in Aboriginal Australia.* New York: Palgrave Macmillan.

Calma, T. (2008). *The Role of Social Workers as Human Rights Workers with Indigenous People and Communities.* Sydney: Australian Human Rights Commission. Retrieved from https://www.humanrights.gov.au/news/speeches/role-social-workers-human-rights-workers-indigenous-people-and-communities#fn3

Carson, B., Dunbar, T., Chenhall, R., & Bailie, R. (Eds) (2007). *Social Determinants of Indigenous Health.* Sydney: Allen & Unwin.

Chesterman, J., & Galligan, B. (1997). *Citizens without Rights*. Melbourne: Cambridge University Press.

Cohen, S. (1988). Psychosocial models of social support in the etiology of physical disease. *Health Psychology*, 7, 269–297.

Cohen, S., Gottlieb, B., & Underwood, L. (2000). Social relationships and health. In S. Cohen, L. Underwood & B. Gottlieb (Eds), *Measuring and Intervening in Social Support* (pp. 3–25). New York: Oxford University Press.

Cohen, S., & Syme, S.L. (1985). *Social Support and Health.* San Francisco: Academic Press.

Danalis, J. (2009). *Riding the Black Cockatoo*. Sydney: Allen & Unwin.

Deci, E.L., & Ryan, R.M. (2000). The 'what' and 'why' of goal pursuits: human needs and the self-determination of behavior. *Psychological Inquiry*, 11, 227–268. doi:10.1207/S15327965PLI1104_01

Deci, E.L., & Ryan, R.M. (2008). Facilitating optimal motivation and psychological well-being across life's domains. *Canadian Psychology*, 49, 14–23. doi:10.1037/0708-5591.49.1.14

DIBP (Department of Immigration and Border Protection) (2017). *A History of the Department of Immigration: Managing Migration to Australia*, 2nd edn. Canberra: Commonwealth of Australia.

Dockery, A.M. (2011). *Traditional Culture and the Wellbeing of Indigenous Australians: An Analysis of the 2008 NATSISS.* Centre for Labour Market Research Discussion Paper Series 2011/01. Perth: Curtin Business School, Curtin University.

DoH (Department of Health (2015). *Implementation Plan for the National Aboriginal and Torres Strait Islander Health Plan 2013–2023*. Canberra: Australian Government. Retrieved from http://www.health.gov.au/internet/main/publishing.nsf/Content/AC51639D3C8CD4ECCA257E8B00007AC5/$File/DOH_ImplementationPlan_v3.pdf

DoH (Department of Health) (2017). *My Life My Lead: Opportunities for Strengthening Approaches to the Social Determinants and Cultural*

Determinants of Indigenous Health. Report on the National Consultations. Retrieved from http://www.health.gov.au/internet/main/publishing.nsf/Content/D2F6B905F3F667DACA2580D400014BF1/$File/My%20Life%20My%20Lead%20Consultation%20Report.pdf

DPMC (Department of Prime Minister and Cabinet) (2018). *Closing the Gap: Prime Minister's Report 2018.* Canberra: Commonwealth of Australia. Retrieved from https://closingthegap.pmc.gov.au/sites/default/files/ctg-report-2018.pdf

Dwyer, J., O'Donnell, K., Willis, E., & Kelly, J. (2016). Equitable care for Indigenous people: every health service can do it. *Asia Pacific Journal of Health Management*, 11(3), 11–17.

Eckermann, A., Dowd, T., Chong, E., Nixon, L., Gray, R., & Johnson, S. (2010). *Binaŋ Goonj: Bridging Cultures in Aboriginal Health*, 3rd edn. Sydney: Elsevier Australia.

Elkin, A.P. (1951). Reaction and interaction: a food-gathering people and European settlement in Australia. *American Anthropologist*, 53(2), 164–186. doi:10.1525/aa.1951.53.2.02a00020

Fanon, F. (1967). *A Dying Colonialism.* New York: Grove Press.

Fisher, M., Battams, S., McDermott, D., Baum, F., & Macdougall, C. (2018). How the social determinants of Indigenous health became policy reality for Australia's National Aboriginal and Torres Strait Islander Health Plan. *Journal of Social Policy*. doi:10.1017/S0047279418000338

Fitzpatrick, S. (2011). What's stopping us now? Envisioning a transformed Australia through critical reflection. *Journal of Australian Indigenous Issues*, 14(2–3), 199–218.

Fitzpatrick, S. (2003). Imagining a truth commissioned for Australia. In C. Schraner (Ed.), *Peace Year Book* (pp. 52–59) Sydney: People for Nuclear Disarmament.

FNNCC (First Nations National Constitutional Convention) (2017). *Uluru Statement from the Heart.* Retrieved from https://www.referendumcouncil.org.au/event/first-nations-regional-dialogue-in-uluru

Fogarty, W., Bulloch, H., McDonnell, S., & Davis, M. (2018). *Deficit Discourse and Indigenous Health.* Melbourne: Lowitja Institute. Retrieved from https://www.lowitja.org.au/sites/default/files/docs/deficit-discourse.pdf

Foley, G (1991). Redfern Aboriginal Medical Service: 20 years on. *Aboriginal and Islander Health Worker Journal*, 15(4), 4–8.

Fook, J. (2009). Critical reflection: overview and latest ideas. *Australian Association for Social Work and Welfare Education Forum,* 1 October. Melbourne.

Gapps, S. (2018). *The Sydney Wars: Conflict in the Early Colony 1788–1817.* Sydney: NewSouth Publishing.

Gillor, G.I. (2012). *Taking Control: A Case Study of the National Aboriginal and Islander Health Organisation (NAIHO).* Penrith: University of Western Sydney.

Gooda, M. (2014). *Social Justice and Native Title Report.* Sydney: Australian Human Rights Commission.

Grant, M., Wronski, I., Murray, R.B., & Couzos, S. (2008). Aboriginal health and history. In S. Couzos & R. Murray (Eds), *Aboriginal Primary Health Care: An Evidence-based Approach* (pp. 1–28). Melbourne: Oxford University Press.

Haswell, M., Blignault, I., Fitzpatrick, S., & Jackson Pulver, L. (2013). *The Social and Emotional Wellbeing of Indigenous Youth: Reviewing and Extending the Evidence and Examining the Implications for Policy and Practice*. Sydney: University of New South Wales, Muru Marri, School of Public Health and Community Medicine.

Haswell, M.R., Kavanagh, D., Tsey, K., Reilly, L., Cadet-James, Y., Laliberte, A. … Doran, C. (2010). Psychometric validation of the Growth and Empowerment Measure (GEM) applied with Indigenous Australians. *Australian and New Zealand Journal of Psychiatry*, 44(9), 791–799. doi:10.3109/00048674.2010.482919

Haswell, M.R., Williams, M., Blignault, I., Grand Ortega, M., & Jackson Pulver, L. (2014). *Returning Home, Back to Community from Custodial Care: Learnings from the First Year Pilot Project Evaluation of Three Sites around Australia.* Sydney: University of New South Wales.

Havemann, P. (2001). *Settling the Anglo-Commonwealth: Indigenous Peoples' Rights in Australia, Canada, and New Zealand.* Auckland: Oxford University Press.

Hilton, B.T. (2011). Frantz Fanon and colonialism: a psychology of oppression. *Journal of Scientific Psychology*, December, 45–59.

Holland, C. (2018). *Close the Gap 2018: A Ten-year Review. The Closing the Gap Strategy and Recommendations for Reset.* Sydney: Close the Gap Steering Committee for Indigenous Health Equality.

HREOC (Human Rights and Equal Opportunity Commission) (1997). *Bringing Them Home: Report of the National Inquiry into the Separation of Aboriginal and Torres Strait Islander Children from their Families*. Sydney: Human Rights and Equal Opportunity Commission.

ICPHC (International Conference on Primary Health Care) (1978). *Declaration of Alma-Ata.* International Conference on Primary Health Care. Alma-Ata, USSR. 6–12 September. Retrieved from http://www.who.int/publications/almaata_declaration_en.pdf

Jackson Pulver, L. (2003). An argument on culture safety in health service delivery: towards better health outcomes for Aboriginal peoples. PhD dissertation. University of Sydney. Retrieved from https://www.researchgate.net/publication/279462144_An_argument_on_culture_safety_in_health_service_delivery_towards_better_health_outcomes_for_Aboriginal_peoples

Kelaher, M.A., Ferdinand, A.S., & Paradies, Y. (2014) Experiencing racism in health care: the mental health impacts for Victorian Aboriginal communities. *Medical Journal of Australia*, 201(1), 44–47. doi:10.5694/mja13.10503

Madden, R., & Jackson Pulver, L. (2009). Aboriginal and Torres Strait Islander population: more than reported. *Australian Actuarial Journal*, 15(2), 181–208. Retrieved from https://www.actuaries.asn.au/Library/AAJ_Vol15_Iss2_web.pdf

Markham, F., & Biddle, N. (2018). *Income, Poverty and Inequality.* Census Paper No. 2. Canberra: Centre for Aboriginal Economic Policy Research. Retrieved from http://caepr.cass.anu.edu.au/sites/default/files/docs/CAEPR_Census_Paper_2.pdf

Marmot, M. (2005). Social determinants of health inequalities. *Lancet*, 365, 1099–1104. doi:10.1016/S0140-6736(05)71146–6

Marmot, M. (2011). Social determinants and the health of Indigenous Australians. *Aboriginal and Islander Health Worker Journal*, 35(3), 21–22.

Marmot, M.G., Smith, G.D., Stansfeld, S., Patel, C., North, F., Head, J. … Feeney, A. (1991). Heath inequalities among British civil servants: the Whitehall II Study. *Lancet*, 337, 1387–1393. doi:10.2190/4C1A-G146-71C6-CG7C

Mazel, O. (2016). Self-determination and the right to health: Australian Aboriginal Community Controlled Health Services. *Human Rights Law Review*, 16, 323–355. doi:10.1093/hrlr/ngw010

McInerney, M. (2017). *When the (Non-Indigenous) Doctor didn't know Best: Researching Indigenous Health Priorities*. Retrieved from https://croakey.org/when-the-non-indigenous-doctor-didnt-know-best-researching-indigenous-health-priorities/

McPhail-Bell, K., Fredericks, B., & Brough, M. (2013). Beyond the accolades: a postcolonial critique of the foundations of the Ottawa Charter. *Global Health Promotion*, 20(2), 22–29. doi:10.1177/1757975913490427

Memmott, P., Long, S., & Thomson, L. (2006). *Indigenous Mobility in Rural and Remote Australia.* Melbourne: Australian Housing and Urban Research Institute.

Mohamed, J., & Sweet, M. (2017). *The Impact of Colonisation on the Health Outcomes for Aboriginal and Torres Strait Islander Peoples*. Paper presented at the New South Wales Nurses and Midwives' Association Professional Day 2017. 26 July. Retrieved from http://www.nswnma.asn.au/podcasts-and-powerpoints-professional-day-2017/

Moodie, P. (1973). *Aboriginal Health.* Canberra: ANU Press.

Muru Marri with Blignault, I., & Arkles, R. (2015). *Collective Healing for Members of the Stolen Generations: Summary Report*. Canberra: Healing Foundation.

Muru Marri with Blignault, I., Jackson Pulver, L., Fitzpatrick, S., Arkles, R., Williams, M., Haswell, M., & Grand-Ortega, M. (2014). *A Resource for Collective Healing for Members of the Stolen Generations: Planning, Implementing and Evaluating Effective Local Responses*. Canberra: Healing Foundation. Retrieved from https://healingfoundation.org.au/

NACCHO (National Aboriginal Community Controlled Health Organisation) (2011). *Constitution for the National Aboriginal Community Controlled Health Organisation*. Retrieved from https://www.naccho.org.au/

NACCHO (National Aboriginal Community Controlled Health Organisation) (2013). *NACCHO 10 Point Plan 2013–2030: Investing in Health Futures for Generational Change.* Retrieved from https://www.naccho.org.au/naccho-healthy-futures-10-point-plan-2013-2030/

NAHSWP (National Aboriginal Health Strategy Working Party) (1989). *A National Aboriginal Health Strategy.* Canberra: National Aboriginal Health Strategy Working Party.

Nakata, M. (2007). The cultural interface. *Australian Journal of Indigenous Education*, 36(Suppl.), 7–14.

NCAFP (National Congress of Australia's First Peoples) (2016). *The Redfern Statement.* http://nationalcongress.com.au/wp-content/uploads/2017/02/The-Redfern-Statement-9-June-_Final.pdf

NCAFP (National Congress of Australia's First Peoples) (2018). *National Congress Intervention at the United Nations.* Press release, 24 April. Retrieved from https://nationalcongress.com.au/wp-content/uploads/2018/04/National-Congress-UN-Intervention-24-April-2018.pdf

NHMRC (National Health and Medical Research Council) (2003). *Values and Ethics: Guidelines for Ethical Conduct in Aboriginal and Torres Strait Islander Health Research.* Canberra: National Health and Medical Research Council.

Paradies, Y. (2007). Racism. In B. Carson, T. Dunbar, R.D. Chenhall & R. Bailie (Eds), *Social Determinants of Indigenous Health* (pp. 65–80). Sydney: Allen & Unwin.

Pascoe, B. (2014). *Dark Emu: Black Seeds. Agriculture or Accident?* Broome: Magabala Books.

Quayle, A., Sonn, C.C., & van den Eynde, J. (2016). Narrating the accumulation of dispossession: stories of Aboriginal Elders. *Community Psychology in Global Perspective*, 2(2), 79–96. doi:10.1285/i24212113v2i2p79

Rasmussen, M., Xiaosen, G., Yong, W., Lohmueller, K.E., Rasmussen, S., Albrechtsen, A. … Willerslev, E. (2011). An Aboriginal Australian genome reveals separate human dispersals into Asia. *Science*, 344(6052), 94–98. doi:10.1126/science.1211177

Reynolds, H. (1999). *Why Weren't we Told? A Personal Search for the Truth about our History.* Melbourne: Viking.

Richmond, C., Ross, N.A., & Egeland, G.M. (2007). Societal resources and thriving health: a new approach for understanding the health of Indigenous Canadians. *American Journal of Public Health*, 97(10), 1827–1833. doi:10.2105/AJPH.2006.096917

Ritte, R., Panozzo, S., Johnston, L., Agerholm, J., Kvernmo, S., Rowley, K., & Arabena, K. (2016). An Australian model for the First 1000 Days. *Global Health, Epidemiology and Genomics*, 1(e11), 1–10. doi:10.1017/gheg.2016.7

Saggers, S., & Gray, D. (1991). *Aboriginal Health and Society: The Traditional and Contemporary Aboriginal Struggle for Better Health.* Sydney: Allen & Unwin.

Saggers, S., & Gray, D. (2007). Defining what we mean. In B. Carson, T. Dunbar, R.D. Chenhall & R. Bailie (Eds), *Social Determinants of Indigenous Health* (pp. 1–18). Sydney: Allen & Unwin.

Sanders, W. (2013). Changing agendas in Australian Indigenous policy: federalism, competing principles and generational dynamics. *Australian Journal of Public Administration*, 72(2), 156–170. doi:10.1111/1467-8500.12014

Santrock, J.W. (2007). *Child Development*, 11th edn. Boston: McGraw-Hill.

Schulz, A.J., Israel, B.A., Zimmerman, M.A., & Checkoway, B.N. (1995). Empowerment as a multi-level construct: perceived control at the individual, organisational and community levels. *Health Education Research*, 10(3), 309–327.

Schwarzer, R., & Knoll, N. (2007). Functional roles of social support within the stress and coping process: a theoretical and empirical overview. *International Journal of Psychology*, 42(4), 243–252. doi:10.1080/00207590701396641

Schwarzer, R., & Leppin, A. (1991). Social support and health: a theoretical and empirical overview. *Journal of Social and Personal Relationships*, 8, 99–127. doi:10.1177/0265407591081005

Seccombe, M. (2018). Gap not closing on Indigenous disadvantage. *Saturday Paper*, 31 March, 198. Retrieved from https://www.thesaturdaypaper.com.au/news/politics/2018/03/31/gap-not-closing-indigenous-disadvantage/15224148006024

Sheaff, M. (2005). *Sociology and Health Care: An Introduction for Nurses, Midwives and Allied Health Professionals*. Maidenhead: Open University Press.

Sheehan, N. (2012). *Stolen Generations Education: Aboriginal Cultural Strengths and Social and Emotional Wellbeing*. Brisbane: Link-Up (Qld).

Smith, L.T. (2012). *Decolonizing Methodologies: Research and Indigenous Peoples* 2nd edn. London: Zed Books.

Smylie, J., Anderson, A., Ratima, M., Crengle, S., & Anderson, M. (2006). Indigenous health performance measurement systems in Canada, Australia, and New Zealand. *Lancet*, 367(9527), 2029–2031. doi:10.1016/S0140-6736(06)68893-4

SNAICC (Secretariat of National Aboriginal and Islander Child Care) (2011). *Growing Up Our Way: Practices Matrix.* Melbourne: Secretariat of National Aboriginal and Islander Child Care.

Soutphommasane, T. (2017). *The Many Faces of Racism.* ABS Religion and Ethics. Retrieved from http://www.abc.net.au/religion/articles/2017/11/02/4759290.htm

Spurling, G.K.P. (2017). Computerised Aboriginal and Torres Strait Islander health assessments in primary health care research. PhD dissertation. University of Queensland, Brisbane. doi:10.14264/uql.2017.902

Stanner, W.E.H. (1969). *The Great Australian Silence*. Sydney: Australian Broadcasting Commission.

Stansfeld, S. (2006). Social support and social cohesion. In M. Marmot & R. Wilkinson (Eds), *Social Determinants of Health*, 2nd edn (pp. 149–170). Oxford: Oxford University Press.

Sullivan, P. (2011). *Belonging Together: Dealing with the Politics of Disenchantment in Australian Indigenous Policy*. Canberra: Aboriginal Studies Press.

Sweet, M., Geia, L., Dudgeon, P., McCallum, K., Finlay, S. … Ricketson, M. (2017). Outlining a model of social journalism in health. *Australian Journalism Review*, 39(2), 91–106.

Syme, S.L. (2004). Social determinants of health: the community as an empowered partner. *Preventing Chronic Disease: Public Health Research Practice and Policy*, 1(1), 1–5. Retrieved from https://www.cdc.gov/pcd/issues/2004/jan/pdf/03_0001.pdf

Taylor, S.E., Welch, W., Kim, H.S., & Sherman, D.K. (2007). Cultural differences in the impact of social support of psychological and biological stress responses. *Psychological Science*, 18, 831–837. doi:10.1111/j.1467-9280.2007.01987

Thorpe, A., Arabena, K., Sullivan, P., Silburn, K., & Rowley, K. (2016). *Engaging First Peoples: A Review of Government Engagement Methods for Developing Health Policy.* Melbourne: Lowitja Institute. Retrieved from https://www.lowitja.org.au/sites/default/files/docs/Engaging-First-Peoples.pdf

Treloar, C., Jackson, C., Gray, R., Newland, J., Wilson, H., Saunders, V. … Brener, L. (2016) Multiple stigmas, shame and historical trauma compound the experience of Aboriginal Australians living with hepatitis C. *Health Sociology Review*, 5(1), 18–32. doi:10.1080/14461242.2015.1126187

Tripcony, P. (2000). *The Most Disadvantaged? Indigenous Education Needs* (RC 023 888). National Education and Employment Forum, Brisbane. Retrieved from https://files.eric.ed.gov/fulltext/ED475373.pdf

Tsey, K., Whiteside, M., Haswell-Elkins, M., Bainbridge, R., Cadet-James, Y., & Wilson, A. (2010). Empowerment and Indigenous Australian health: a synthesis of findings from Family Wellbeing formative research. *Health and Social Care in the Community*, 18(2), 169–179. doi:10.1111/j.1365-2524.2009.00885.x

Uchino, B.N., Uno, D., & Holt-Lunstad, J. (1999). Social support, physiological processes, and health. *Current Directions in Psychological Science*, 8, 218–221. doi:10.1111/1467-8721.00034

UN (United Nations) (2008). *United Nations Declaration on the Rights of Indigenous Peoples*. Retrieved from http://www.un.org/esa/socdev/unpfii/documents/DRIPS_en.pdf

Vickery, J., Faulkhead, S., Adams, K., & Clarke, A. (2004). In I. Anderson, F. Baum & M. Bentley (Eds), *Beyond Bandaids: Exploring the Underlying Social Determinants of Aboriginal Health Workshop* (pp. 19–36), Adelaide, July. Darwin: Cooperative Research Centre for Aboriginal Health. Retrieved from https://www.lowitja.org.au/beyond-bandaids

Virdun, C., Gray, J., Sherwood, J., Power, T., Phillips, A., Parker, N., & Jackson, D. (2013). Working together to make Indigenous health care curricula everybody's business: a graduate attribute teaching innovation report. *Contemporary Nurse*, 46(1), 97–104. doi:10.5172/conu.2013.46.1.97

Wallerstein, N. (1992). Powerlessness, empowerment, and health: implications for health promotion. *American Journal of Health Promotion*, 6(3), 197–205. doi:10.4278/0890-1171-6.3.197

Walter, M., & Andersen, C. (2013). *Indigenous Statistics: A Quantitative Research Methodology*. Walnut Creek: Left Coast Press.

Waterworth, P., Pescud, M., Braham, R., Dimmock, J., & Rosenberg, M. (2015). Factors influencing the health behaviour of Indigenous Australians: perspectives from support people. *PLoS ONE*, 10(11), 1–17. doi:10.1371/journal.pone.0142323

Weber, M.L. (1998). *She Stands Alone: A Review of the Recent Literature on Women and Social Support.* Winnipeg: Prairie Women's Health Centre of Excellence. Retrieved from http://www.pwhce.ca/pdf/weber.pdf

Whiteside, M., Tsey, K., & Cadet-James, Y. (2011). A theoretical empowerment framework for transdisciplinary team building. *Australian Social Work*, 64(2), 228–232. doi:10.1080/0312407X.2010.537351

WHO (World Health Organization) (1986). *The Ottawa Charter for Health Promotion.* Retrieved from http://www.who.int/healthpromotion/conferences/previous/ottawa/en/index.html

Wilkins, J. (2009). *Myth 7: Darwin thought that Australian Aborigines were Closer to Apes than to Europeans.* Blog post. Retrieved from http://scienceblogs.com/evolvingthoughts/2009/03/01/myth-7-darwin-thought-that-aus/

Wilkinson, R.G., & Marmot, M. (1998). *Social Determinants of Health: The Solid Facts.* Geneva: World Health Organization, Regional Office for Europe, WHO Centre for Urban Health (Europe) & International Centre for Health and Society. Retrieved from http://www.who.int/iris/handle/10665/108082

Williams, M. (2018). Ngaa-bi-nya evaluation framework. *Evaluation Journal of Australasia*, 18(1), 6–20. d*oi:10.1177/1035719X18760141*

Wolfe, P. (2006). Settler colonialism and the elimination of the native. *Journal of Genocide Research*, 8(4), 387–409. doi:10.1080/14623520601056240

Yunkaporta, T., & McGinty, S. (2009). Reclaiming Aboriginal knowledge at the cultural interface. *Australian Educational Researcher*, 36(2), 55–72. doi:10.1007/BF03216899

Zubrick, S.R., Shepherd, C., Dudgeon, P., Gee, G., Paradies, Y., Scrine, C., & Walker, R. (2014). Social determinants of social and emotional wellbeing. In P. Dudgeon, H. Milroy, & R. Walker (Eds), *Working Together: Aboriginal and Torres Strait Islander Mental Health and Wellbeing Principles and Practice*, 2nd edn (pp. 93–112). Canberra: Department of Health. Retrieved from https://www.telethonkids.org.au/

Chapter 9

Gender and Sexuality as Social Determinants of Health

Tinashe Dune and Pranee Liamputtong

Topics covered

This chapter covers the following topics:

- definitions of gender, sexuality and gender diversity
- social and cultural influences on gender and sexuality
- gender and sexuality as social determinants of health
- impact of gender and sexuality-based inequality on health outcomes
- relationship between gender, sexuality and other social determinants of health

Key terms

biological sex
gender
LGBTIQ
sex
sexual diversity
sexual inequality
sexuality

Introduction

When a child is born they are generally categorised as either male or female, based on their genitals or **sex**. We assume that a person born with a penis will be a boy and a person with a vulva will be a girl. For many societies and people, this dichotomy is assumed as obvious, linear and of little concern or further thought—there is, however, much more to this story (Stuber 2016).

Gender
Socially and culturally constructed categories reflecting what it means to be 'masculine' and 'feminine', and associated expectations of the roles and behaviours of men and women.

Sex
A biological construct based on biological characteristics that enable sexual reproduction.

Notably, every society attaches expectations to **gender**. Such expectations can be seen in statements like, 'boys will be boys, and girls will be girls'. This expectation is the result of a series of socio-cultural constructs assumed to be natural characteristics of masculinity or femininity (Dune & Shuttleworth 2009; Watts 2015; Stuber 2016). That is, how boys and men should think, behave and be treated and how girls and women are expected to think, behave and be treated. For instance, the classic cues of masculinity—aggressive posture, self-confidence, a tough appearance—and the traditional signs of femininity—gentleness, passivity, strong nurturing instincts—are often considered 'normal' (Blau 2012; Kenschaft et al. 2015; Watts 2015). However, any of these characteristics can be, and often are, displayed by persons of either gender (Jones et al. 2015). Cross-gender behaviours are often ignored by observers, unless they are very apparent and labelled as inappropriate gender role behaviours (Dune 2012a). Although these behaviours are closely linked to sexual status in the minds and experiences of most people, research shows that dominant persons of either gender tend to use influence tactics and verbal styles usually associated with men and masculinity, while subordinate persons of either gender tend to use those considered to be the province of women. However, there is more to understanding gender than the restrictive dichotomy of being a man or a woman (Deutsch 2007; Stuber 2016).

Sexuality
The means by which people experience and express themselves as sexual beings. Human sexuality is characterised by the interaction between biological, physical, psychological, societal and cultural aspects, to name a few key factors.

Biological sex
The biologic character or quality that distinguishes male and female from one another as expressed by the person's gonadal, morphologic (internal and external), chromosomal and hormonal characteristics.

Constructions of gender are also linked to constructions of **sexuality**, with women being perceived as the lesser and opposite to men, thus making them 'natural' sexual partners (Dune 2012b). But sexuality goes far beyond **biological sex**, intercourse or procreation processes, as exemplified by the diversity that exists across all these, and many more, aspects of gender and sexuality (Butler 2006; Stuber 2016). Importantly, societal constructions of gender and sexuality often restrict or penalise experiences and manifestations of gender or sexuality that diverge from what is expected (Jones et al. 2015; Moolchaem et al. 2015). Notably, however, expectations of being typical or punishment for being atypical determine how we experience health and well-being. That is, gender and sexuality are key social determinants of health that determine the ways in which a society defines and therefore perceives and treats a person across their life-span (Austin et al. 2017; Booker et al. 2017; Gustafsson et al. 2017; Marti-Pastor et al. 2018; see also Chapters 1, 2, 7, 10 & 14 in this volume).

In this chapter, we will bring readers through several important issues relevant to gender and sexuality. We will first discuss gender and sexuality, acknowledging the range of diversity within these concepts and their impacts on health and well-being. We also discuss the role of gender and sexuality through a case example which explores social constructions related to health outcomes.

Gender, sexuality and diversity

Many societies tend to use the terms 'gender' and 'sex' interchangeably. However, gender is not the same as sex (Watts 2015; Stuber 2016). As mentioned, gender is assumed to begin and align with the assignment of sex (male or female). Gender is, however, developed or defined by a complex interrelationship between three dimensions (Gender Spectrum 2018):

- our body—our sex as well as our experience of our own body, how society genders bodies, and how others interact with us based on our body
- our identity—our deeply held, internal sense of self as male, female, a blend of both or neither; who we internally know ourselves to be
- gender expression—how we present our gender in the world and how society, culture, community and family perceive, interact with and try to shape our gender. Gender expression is also related to gender roles and how society uses those roles to try to enforce conformity to current gender norms.

These dimensions can vary significantly, and a person's comfort in their gender is related to the degree to which these three dimensions feel in harmony. Useful details about the dimensions are provided by Gender Spectrum (2018), an organisation aiming to create a gender-inclusive world (see https://www.genderspectrum.org/quick-links/understanding-gender/).

In western societies, there is a limited language for gender. As a result, it may take a person quite some time to discover, create and then communicate their gender in a way that is most relevant to them. This is becoming easier, however, with various descriptors for gender identities rapidly expanding. Youth often lead the way in this regard as many are willing to challenge rigid frameworks of gender and no longer feel bound to identify strictly with one of two genders. This has resulted in a growing vocabulary for gender, involving not just a tokenistic use of words but a more nuanced understanding of the experience of gender itself. Consequently, young people see gender as a spectrum rather than as a binary concept (Jones et al. 2015).

This indicates that while gender is a social determinant of health, norms around gender change across societies and over time, resulting in increased flexibility. For instance, even the seemingly unchangeable notion that pink is for girls and blue is for boys is actually quite new. Before the mid-20th century, pink was associated with boys' clothing and blue with girls' clothing (Paoletti 2012). There is obviously some way to go to move away from dichotomous understanding and expectations based on gender. Given that these expectations around gender can be so rigid, we too easily accept that what someone wears, or how they move, talk or express themselves, tells us something about who they are and how we should treat them—for better or for worse.

Stop and Think

Raine is 12 years old and has never been sure about whether to be a boy or a girl. This is because Raine was born with some female and some male reproductive organs, and was assigned as intersex at birth. Intersex people used to be called hermaphrodites, a term no longer accurate to use when referring to humans (Dreger et al. 2005). In the past, when many intersex people were born their sex was decided by health professionals and parts of their bodies were surgically removed to make their bodies conform with the sex they had been assigned. It was also assumed that if their body appeared aligned to the assigned sex, they would have an easier time adhering to the gender norms associated with their sex (Dreger et al. 2005). However, sometimes mistakes were made—children were assigned one sex then their body developed in line with the other (Matta 2005). However, reconstructive procedures were often impossible. These days, children like Raine are assigned as intersex, allowing them (and their carers) to explore and decide on their gender and to see how their reproductive and sex organs develop throughout puberty before any surgical or hormonal interventions are suggested (Chase 2013).

- What impact do you think being intersex has on Raine's gender identity and gender expression across the life-span?
- What impact might there be in the family, how they raise Raine and how they interact with other people?

Gender diversity

Gender diversity is not a recent concept. It has existed throughout history and all over the world. Given that gender deeply influences every part of our lives, when this central aspect of self is narrowly defined and rigidly enforced, individuals who exist outside its norms face immeasurable challenges (Dune & Armstrong 2015). Even those who vary only slightly from the norm can become targets, perceived as deviant and stigmatised (see Chapter 4).

Given that gender is a culmination of the body, identity and expression there are many different ways that people can describe themselves. People who identify as having no specific gender may use terms such as 'gender-queer', 'gender-neutral', 'gender-fluid' or 'gender-diverse' to indicate they feel they do not fit into traditional gender categories of male or female (Dune et al. 2017b). Some communities, such as Aboriginal or Torres Strait Islander people, may use culturally specific terms such as sistergirl or brotherboy. Further, gender-diverse people may be gay, lesbian, bisexual or heterosexual, may choose to identify as queer or describe their sexual identity in other terms (Jones et al. 2015).

Gender and sexual orientation

A final distinction is the difference between gender and sexual orientation, which are often incorrectly thought to be the same thing. Gender and sexual orientation are two distinct aspects of our identity. Gender refers to how we see ourselves, and is personal. Sexual orientation is interpersonal, and refers to who we are physically, emotionally and/or intimately attracted to (Krane et al. 2004; Krane & Symons 2014; Stuber 2016).

It is important to distinguish between these two concepts because assumptions can too easily be made about someone on the basis of either. For example, when someone's gender expression is inconsistent with societal expectations, they are frequently assumed to be homosexual. The boy who loves to play with dolls is assumed to be gay, and the adolescent girl who prefers a short haircut may be assumed to be a lesbian. Confusing gender and sexual orientation can interfere with a person's ability to understand and articulate aspects of their own gender, which can cause a great deal of unnecessary mental and physical distress (Frock 2000; Munro et al. 2013).

Case Example 9.1

LGBTIQ older people

Described as 'an invisible minority', the concerns and well-being of ageing **LGBTIQ** individuals can often be overlooked (Blando 2001). Ageing individuals are often perceived as desexualised (asexual) and the effects of homophobia are compounded when an individual's LGBTIQ identity is revealed (Hinrichs & Vacha-Haase 2010). Discrimination (both actual and expected) is identified as one of many sources of concern for ageing LGBTIQ individuals (MMMI & LGAIN 2010). Further, when asked about their attitudes towards engaging with health and social service providers as they age, a higher proportion of lesbian women in comparison to gay men expressed doubt about potential access to non-discriminatory treatment (MMMI & LGAIN 2010). It has been identified that actual and/or expected discrimination is one of three major barriers hindering LGBTIQ individuals' disclosure of information when dealing with healthcare services (Koh et al. 2014). Additionally, a study by Khan and colleagues (2008) revealed that over half of the healthcare professionals surveyed were uncomfortable dealing with issues relating to gay and lesbian individuals (e.g. STIs). This presents a valid reason to assess the needs and experiences of ageing LGBTIQ individuals in accessing health, social, aged care and retirement services.

Similarly, it has been argued that both staff and residents of aged care are potential sources of sexuality-related discrimination (Johnson et al. 2005). A study by Hinrichs and Vacha-Haase (2010) found that aged care staff members tended to rate romantic relationships relating to same-sex couples more negatively than those of opposite-sex couples. Another study by Villar and colleagues (2015) interviewed heterosexual aged care residents about their reactions towards another resident's hypothetical coming-out. Their findings indicated that most residents would behave negatively towards the homosexual resident, in the form of maintaining distance from the resident, and even extreme rejection. Along with Hinrichs and Vacha-Haase's findings (2010), this supports Johnson et al.'s (2005) assertion that both staff and residents are sources of discrimination. It is no surprise that ageing LGBTIQ individuals often express a desire for either LGBTIQ-exclusive or LGBTIQ-friendly aged care services (Johnson et al. 2005).

LGBTIQ
An abbreviation for those who identify as lesbian, gay, bisexual, transgender, intersex and/or queer.

Relative to this, a study by Horner et al. (2012) examined aged care and retirement services in relation to their inclusion/addressing of LGBTIQ issues. It was revealed that few accommodated the specific needs of LGBTIQ individuals. In a recent interview study by Barrett and colleagues (2015), participants reported that the lack of LGBTIQ-inclusive services forces them to enter a heteronormative context and go back into the 'closet'. Given these concerning findings regarding LGBTIQ-inclusive policies and practices in regards to health, social, aged care and retirement services (Johnson et al. 2005; Koh et al. 2014), it can be argued that a synthesised examination of all these services is required in order to obtain an up-to-date overview and provide recommendations for addressing the issues.

There are a number of reviews that focus on the health, social, aged care and/or retirement service experiences of LGBTIQ individuals (Brotman et al. 2003; Addis et al. 2009; GRAI & CHIRI 2010; Alencar Albuquerque et al. 2016). However, no synthesised report exists on the access of health, social, aged care and retirement services in relation to ageing LGBTIQ women specifically—a 'triple minority' (Deevey 1990) in relation to their age, gender and sexual orientation.

Stop and Think

In light of increases in the ageing population (UNDESA 2016) and increased average life expectancy (AIHW 2018a):

- What might be key issues for ageing LGBTIQ people when accessing health, social and aged care services?

Role of culture and society in gender and sexuality

Where do all these expectations about gender and sexuality come from? They are dictated by cultural norms of society (see Chapter 3 for culture as a social determinant of health). Some scholars call these social scripts or schemas—sets of rules that guide the individual within collective life—meaning that they dictate the requirements needed to fulfil specific roles, including the process by which a person enters those roles and how they should behave within them (Dune 2012b; Watts 2015). Interpersonally, individuals try to act out what has been culturally scripted (Dune 2013). So, while people are born female or male (or intersex), they learn to be girls and boys who grow into women and men. These learned cultural scripts make up gender norms, roles and stereotypes.

Gender norms

Gender norms are socio-culturally defined expectations on how to appropriately perform gender roles (Ellemers 2018). It is a type of socio-cultural regulation (to encourage socially desirable behaviour). The expectation that an individual fulfils the norms provides societies with a way to control, dictate and moderate how people behave within a society. For instance, in western societies it is the norm that men hold more positions of power and dominance (e.g. politicians, CEOs of companies, high-level roles in the military) and women hold positions as nurturers, submissive to the demands of others (e.g. childcare workers, nurses, stay-at-home mums) (Watts 2015; Ellemers 2018). Obviously, these norms are generalisations that do not represent a large minority of women who run companies or men who stay at home to mind children. While times are changing, the persistence of gender norms is evident in popular culture (e.g. music videos, magazine covers, social media). Gender norms persist because societies encourage adherence to them using gender stereotypes to maintain perceptions and expectations of men and women (Butler 2006; Yu et al. 2017; Ellemers 2018).

Gender stereotypes

Stereotypes echo prevailing assumptions about individuals of specific social groups (Ellemers 2018). Gender stereotypes are quite stable elements within a society's social structures (Eisenchlas 2013; Ellemers 2018). A stereotype is an undifferentiated and generalised attribution of certain characteristics to all members of a group. For example, a statement like 'boys will be boys' signifies that boys will be aggressive, promiscuous and career-focused. Girls who display these traits are often dubbed 'tomboys', unfriendly and, in the case of promiscuity, sluts. Although gender stereotypes are changing, they continue to fulfil the function of maintaining a hierarchical-unequal relationship between men and women while completely ignoring gender diversity. Just think of statements such as, 'you throw like a girl' or 'man up'. What do these tell us? Prejudice towards one gender (most often women) or rejection of any variation is called sexism. Just as with racism, sexism is the manifestation of intolerance (Walter 2011; Bates 2014).

These outputs of gender stereotypes offer a partial explanation of the persistence of gender discrimination, despite evolving gender roles and gender norms (Ellemers 2018). Gender stereotypes, according to Ellemers (2018, p. 278), 'exaggerate the perceived implications of categorizing people by their gender and offer an oversimplified view of reality'. Gender stereotypes 'reinforce perceived boundaries between women and men', and thus 'justify the symbolic and social implications of gender for role differentiation and social inequality'.

Gender roles

Gender roles are social roles associated with perceptions of masculinity and femininity (Krane et al. 2004; Eagly 2009; Watts 2015). While gender roles are only one of many social roles, they often lead to the perception of particular traits or behaviours as natural (biologically derived, or historically confirmed and therefore valid) to being a woman or a man (Watts 2015). Notably, western gender roles do not consider gender diversity in gender role scripting. It is perceived that men are dominating and women are submissive; men are (and should be) the primary breadwinners and women are (and should be) the primary caregivers. The script dictates that women should want to have and care for children while men should want to have careers outside the home and distance themselves from domestic activities (Ellemers 2018). Of course, times are changing and gender role expectations are adapting to modern life. However, the persistence of these gender roles is present in the ways we structure and perceive work, leisure, parenting and remuneration structures, to name a few (Watts 2015). Inevitably, with presumably fixed gender norms, stereotypes and roles come scripts and expectations about how individuals understand, express and engage in their sexual lives.

Sexual scripts

Sexual scripts refer to an understanding of how males and females are presumed to act in sexual situations (Masters et al. 2013). In thinking about their sexual experiences, people may contemplate how they fit or do not fit into gender expectations. Cultural schemas, therefore, instruct individuals on the topics of time, place, gestures, utterance and what people engaging in sexual behaviour are supposed to be feeling: 'qualities of instruction that make most of us far more committed and rehearsed at the time of our initial sexual encounters than most of us realize' (Simon & Gagnon 1986, p. 105). For example, being a 'man' in a western culture may mean fulfilling the expectation that one is the sexual aggressor, knows what their partner enjoys, and is able to perform flawlessly (Dune & Shuttleworth 2009).

Interpersonal scripts define people as being both actors and agents in the formulation of sexual rules. The construct of interpersonal scripts reinforces the relevance of cultural schemas, because people act out their perceptions of appropriate identities and the desired expectations from playing such roles (Dune 2012b). By legitimising and lowering uncertainty for oneself and others involved in a sexual encounter, a person who has been scripted as the sexual aggressor could be reinforced by their partner who is habituated to play the passive role—the role often relegated to women (Tinarwo & Pasura 2014). Although individuals may experience sexual feelings throughout the interaction, they may only express or allow themselves to become aware of feelings that are 'appropriate' to the situation. This can cause 'inappropriate' thoughts to halt, or be repressed (Dune & Shuttleworth 2009). Presumably, individuals must think about how they are going to express and execute these scripts with others through the interplay of interpretation and mental rehearsal of sexual expectations.

Private scripts are a significant factor in personal mental processes which involve inner dialogue (Dune 2012c). They influence the way individuals internalise the script of what is sexually desirable and how they fit into that scenario. As described by Simon and Gagnon (2003, p. 99), private scripts are 'the symbolic reorganization of reality in ways that make it complicit in realizing more fully the actor's many-layered and sometimes multicoated wishes'. Despite the mental world of private desires and wishes, an individual's thoughts are socially bound (Simon & Gagnon 1987). For example, a man who is expected to be sexually aggressive may wish to be cuddled and submissive but may not ask for such things (Butler 2006).

Stop and Think

- Is it possible to understand your own gender and sexuality without the influence of society or culture?
- What societal or cultural norms are assumed in the statement 'boys will be boys, and girls will be girls'?
- What impact do social and cultural scripts have on how we understand gender and sexuality?
- Where do gender and sexual diversity fit within gender and sexual scripts in western cultures?

Sexual diversity
All the diversities of sex characteristics, sexual orientations and gender identities, without the need to specify each of the identities, behaviours or characteristics that form this plurality.

Gender and sexuality as social determinants of health

Given how closely tied gender, sexuality and social expectations are, it is no surprise that gender and sexuality are determinants of health. This relationship has been acknowledged by the World Health Organization (2002, p. 2) in the Madrid Statement:

> To achieve the highest standard of health, health policies have to recognize that women and men, owing to their biological differences and their gender roles, have different needs, obstacles and opportunities.

As implied in this statement, women and men have different lives and, therefore, health experiences due to the biological, psychological, economic, social, political and cultural attributes and opportunities associated with being male and female. According to the Australian Department of Health, these differences impact health status. For instance, some biological experiences, such as pregnancy and breastfeeding, affect only women. Other health conditions, such as depression, are more prevalent among women (Kessler 2003; Schofield 2015; Kuehner 2017) and suicide is more prevalent among men (Elliott & Masters 2009; Platt 2016, 2017; ABS 2016).

The Madrid Statement recognises that many social and cultural constructions of gender determine health outcomes for both men and women (WHO 2002). Similarly, the Public Health Association of Australia and many other human rights-based organisations acknowledge that gender- and sexuality-diverse individuals experience prejudice and discrimination because they are perceived to deviate from socio-cultural gender norms/roles and sexual scripts. As a result, they experience poorer physical and mental health outcomes than people whose gender identity and/or sexuality fall within socio-cultural expectations (Andrinopoulos & Hembling 2014; Jones et al. 2015; Moolchaem et al. 2015). As with gender, there is a socio-cultural hierarchy with regards to sexuality and sexual orientation which reinforces the privilege and power of some people (most often heterosexual men) while denigrating other groups of people (Connell 1987). This underpins processes of inequality and therefore inequity, which exacerbates poor health outcomes (Harcourt 2006; Logie 2012; Andrinopoulos & Hembling 2014; Karban & Sirriyeh 2015; Austin et al. 2017; Booker et al. 2017; Marti-Pastor et al. 2018).

Case Example 9.2

Social determinants of health for MSM and transgender women

Carmen Logie (2012, p. 1245) contends that 'social injustices are endangering the health of sexual minorities'. Sexual orientation was not included in the social determinants of health conceptual framework devised by the WHO Committee on the Social Determinants of Health (CSDH 2008), nor discussed anywhere in the document. She calls for recognition of sexual orientation as one of the social determinants of health, so that inequities and social justice among sexual minorities can be addressed.

Globally, empirical research has revealed that in comparison to heterosexual individuals, members of sexual minority groups are disproportionately influenced by mental health problems, substance use problems and HIV (Beyrer et al. 2012; Baral et al. 2013; Moolchaem et al. 2015; Hsieh & Ruther 2016; Arístegui et al. 2018; Felson & Adamczyk 2018; Marti-Pastor et al. 2018). A major reason for disparities in health for sexual minorities is 'sexual stigma' which refers to 'negative regard, inferior status, and relative powerlessness that society collectively accords to any non-heterosexual behaviour, identity, relationship, or community' (Herek 2007, pp. 906–907). Sexual stigma 'devalues people who are homosexual, bisexual, or hold nonconforming gender identities' (Andrinopoulos & Hembling 2014, p. 1). It affects health and well-being, as it leads to unequal access to healthcare, an emotional burden and internalised feelings of shame which impact on health-related behaviour (Logie 2012; Ngamake et al. 2016; Arístegui et al. 2018; see also Chapter 4).

Sexual stigma may also affect the social conditions of sexual minority groups. They may not have access to social capital such as power, prestige, money, social support and social networks which can help them to avoid health problems or reduce the consequences of health issues. Limited or no access to these social capitals may in turn disturb 'livelihood strategies'—the choices and activities individuals make in order to obtain basic necessities of life including food and shelter. Transgender women and men who have sex with men (MSM) who have constrained economic opportunities may end up in sex work and/or become homeless. These life circumstances, sex work and homelessness affect health and well-being as they increase the vulnerability to health risks.

Adapted from Andrinopoulos and Hembling (2014, pp. 1–2).

Impact of gender- and sexuality-based inequity on health outcomes

Health inequities are avoidable inequalities in health between groups of people. These inequalities are determined by the social and economic conditions in which people live (CSDH 2008, 2014; see also Chapters 1, 7 & 14). Relevant to this chapter are gender and sexuality-based inequities and their impact on health outcomes.

Gender inequality and health

In addition to the gendered hierarchies described above, many groups of women experience additional barriers to health resulting from prejudice towards their ethnicity or religion. In this way, gender, among other social determinants, has a compounding effect on health outcomes (see Chapter 1). This section looks at sexual and reproductive health as a socially determined health outcome and its relationship to gender.

According to the WHO (2006), sexual health can be defined as 'a state of physical, emotional, mental and social well-being in relation to sexuality'. Sexual health necessitates 'a positive and respectful approach to sexuality and sexual relationships'. It should be possible for everyone to enjoy pleasurable and safe sexual experiences, 'free of coercion, discrimination and violence' (AMA 2014, p. 1). Reproductive health signifies that individuals are able to have 'a responsible, satisfying and safe sex life' and that 'they have the capacity to reproduce and the freedom to decide if, when and how often to do so' (AMA 2014, p. 1). These concepts suggest that all individuals, regardless of their gender, ethnicity, social position and sexuality, should enjoy healthy sexual and reproductive health. However, this is not the case. There appear to be inequalities among population groups.

Recent evidence indicates an increasing prevalence of sexually transmitted infections (STIs) in Australia (AIHW 2018a). Gonorrhoea and syphilis incidences are increasing (Kirby Institute 2017). Over the past five years, gonorrhoea has expanded by 63 per cent; the increase occurred among young heterosexual individuals in major cities. Indigenous peoples are five times more likely than non-Indigenous Australians to experience teenage pregnancy and more at risk of contracting an STI (SHINE SA 2008; Kirby Institute 2017). Among Indigenous peoples, chlamydia and gonorrhoea rates were three and seven times greater than the non-Indigenous group. The gaps were larger in remote and regional areas. There has been a sharp increase in syphilis among young Indigenous peoples in remote and regional areas of northern Australia since 2011. These findings highlight social inequities that manifest spatially.

Teenage pregnancy is substantially more common in geographically remote and socio-economically disadvantaged communities (Hoffman & Vidal 2017; AIHW 2018b). Such environments often have limited resources to support the development of recreational, social, health and well-being facilities that are easily accessible to the majority of inhabitants, compared to those in more affluent and urban locations (Cohen et al. 2003; Crouch et al. 2019). This is because inequality exacerbates and even fuels many of the sexual and reproductive health (SRH) issues faced by disadvantaged populations (Landsbergis et al. 2014).

Extensive research notes that inequity of access to SRH services is likely to be compounded by a range of factors within disadvantaged communities; for instance, people who live in areas where many inhabitants do not make enough money to match inflation (Kline & Moretti 2014) and are more likely to have poor education outcomes. Those who do not have the opportunity, for various reasons, to finish high school (where more comprehensive forms of SRH are taught) are more likely to become young (teen) parents and have little time to return to school, find adequate employment, pay childcare fees or buy enough to eat (Mortimer 2012; Ford & Moore 2013). Further, protective health behaviours may be difficult to maintain when money is tight (Burbank et al. 2015; see also Chapter 7).

Many ethnic groups have distinctive ideologies concerning sexual behaviour and related healthcare (Dune et al. 2015; Meldrum et al. 2014, 2016). As such, simply living within a short distance of a relevant health service may not translate into meaningful protection against problems. Additionally, while cultural competency among healthcare providers is fundamental (Olson et al. 2016), it is unlikely to be a panacea given that the focus is on treatment rather than prevention (see Chapter 3).

People living in areas of disadvantage may suffer generational precedent. For instance, Ferraro and Cardoso (2013) indicate that if a girl's mother had children as a teenager the girl is three times more likely to be a teen mother herself. Further, according to Mortimer (2012), if young people have parents who had offspring during adolescence those children are less likely to achieve well at school or to advance past secondary education (see also Martin 2012; Assini-Meytin & Green 2015). Summarily, inequality within the context of the built environment is linked to the uneven distribution of resources and different living standards; for example, differences in income, unemployment, education and social capital (Ezcurra & Rodríguez-Pose 2013; see also Chapter 7).

Case Example 9.3

Caught between two worlds: sexuality and young Muslim women in Australia

Culture, society and tradition have 'a significant impact on sexuality and sexual health' (Sathyanarayana Rao et al. 2012, p. 2). Sexuality, culture and gender are historically linked with religion. Research suggests that young Muslim women living in Australia often attempt to balance the expectations of Islamic religion (based on the revelations received by the Prophet Muhammad), Muslim culture (a broad and diverse culture of people who are adherent to Islam) and the Australian culture (a broad and diverse western culture) (Muhammad 2010). This attempt to live in two cultures, with the added influence of religion, has the potential to adversely affect the development of young Muslim women's sexuality and sexual health outcomes.

Meldrum, Liamputtong and Wallersheim (2014, 2016) qualitatively examined the influence of Islam, Muslim culture and Australian culture on the sexuality of young Muslim women in Melbourne. Their findings revealed a marked influence of religion and culture on the sexuality of young Muslim women. The studies highlight the challenges that young Muslim women face in regards to balancing Muslim culture, Australian culture and Islamic religion.

Constructs surrounding sexuality held by Muslims are often informed by cultural underpinnings rather than Islamic perspectives. The participants in these studies explained how both Islamic religion and Muslim culture influenced their sexuality. Some participants noted that often Muslim culture is justified by Islam in regards to a woman's sexuality. For example, one participant said that her brother is allowed to express his sexuality externally, yet if she did so she would be judged by her family, friends and the community. This example highlights the dominance and power of religious institutions on the attitudes and behaviours of groups and individuals. Many cultural values stem from the roots of a religion, but individuals and groups often adapt culture in a way that suits the best interests of the most dominant group. This perspective confirms the experiences of some participants and has the potential to further complicate the ways in which young Muslim women give meaning to and experience their sexuality in Australia.

Balancing Islam, Muslim culture and Australian culture with regards to sexuality leads to similar experiences among participants regardless of where they were born. The institutionalisation of sexuality can often provide conflicting influences among those who are committed to Islam and Muslim culture, yet often subjected to the dominant sexualised culture in Australia. The findings of the studies suggest that religion, as well as culture, has a significant impact on the ways young Australians make sense of and express their sexuality. Many participants explained how they struggle to have grounded attitudes towards sexuality as a result of the numerous, and often contradictory, influences to which they are exposed.

This study contributes to knowledge about the lived experiences of young Muslim women in Australia regarding meanings of sexuality and the difficulty of balancing the influences of religion and culture. This knowledge can be useful for the provision of sexual healthcare that reflects a culturally and religiously sensitive approach for young Muslim women in Australia and elsewhere.

Sexuality-based inequality and health

Sexual inequality
Unequal treatment or perceptions of individuals wholly or partly due to their gender or sexuality. It arises from perceived differences in societally prescribed gender roles and sexual norms. Socio-cultural gender and sexuality systems are often dichotomous, hierarchical and detrimental to the functioning of men, women and gender-diverse individuals.

People who identify as gender- or sexually diverse often experience prejudice and discrimination (Minichiello & Dune 2012; Andrinopoulos & Hembling 2014; Jones et al. 2015; Moolchaem et al. 2015; Austin et al. 2017; Booker et al. 2017; Gonzales & Henning-Smith 2017; Seelman et al. 2017). Thus, **sexual inequality** occurs among these individuals. This is because people who identify as gender- and/or sexually diverse continue to endure a high level of societal intolerance (Harcourt 2006). This lack of acceptance is sometimes referred to as homophobia. It results in inequality and inequity across all areas of life, and therefore health.

Homophobia is the fear or dislike of people who are lesbian, gay or bisexual. When this fear and dislike is directed at bisexual people, it is called biphobia. Transphobia is the fear of and discrimination against transgender people and people thought to be transgender, regardless of their actual gender identity. These prejudicial perspectives can lead to bias and even violence towards gender- and sexually diverse people, and create many barriers to good health outcomes (Jones et al. 2015; Moolchaem et al. 2015).

Healthcare providers are not immune to holding prejudicial or discriminatory beliefs about LGBTIQ people. As a result, identifying specific healthcare providers who are LGBTIQ-inclusive can be a stumbling block to care. For some individuals, hiding their identities when they seek health support is the only way they can access care (Minichiello et al. 2014). Given the potentially constant exposure to prejudice that gender- and sexually diverse people face, they are more likely to experience high rates of depression and substance abuse, bullying and domestic violence and are more likely to have attempted or completed suicide than their gender-conforming and heterosexual counterparts (Hillin et al. 2007; Logie 2012; Andrinopoulos & Hembling 2014; Moolchaem et al. 2015; Kenschaft et al. 2016). As noted by Minichiello and Dune (2012), due to practitioners' inexperience, lack of skills or negative attitudes, more than half of Australian GPs (54–60 per cent) were uncomfortable caring for gay and lesbian clients. Becoming open, supportive and non-judgmental is imperative in addressing the health needs of non-heterosexual clients.

Another reason healthcare providers may not know that a gender- or sexually diverse person is seeking care is that health forms rarely provide alternate options for 'gender' or 'sex' (Jones et al. 2015). Further, such forms often use the terms interchangeably. This makes research on the experiences of gender- and sexually diverse people, and comparisons to other population groups, difficult as there is no data to identify them. This lack of inclusion at both the population and healthcare system levels systematically erases gender- and sexually diverse individuals from the healthcare discourse (Frock 2000; Johnson et al. 2005; Hinrichs & Vacha-Haase 2010; Logie 2012).

Case Example 9.4

Crossing the gender line: the lived experience of transgender individuals

Moolchaem and colleagues (2015) conducted a metasynthesis to examine the lived experience of transgender individuals around the globe. The authors point out that although the transgender phenomenon tends to be viewed as an identity condition rather than a disorder, transgender individuals seem to have a heightened vulnerability to mental health problems resulting from social stigma. Transgender people tend to experience discrimination, stigmatisation, physical and mental violence, psychological distress and physical health problems. Transgender persons encounter not only abuse, discrimination and barriers to receiving healthcare, but are also vulnerable to developing substance abuse problems and HIV infection.

Results from the individual studies reveal five major themes: crossing gender and physical problems in life; experiencing psychological distress; encountering discrimination and social exclusion; having relationships matter; and dealing with difficulties in life. Despite the negative experiences they have encountered, transgender people attempt to find ways to help them deal with their difficulties.

This metasynthesis depicts a clearer picture of the lived experiences of transgender individuals, reflecting the physical, mental, social and spiritual aspects that vitally affect their health and well-being. All aspects of these experiences also influence one another. For example, the review shows that experiencing gender nonconformity, which may lead to the feeling of discomfort of being in the wrong body, tends to stigmatise transgender individuals. This may lead individuals to transition to their desired gender. Transitioning gender identity is crucial for transgender people's lives as it may result in positive or negative outcomes—congruence between inner identity and body appearance, or facing rejection from people around them. Transitioning methods involve medical and surgical procedures, which could affect their health. As a consequence of 'coming out' and transitioning, transgender people have been considered outsiders, leading them to experience discrimination, social exclusion and violence. These experiences may preclude transgender persons from proper healthcare access and social welfare, thus affecting their health and well-being.

Based on these findings, the authors contend that healthcare providers, social workers and health promoters need to understand these lived experiences from the perspective of transgender persons. Respect for and sensitivity to the diversity of individuals and their gender identities should be observed. To enrich the health and well-being of transgender individuals, a holistic program of care and support should be created, incorporating the physical, mental, social and spiritual aspects of transgender persons into health programs, with specific transgender support groups as well as transgender clinics. Transgender individuals, as well as their partners, need health education related to their health problems, and, most importantly, healthcare providers may need specialised education in transgender issues in order to reduce stigma and social exclusion in healthcare. When considering future health policies, governments need to consider the specific needs and concerns relating to the health and well-being of these vulnerable people.

Stop and Think

Individuals who identify as male after being categorised as female at birth are referred to as FTM (female to male), transmen or men, regardless of whether they have had sex reassignment surgery or not. Similarly, those who identify as female after being categorised as male are called MTFs (male to female), transwomen or women (Kenschaft et al. 2016, p. 9).

As discussed above, individuals who are transgender, gender-queer or otherwise gender-nonconforming are likely to experience high levels of social stigma. They may be subjected to verbal harassment, physical and sexual violence, discrimination by others, rejection by their families, and exclusion from homeless shelters or other facilities that settle people by gender.

Evidence suggests that transwomen are particularly at risk in comparison to transmen. In the US in 2014, 13 transwomen were murdered in hate crimes, 12 of whom were transwomen of colour. There are no reports of hate crime murders of transmen in most years (NCAVP 2015). A study of transgender people's experiences in the workplace found that many transwomen encountered harassment, demotion and termination, but transmen received more respect and enjoyed more authority. Transmen also earned more pay than transwomen.

- Why do you think social stigma, discrimination and hate crimes happen to transgender individuals in a western society like the US?
- Does or will this happen in Australia or other western societies? Why?

Case Example 9.5

The impact of sexuality-based inequity

Homosexuality has existed for centuries. But how it is defined and labelled—a sin, an act against morality, a physical illness, a psychiatric condition and, more recently, a life-style—has changed considerably over time. These socially imputed definitions of homosexuality have had a significant impact on individuals.

This example looks through the eyes of a boy born at the beginning of the 20th century, who has 'special' romantic and sexual feelings for other boys. When his parents become aware of their son's feelings when he is aged 18, he is rushed to a physician, who, as the expert of the day on such matters, explains that the boy has a biological condition requiring a surgical intervention—lobotomy. Luckily for this boy, the operation is not performed. But he may have been subjected to cold sitz baths (soaking the pelvis and genitals in cold water mixed with essential oils to draw out 'infection'), sterilisation, medical castration or the sectioning of his pudic nerve.

Despite the treatment, his feelings and attraction towards boys remain. Fifty years later, the problem is regarded as a 'mental illness' and he seeks treatment from psychiatrists, who subject him to (unsuccessful) aversion therapy. In his late 80s, he is watching the Sydney Mardi Gras parade on national television. He is shocked by the goodwill messages from parents and politicians, and the platoon of openly gay doctors, psychiatrists and police officers who lobby for equal rights.

As he reflects on his life, including several attempts of suicide, he cannot help but conclude that time has made an enormous difference in how homosexuality has been defined. Unfortunately for him, he was socialised into accepting that homosexuality was a problem and he internalised homophobic attitudes, which had a profound influence on how he lived his life.

Adapted from Minichiello & Dune (2012)

Stop and Think

Consider the case example.

- What issues do you think this man might encounter when trying to access health services?
- How might he interact with healthcare providers, given his experiences?
- What could be done to assist this man in accessing healthcare and achieving his health goals?

Reflection Exercise

Gender equality in health, according to the WHO (2015), 'means that women and men ... in all their diversity, have the same conditions and opportunities to realise their full rights and potential to be healthy, contribute to health development and benefit from the results'. Consider the first three points in light of this statement:

- Certain groups of people who are seen as 'different' continue to be systematically excluded from the most basic principles of justice and equality. In Africa, homosexuality remains illegal in 38 of the continent's 53 nations and punishable in others. In recent times, there have been shocking headlines about gross human rights violations against LGBTI people in many African countries.
- Same-sex marriages are seen as a threat to heterosexual marriage, despite the fact there is no evidence to support the belief that same-sex unions would sabotage heterosexual marriages.
- LGBTIQ individuals are considered unfit to be parents or to not make good parents, although there is no evidence to suggest that the children of LGBTIQ parents have a higher incidence of an emotional burden than do the children of heterosexual parents.
- What does the WHO statement say about gender diversity, sexuality and equality? What implications does the statement have for those who belong to sexual minority groups?

As discussed in this chapter, not all genders experience gender equality. Certain gender groups are still discriminated against, and this is worsened when gender is combined with sexuality and other social diversities such as ethnicity and social class. Healthcare and social care providers must take into account gender differences and diversity when providing care to these individuals. Sensitivity and respect play a significant role in the provision of healthcare and social care. Without these, we will continue to see inequality in healthcare and social care among gender-diverse groups.

Summary

Gender norms are socio-culturally defined guidelines on how to appropriately perform gender roles. They are a type of socio-cultural regulation to encourage socially desirable behaviour, offering a 'pattern' of what individuals—as members of a group, or representing a particular social position—should do in given circumstances. In order to encourage adherence to gender norms, stereotypes are used to maintain perceptions and expectations of men and women. While gender is a social determinant of health, norms around gender change across societies and over time, resulting in increased flexibility. However, expectations around gender can be so rigid that we too easily accept that what someone wears, or how they move, talk or express themselves, indicates who they are and how we should treat them. It is important to recognise that social and cultural constructions of gender determine health outcomes for both men and women. We must also acknowledge that gender- and sexuality diverse individuals experience prejudice and discrimination because they are perceived to deviate from socio-cultural gender norms/roles and sexual scripts. As with gender, there is a socio-cultural hierarchy of sexuality and sexual orientation which reinforces the privilege and power of some people while denigrating other groups of people. This underpins processes of inequality and therefore inequity, which exacerbate poor health outcomes across identities and across the life-span.

Tutorial exercises

1. From your own experiences and from what you have read, seen or heard, list at least five ways that gender inequality benefits women and at least five ways that it benefits men. From your lists, who benefits more from gender inequality? Why? Then compare your lists with your classmates. Are they similar or different? What is a possible explanation for the similarity or differences? Discuss as a group in the class.
2. It has been suggested that movies are a mirror of society. With some creative liberties, they reflect the issues, problems and thinking of contemporary society. As gender stereotypes are present in many aspects of society, these appear in movies as well. As a group, look for such stereotypes and bias in a TV series like *Modern Family, Two and a Half Men* and *The Big Bang Theory*. As a group, discuss what you see and why it occurs.
3. There is a belief that allowing transpeople to use the bathroom or locker room that matches their gender identity is dangerous and could expose others in the bathroom or locker toom to sexual assault—although there is no evidence to support this claim. Generally, transgender people prefer to use the facility that corresponds with their gender identity, not the one that matches the gender they were assigned at birth. What are your views about this? Where might danger lie? Discuss in class.
4. What do the laws on same-sex marriage in Ireland, New Zealand and Australia indicate about the sexual and reproductive health rights of individuals regardless of their sexuality? How does this relate to social determinants of health? Discuss as a group.

Further reading

Gender Spectrum (2018). *Understanding Gender*. Retrieved from https://www.genderspectrum.org/quick-links/understanding-gender/

Jones, T., de Bolger, A.D.P., Dune, T., Lykins, A., & Hawkes, G. (2015). *Female-to-male (FTM) Transgender People's Experiences in Australia: A National Study*. Dordrecht, d: Springer.

Kenschaft, L., Clark, R., & Ciambrone, D. (2016). *Gender Inequality in our Changing World: A Comparative Approach*. Abingdon: Routledge.

Kim, J.H. (2012). *Murdering Miss Marple: Essays on Gender and Sexuality in the New Golden Age of Women's Crime Fiction*. Jefferson, NC: McFarland & Co.

Murphy, K.P., & Spear, J.M. (2011). *Historicising Gender and Sexuality*. Chichester: Wiley.

Ozyegin, G. (2016). *Gender and Sexuality in Muslim Cultures*. London: Routledge.

Stuber, J. (2016). *Exploring Inequality: A Sociological Approach*. New York: Oxford University Press.

Watts, J.H. (2015). *Gender, Health and Healthcare: Women's and Men's Experience of Health and Working in Healthcare Roles*. Abingdon: Routledge.

White, M.K., White, J.M., & Korgen, K.O. (2014). *Sociologists in Action on Inequalities: Race, Class, Gender, and Sexuality*. Thousand Oaks, CA: Sage.

Websites

https://www.youtube.com/watch?v=M8EiCCTto9U

This animated video shows gender inequality across the globe. It focuses on how girls are perceived and treated in societies and the impacts on girls when gender inequality is combined with poverty.

https://www.youtube.com/watch?v=FigeKLGSsRk

Gender stereotyping happens in everyday life and has great impact on girls and boys as they grow into women and men.

https://www.youtube.com/watch?reload=9&v=PTlmho_RovY

In this video, Jean Kilbourne talks about how advertising traffics in distorted and destructive ideals of femininity, which she has termed 'Killing Us Softly'. She discusses many damaging gender stereotypes, images and messages that all too often reinforce unrealistic, and unhealthy, perceptions of beauty, perfection and sexuality.

https://www.youtube.com/watch?v=NXhQVwo_OdM

Paul Vasey, a neuroscientist, discusses how society and culture can influence biology, particularly homosexuals in cultures where there is no societal stereotype of 'gay' with which to identify. He talks about his experiences when studying the fa'afafine in Samoa, who show this different perspective on sexuality.

https://www.youtube.com/watch?v=lZsnPmuYp9c

Sexuality and gender play a significant role in forming identity, but for much of human history their process of determination has been unclear. How does sexual orientation develop? What is it? Can it be changed? What is the relationship between sexuality and gender? How do biology and culture interact to produce it? In this video, a panel of experts discusses some of these issues.

https://www.youtube.com/watch?v=OIsyVZCB3KM

Sexual and reproductive health and rights are fundamental human rights. Having access to those rights will lead to great changes in the lives of women and girls around the globe. This animation illustrates, in the stories of two girls, what happens when women and girls are given power to decide for themselves and are in control of their own bodies.

https://www.youtube.com/watch?v=lrYx7HaUlMY

As a transgender woman, Paula Stone Williams has lived on both sides of gender. In this insightful and humorous talk, she says that the differences between being a male and female are massive, and shares her wisdom with the audience.

http://www.worldbank.org/en/news/video/2017/03/01/video-blog-to-fight-discrimination-we-need-to-fill-the-lgbti-data-gap

Discrimination and exclusion based on sexual orientation and gender identity (SOGI) is a serious development issue. The World Bank's Senior Director Ede Ijjasz-Vasquez and SOGI Advisor Clifton Cortez discuss the urgent need to fill the LGBTI data gap. They also explain why inclusion is crucial for development, and what can be done to end poverty and inequality for LGBTI and other excluded individuals.

https://www.youtube.com/watch?v=LX74Bg8xPcE

What happens when sexuality clashes with cultural, religious or political beliefs? This video shows a fiery and emotional debate about the different struggles about gay marriage, which recently became legal in Australia. It is from the SBS 'Insight' program, http://www.sbs.com.au/insight

References

ABS (Australian Bureau of Statistics) (2016). *Australia's Leading Causes of Death, 2016*. Retrieved from http://www.abs.gov.au/ausstats/abs@.nsf/Lookup/by%20 Subject/3303.0~2016~Main%20Features~Australia%27s%20leading%20causes%20 of%20death,%202016~3#

Addis, S., Davies, M., Greene, G., MacBride-Stewart, S., & Shepherd, M. (2009). The health, social care and housing needs of lesbian, gay, bisexual and transgender older people: a review of the literature. *Health and Social Care in the Community*, 17(6), 647–658. doi:10.1111/j.1365-2524.2009.00866.x

AIHW (Australian Institute of Health and Welfare) (2018a). *Australia's Health 2018*. Retrieved from https://www.aihw.gov.au/getmedia/7c42913d-295f-4bc9-9c24-4e44eff4a04a/aihw-aus-221.pdf.aspx?inline=

AIHW (Australian Institute of Health and Welfare) (2018b). *Teenage Mothers in Australia*. Retrieved from https://www.aihw.gov.au/getmedia/6976ff0b-4649-4e3f-918f-849fc29d538f/aihw-per-93.pdf.aspx?inline=true

Alencar Albuquerque, G., de Lima Garcia, C., da Silva Quirino, G., Alves, M.J.H., Belém, J.M., dos Santos Figueiredo, F.W. … Adami, F. (2016). Access to health services by lesbian, gay, bisexual, and transgender persons: systematic literature review. *BMC International Health and Human Rights*, 16(1), 2. doi:10.1186/s12914-015-0072-9

AMA (Australian Medical Association) (2014). *Sexual and Reproductive Health, 2014*. Retrieved from https://ama.com.au/position-statement/sexual-and-reproductive-health-2014

Andrinopoulos, K., & Hembling, J. (2014). *Social Determinants of Health for Men who have Sex with Men and Transgender Women in San Salvador*. Chapel Hill, NC: MEASURE Evaluation.

Arístegui, I., Radusky, P.D., Zalazar, V., Lucas, M., & Sued, O. (2018). Resources to cope with stigma related to HIV status, gender identity, and sexual orientation in gay men and transgender women. *Journal of Health Psychology*, 23(2), 320–331.

Assini-Meytin, L.C., & Green, K.M. (2015). Long-term consequences of adolescent parenthood among African-American urban youth: a propensity score matching approach. *Journal of Adolescent Health*, 56(5), 529–535.

Austin, S.B., Gordon, A.R., Ziyadeh, N.J., Charlton, B.M., Katz-Wise, S.L., & Samnaliev, M. (2017). Stigma and health-related quality of life in sexual minorities. *American Journal of Preventive Medicine*, 53(4), 559–566.

Baral, S.D., Poteat, Y., Strömdahl, A., Wirtz, L., Guadamuz, T.E., & Beyrer, C. (2013). Worldwide burden of HIV in transgender women: a systematic review and meta-analysis. *Lancet Infectious Disease*, 13, 214–222.

Barrett, C., Whyte, C., Comfort, J., Lyons, A., & Crameri, P. (2015). Social connection, relationships and older lesbian and gay people (1). *Sexual and Relationship Therapy*, 30(1), 131–142. doi:10.1080/14681994.2014.963983

Bates, L. (2014). *Everyday Sexism*. London: Simon & Schuster.

Beyrer, C., Baral, S.D., van Griensven, F. et al. (2012). Global epidemiology of HIV infection in men who have sex with men. *Lancet*, 380, 367–377.

Blando, J. (2001). Twice hidden: older gay and lesbian couples, friends, and intimacy. *Generations*, 25(2), 87–89.

Blau, F.D. (2012). *Gender, Inequality, and Wages*. Oxford: Oxford University Press.

Booker, C.L., Rieger, G., & Ungar, J.B. (2017). Sexual orientation health inequality: evidence from *Understanding Society*, the UK Longitudinal Household Study. *Preventive Medicine*, 101, 126–132.

Brotman, S., Ryan, B., & Cormier, R. (2003). The health and social service needs of gay and lesbian elders and their families in Canada. *Gerontologist*, 43(2), 192–202. doi:10.1093/geront/43.2.192

Burbank, V., Senior, K., & McMullen, S. (2015). *Precocious Pregnancy, Sexual Conflict, and Early Childbearing in Remote Aboriginal Australia*. Paper presented at the Anthropological Forum.

Butler, J. (2006). Performative acts and gender constitution: an essay in phenomenology and feminist theory. In M. Arnot & M. Mac an Ghaill (Eds), *The RoutledgeFalmer Reader in Gender and Education* (pp. 73–83). London: Routledge.

CEF (Colorado Education Fund) (2014). *Transparent: The State of Transgender Health in Colorado*. Retrieved from http://www.one-colorado.org/wp-content/uploads/2014/11/OC_Transparent_Download2mb.pdf

CESCR (Committee on Economic, Social and Cultural Rights) (2016). *General Comment No. 22 (2016) on the Right to Sexual and Reproductive Health (Article 12 of the International Covenant on Economic, Social and Cultural Rights)*.

Retrieved from https://www.ilga-europe.org/resources/news/latest-news/united-nations-sends-strong-support-lgbti-peoples-right-sexual-and-reproductive-health

Chase, C. (2013). Hermaphrodites with attitude: mapping the emergence of intersex political activism. In S. Stryker & A. Aizura (Eds), *The Transgender Studies Reader* (pp. 316–330). London: Routledge.

Cohen, D.A., Mason, K., Bedimo, A., Scribner, R., Basolo, V., & Farley, T.A. (2003). Neighborhood physical conditions and health. *American Journal of Public Health*, 93(3), 467–471.

Connell, R. (1987). *Gender and Power: Society, the Person, and Sexual Politics*. Palo Alto: Stanford University Press.

Connell, R., & Pearse, R. (2015). *Gender Norms: Are They the Enemy of Women's Rights?* Retrieved from http://www.unrisd.org/beijing+20-connell-pearse

Crouch, A., Bourke, L., & Pierce, D. (2019). The health of rural peoples. In. P. Liamputtong (Ed.), *Public Health: Local and Global Perspectives*, 2nd edn (Chapter 21). Melbourne: Cambridge University Press.

CSDH (Commission on Social Determinants of Health) (2008). *Closing the Gap in a Generation: Health Equity through Action on the Social Determinants of Health. Final Report of the Commission on Social Determinants of Health*. Geneva: World Health Organization.

CSDH (Commission on Social Determinants of Health) (2014). *Closing the Gap in a Generation: Health Equity through Action on the Social Determinants of Health. Final Report of the Commission on Social Determinants of Health*. Geneva: World Health Organization.

Deevey, S. (1990). Older lesbian women an invisible minority. *Journal of Gerontological Nursing*, 16(5), 35–39.

Deutsch, F.M. (2007). Undoing gender. *Gender and Society*, 21(1), 106-127.

DoH (Department of Health) (2009). *Development of a New National Women's Health Policy*. Consultation Discussion Paper. Retrieved from http://www.health.gov.au/internet/publications/publishing.nsf/Content/whdp-09

Dreger, A.D., Chase, C., Sousa, A., Gruppuso, P.A., & Frader, J. (2005). Changing the nomenclature/taxonomy for intersex: a scientific and clinical rationale. *Journal of Pediatric Endocrinology and Metabolism*, 18(8), 729–734.

Dune, T. (2012a). Sexual expression, fulfilment and haemophilia: reflections from the 16th Australian and New Zealand Haemophilia Conference. *Haemophilia*, 18(3), e138–e139.

Dune, T. (2012b). *Constructions of Sexuality and Disability: Implications for People with Cerebral Palsy*. Saarbrücken: Lambert Academic Publishing.

Dune, T. (2012c). Understanding experiences of sexuality with cerebral palsy through sexual script theory. *International Journal of Social Science Studies*, 1(1), 1–12.

Dune, T.M. (2013). Sexuality in chronic illness and disability. In E. Chang & A. Johnson (Eds), *Chronic Illness and Disability: Principles for Nursing Practice* (pp. 115–132). Sydney: Elsevier.

Dune, T., & Armstrong, A.C. (2015). #NewWSUnites: reflections on institutionalising acceptance and diversity through Sydney's Gay and Lesbian Mardi Gras Parade. *Journal of Social Inclusion*, 6(2), 92–98.

Dune, T.M., & Shuttleworth, R.P. (2009). 'It's just supposed to happen': the myth of sexual spontaneity and the sexually marginalized. *Sexuality and Disability*, 27(2), 97–108.

Dune, T., Astell-Burt, T., & Firdaus, R. (2017a). The built environment and sexual and reproductive health. *Australian and New Zealand Journal of Public Health*, 41(5), 458–459.

Dune, T., Mapedzahama, V., Hawkes, G., Minichiello, V., & Pitts, M. (2015). African migrant women's understanding and construction of sexuality in Australia. *Advances in Social Sciences Research Journal*, 2(2), 38–50.

Dune, T.M., Mpofu, E., Evans, D., & Sullivan, G. (2017b). Queering multicultural education. In E.L. Brown & G. Zong (Eds), *Global Perspectives on Gender and Sexuality in Education: Raising Awareness, Fostering Equity, Advancing Justice* (pp. 275–290). US: Information Age.

Eagly, A.H. (2009). The his and hers of prosocial behaviour: an examination of the social psychology of gender. *American Psychologist*, 64, 644–658.

Eisenchlas, S.A. (2013). Gender roles and expectations: any changes online? *Sage Open*, October–December, 1–11. doi:10.1177/2158244013506446

Ellemers, N. (2018). Gender stereotypes. *Annual Review of Psychology*, 69, 275–298.

Elliott, L., & Masters, H. (2009). Mental health inequalities and mental health nursing: practice development. *Journal of Psychiatric and Mental Health Nursing*, 16(8), 762–771. doi:10.1111/j.1365-2850.2009.01453.x

Ezcurra, R., & Rodríguez-Pose, A. (2013). Political decentralization, economic growth and regional disparities in the OECD. *Regional Studies*, 47(3), 388–401.

Felson, J., & Adamczyk, A. (2018). Effects of geography on mental health disparities on sexual minorities in New York City. *Archive of Sexual Behavior*, 47, 1095–1107.

Ferraro, A.A., Cardoso, V.C., Barbosa, A.P., Da Silva, A.A.M., Faria, C.A., De Ribeiro, V.S. … Barbieri, M.A. (2013). Childbearing in adolescence: intergenerational dejà-vu? Evidence from a Brazilian birth cohort. *BMC Pregnancy and Childbirth*, 13(1), 149.

Ford, D.Y., & Moore III, J.L. (2013). Understanding and reversing underachievement, low achievement, and achievement gaps among high-ability African American males in urban school contexts. *Urban Review*, 45(4), 399–415.

Frock, S.D. (2000). *The Relationship between Internalized Homophobia and Psychological Distress in Lesbians.* (61). US: ProQuest Information & Learning. Retrieved from http://ezproxy.uow.edu.au/login?url=http://search.ebscohost.com/login.aspx?direct=true&db=psyh&AN=2000-95014-048&site=ehost-live Available from EBSCOhost psyh database

Gender Spectrum (2018). *Understanding Gender*. Retrieved from https://www.genderspectrum.org/quick-links/understanding-gender/

Gonzales, G., & Henning-Smith, C. (2017). Barriers to care among transgender and gender nonconforming adults. *Milbank Quarterly*, 95(4), 726–748.

GRAI and CHIRI (GLBTI Retirement Association Inc and Curtin Health Innovation Research Institute), 2010, *Best Practice Guidelines: Accommodating older gay, lesbian, bisexual, trans and intersex (GLBTI) people*, Perth: GRAI and CHIRI.

Gustafsson, P.E., Linander, I., & Mosquera, P.A. (2017). Embodying pervasive discrimination: a decomposition of sexual orientation inequalitites in health in a population-based cross-sectional study in Northern Sweden. *International Journal of Equity in Health*, 16, 22. doi:10.1186/s12939-017-0522-1

Harcourt, J. (2006). Current issues in lesbian, gay, bisexual, and transgender (LGBT) health: introduction. *Journal of Homosexuality*, 51(1), 1–11.

Herek, G. (2007). Confronting sexual stigma and prejudice: theory and practice. *Journal of Social Issues*, 63(4), 905–925.

Hillin, A., McAlpine, R., Montague, R., & Markham, R. (2007). Workers' learning needs regarding mental health in aboriginal, same-sex attracted and culturally and linguistically diverse young people. *Australasian Psychiatry*, 15(Suppl.1), S80–S84. doi:10.1080/10398560701701254

Hinrichs, K.L., & Vacha-Haase, T. (2010). Staff perceptions of same-gender sexual contacts in long-term care facilities. *Journal of Homosexuality*, 57(6), 776–789.

Hoffman, H., & Vidal, S. (2017). *Supporting Teen Families: An Assessment of Youth Childrearing in Australia and Early Interventions to Improve Education Outcomes of Young Parents*. Indooroopilly, Qld: Lifecourse Centre.

Horner, B., McManus, A., Comfort, J., Freijah, R., Lovelock, G., Hunter, M., & Tavener, M. (2012). How prepared is the retirement and residential aged care sector in Western Australia for older non-heterosexual people? *Quality in Primary Care*, 20(4), 263–274.

Hsieh, N., & Ruther, M. (2016). Sexual minority health and health risk factors: intersection effects of gender, race, and sexual identity. *American Journal of Preventive Medicine*, 50(6), 746–755. doi:10.1016/j.amepre.2015.11.016

Jackson, C.L., Agénor, M., Johnson, D.A., Bryn Austin, S., & Kawachi, I. (2016). Sexual orientation identity disparities in health behaviors, outcomes, and services use among men and women in the United States: a cross-sectional study, *BMC Public Health*, 16, 807. doi:10.1186/s12889-016-3467-1

Johnson, M.J., Jackson, N.C., Arnette, J.K., & Koffman, S.D. (2005). Gay and lesbian perceptions of discrimination in retirement care facilities. *Journal of Homosexuality*, 49(2), 83–102.

Jones, T., de Bolger, A.D.P., Dune, T., Lykins, A., & Hawkes, G. (2015). *Female-to-Male (FTM) Transgender People's Experiences in Australia: A National Study*. Dordrecht: Springer.

Karban, K., & Sirriyeh, A. (2015). LGBT asylum seekers and health inequalities in the UK 1. *Lesbian, Gay, Bisexual and Trans Health Inequalities: International Perspectives in Social Work*, 187.

Kenschaft, L., Clark, R., & Ciambrone, D. (2015). *Gender Inequality in our Changing World: A Comparative Approach*. London: Routledge.

Kessler, R.C. (2003). Epidemiology of women and depression. *Journal of Affective Disorders*, 74(1), 5–13.

Khan, A., Plummer, D., Hussain, R., & Minichiello, V. (2008). Does physician bias affect the quality of care they deliver? Evidence in the care of sexually transmitted infections. *Sexually Transmitted Infections*, 84(2), 150–151. doi:10.1136/sti.2007.028050

Kirby Institute (2017). *Australia's Annual Report Card on STIs and Blood-borne Viruses*. Retrieved from https://kirby.unsw.edu.au/news/australias-annual-report-card-stis-and-blood-borne-viruses

Kline, P., & Moretti, E. (2014). People, places, and public policy: some simple welfare economics of local economic development programs. *Annual Review of Economics*, 6(1), 629–662.

Koh, C.S., Kang, M., & Usherwood, T. (2014). 'I demand to be treated as the person I am': experiences of accessing primary health care for Australian adults who identify as gay, lesbian, bisexual, transgender or queer. *Sex Health*, 11(3). doi:10.1071/sh14007

Krane, V., Choi, P.Y., Baird, S.M., Aimar, C.M., & Kauer, K.J. (2004). Living the paradox: female athletes negotiate femininity and muscularity. *Sex Roles*, 50(5–6), 315–329.

Krane, V., & Symons, C. (2014). Gender and sexual orientation. In A. Papaioannou & D. Hackfort (Eds), *Routledge Companion to Sport and Exercise Psychology: Global Perspectives and Fundamental Concepts* (pp. 119–135). London: Routledge.

Kuehner, C. (2017). Why is depression more common among women than among men? *Lancet Psychiatry,* 4, 146–158. doi:10.1016/S2215-0366(16)30263-2

Landsbergis, P.A., Grzywacz, J.G., & LaMontagne, A.D. (2014). Work organization, job insecurity, and occupational health disparities. *American Journal of Industrial Medicine*, 57(5), 495–515.

Logie, C. (2012). The case of the World Health Organization's Commission on the Social Determinants of Health to address sexual orientation. *American Journal of Public Health*, 102(7), 1243–1246.

Marti-Pastor, M., Perez, G., German, D., Pont, A., Garin, O., Alonso, J., Gotsens, M., & Ferrer, M. (2018). Health-related quality of life inequalities by sexual orientation: results from the Barcelona Health Interview Survey. *PLOS One*, 13(1), e0191334. https://doi.org/10.1371/journal.pone.0191334

Martin, M.A. (2012). Family structure and the intergenerational transmission of educational advantage. *Social Science Research*, 41(1), 33–47.

Masters, N.T., Casey, E., Wells, E.A., & Morrison, D.M. (2013). Sexual scripts among young heterosexually active men and women: continuity and change. *Journal of Sex Research*, 50(5), 409–420.

Matta, C. (2005). Ambiguous bodies and deviant sexualities: hermaphrodites, homosexuality, and surgery in the United States, 1850–1904. *Perspectives in Biology and Medicine*, 48(1), 74–83.

Meldrum, R., Liamputtong, P., & Wallersheim, D. (2014). Caught between the two worlds: meaning and experiences of sexuality among Muslim young women in Melbourne, Australia. *Sexuality and Culture*, 18, 166–179.

Meldrum, R., Liamputtong, P., & Wallersheim, D. (2016). Sexual health knowledge and needs: young Muslim women in Melbourne. *International Journal of Health Services*, 46(1), 124–140.

Minichiello, V., & Dune, T. (2012). *From Homophobia to Homophilia: The Future Face of Medicine*. Retrieved from https://theconversation.com/from-homophobia-to-homophilia-the-future-face-of-medicine-5899

Minichiello, V., Dune, T., Disogra, C., & Mariño, R. (2014). Male sex work from Latin American perspectives. In T. Dune, C. Disogra & R. Mariño (Eds), *Male Sex Work and Society* (pp. 362–394). New York: Harrington Park Press.

MMMI & LGAIN (Metlife Mature Market Institute & Lesbian Gay Aging Issues Network of the American Society on Aging) (2010). Out and aging: the MetLife study of lesbian and gay baby boomers. *Journal of GLBT Family Studies*, 6(1), 40–57.

Moolchaem, P., Liamputtong, P., O'Halloran, P., & Muhamad, R. (2015). The lived experiences of transgender persons: a meta-synthesis. *Journal of Gay and Lesbian Social Services*, 27, 143–171.

Mortimer, J.T. (2012). Transition to adulthood, parental support, and early adult well-being: recent findings from the youth development study. In A. Booth, S.L. Brown, N.S. Landale, W.D. Manning & S.M. McHale (Eds), *Early Adulthood in a Family Context* (pp. 27–34). New York: Springer-Verlag.

Muhammad, M.Z.A-D. (2010). Perceptions of sex education among Muslim adolescents in Canada. *Journal of Muslim Minority Affairs*, 30(3), 391–407.

Munro, L., Travers, R., St John, A., Klein, K., Hunter, H., Brennan, D., & Chavisa, B. (2013). A bed of roses? Exploring the experiences of LGBT newcomer youth who migrate to Toronto. *Ethnicity and Inequalities in Health and Social Care*, 6(4), 137–150.

NCAVP (National Coalition of Anti-Violence Programs) (2015). *Lesbian, Gay, Bisexual, Transgender, Queer and HIV-affected: Hate Violence in 2014*. New York: National Coalition of Anti-Violencre Programs.

Ngamake, S.T., Walch, S.E., & Raveepatarakul, J. (2016). Discrimination and sexual minority mental health: mediation and moderation effects of coping. *Psychology of Sexual Orientation and Gender Diversity*, 3(2), 213–226.

Olson, R., Bidewell, J., Dune, T., & Lessey, N. (2016). Developing cultural competence through self-reflection in interprofessional education in Australia. *Journal of Interprofessional Care*, 30(3), 347–354.

Paoletti, J.B. (2012). *Pink and Blue: Telling the Boys from the Girls in America*. Bloomington: Indiana University Press.

Platt, S. (2016). Inequalities and suicidal behavior. In R.C. O'Connor & J. Pirkis (Eds), *The International Handbook of Suicide Prevention*, 2nd edn (pp. 258–283). Chichester: John Wiley & Sons.

Platt, S. (2017). Suicide in men: what is the problem? *Trends in Urology and Men's Health*, July/August, 9–12.

Sathyanarayana Rao, T.S., Gopalakrishnan, R., Kuruvilla, A., & Jacob, K.S. (2012). Social determinants of sexual health. *Indian Journal of Psychiatry*, 54(2), 105–107.

Schofield, T. (2015). *A Sociological Approach to Health Determinants*. Port Melbourne: Cambridge University Press.

Seelman, K.L., Colon-Diaz, M.J.P., LeCroix, R.H., Xavier-Brier, M., & Kattari, L. (2017). Transgender noninclusive healthcare and delaying care because of fear: connections to general health and mental health among transgender adults, *Transgender Health*, 2(1), 17–28. doi:10.1089/trgh.2016.0024

SHINE SA (Sexual Health Information Networking and Education South Australia) (2008). *Sexual Health and Wellbeing of Aboriginal People and Communities*. Fact Sheet. Retrieved from http://www.shinesa.org.au

Simon, W., & Gagnon, J.H. (1986). Sexual scripts: permanence and change. *Archives of Sexual Behavior*, 15(2), 97–120.

Simon, W., & Gagnon, J.H. (1987). A sexual scripts approach. In J.H. Geer & W. O'Donohue (Eds), *Theories of Human Sexuality* (pp. 363–383). New York: Springer.

Simon, W., & Gagnon, J. H. (2003). Sexual scripts: origins, influences and changes. *Qualitative Sociology*, 26(4), 491–497.

Stuber, J. (2016). *Exploring Inequality: A Sociological Approach.* New York: Oxford University Press.

Tinarwo, M.T., & Pasura, D. (2014). Negotiating and contesting gendered and sexual identities in the Zimbabwean diaspora. *Journal of Southern African Studies*, 40(3), 521–538. doi:http://dx.doi.org/10.1080/03057070.2014.909258

UNDESA, U. (2016). *Government Survey 2016.* New York: E-Government in Support of Sustainable Development.

USAIDS (2018). *USAID Responds to Gender Inequality and Gender-based Violence.* https://www.usaid.gov/what-we-do/global-health/hiv-and-aids/gender

Villar, F., Serrat, R., Fabà, J., & Celdrán, M. (2015). As long as they keep away from me: attitudes toward non-heterosexual sexual orientation among residents living in Spanish residential aged care facilities. *Gerontologist*, 55(6), 1006–1014.

Walter, N. (2011). *Living Dolls: The Return of Sexism.* London: Virago.

Watts, J.H. (2015). *Gender, Health and Healthcare: Women's and Men's Experience of Health and Working in Healthcare Roles.* Abindon: Routledge.

WHO (World Health Organization) (2002). *Mainstreaming Gender Equity in Health: The Need to Move Forward—Madrid Statement.* Retrieved from http://www.euro.who.int/document/a75328.pdf

WHO (World Health Organization) (2015). *Gender.* Retrieved from http://www.who.int/news-room/fact-sheets/detail/gender

Yu, C., Zuo, X., Blum, R.W., Tolman, D.L., Kågesten, A., Mmari, K., De Meyer, S., Michielsen, K., Basu, S., Acharya, R., Lian, Q., & Lou, C. (2017). Marching to a different drummer: a cross-cultural comparison of young adolescents who challenge gender norms. *Journal of of Adolescent Health,* 61, S48–S54.

Chapter 10

Health throughout the Life Course

Christopher Fox

Topics covered

This chapter covers the following topics:

- definitions of life course, life course determinants, and social gradient
- life course determinants and their effects on health
- life course determinants and the social gradient
- life course determinants and policy

Key terms

cohort
human agency
life and historical times
life course perspective
life event
linked lives
mediating factors
social gradient
social mobility
social protection
timing of lives
trajectory
transition
turning point

Introduction

Life course determinants are considered to be a relatively new approach to exploring health. This approach to understanding health provides the opportunity to understand the interplay between individual experiences and social structures on health inequalities through life (Kendig & Nazroo 2016). Although the concept of such determinants has been known for about 50 years, policy-makers, academics and researchers rarely draw on the approach. Understanding the role of life course determinants in social groups' well-being is important in policy development. Kendig and Nazroo (2016) argue that through understanding the underlying processes which contribute to inequalities (to well-being), better policy development is possible. This understanding can be gained through the application of a life course approach.

Glen Elder, a sociologist, is recognised as one of the early developers of the life course approach and remains its key proponent (Hutchison 2010). Elder was working in the 1960s on data from three early longitudinal studies of children when he identified patterns in the analysis (Elder 1974). The cohorts appeared to have been affected in similar ways when it came to individual and family trajectories. The common factor was that they were children of the 1930s Great Depression. Elder became fascinated with the influence of history, or past events, on family, education and work roles of individuals and communities (Elder 1974).

The life course approach to health draws on several disciplines: psychology, sociology, anthropology, epidemiology and social history to name a few (Elder 1994). As an approach, or theory, it has developed key ideas and concepts. In this chapter, I introduce readers to the life course approach and explore how it can be applied to understanding the determinants of the health of an individual or social group.

Defining the life course perspective

The life course refers to the course of our lives from birth to death. One way of viewing the life course is as a path or road—definitely not straight, but with corners, turns and twists (Hutchison 2010). The life course can be influenced by intragenerational and intergenerational events (Blane 2006); in other words, events that occur within your generation that affect you, or events that occurred in your parents'—even your grandparents'—generation that affect you.

Stop and Think

Draw a map of key events that have affected you, starting from birth. The events may not have happened in a straight line. Some may have happened to someone else but affected you. Some events may have occurred simultaneously. Now connect the events. The path is not likely to be straight and is likely to have branches off it—more like a street directory. This is one way to capture the 'winding road' concept of life course determinants.

The **life course perspective** is also concerned with the impact of one stage of life on another, including events that occur while still in the womb. 'Events' that occurred while you were in the womb can have an impact on your life today, or even in your older age. Decisions and events that occur now could impact on your later life. For example, Delisle's (2002) review of studies of the relationship between birth weight and coronary heart disease reported that babies with a low birth weight had an increased chance of developing that problem at a later stage in life.

Life course perspective
The cumulative effects of events from earlier life on later life.

The life course perspective is also interested in the effects that culture and social structures, or institutions, have on an individual's life. Culture not only refers to ethnicity, but to the cultural groups we belong to and the society in which we live (see also Chapter 3 in this volume). Culture can refer to non-biological aspects of life: the aspects of life that are learnt and/or are symbolic, like the unwritten rules of society, customs and use of language (Willis 2004). Social structures or institutions can refer to organised institutions like the law or education, or phenomena like gender, race, age and sexuality (see Chapter 1). For example, children who have limited exposure to books and reading in early childhood may experience reading difficulties in later childhood (Baydar et al. 1993).

Thus far, we know that life course determinants are about the paths our lives take, that each life stage impacts on a later life stage, and that culture and social institutions also have an influence. These three elements form part of the definition of life course determinants. Blane (2006) suggests that most chronic diseases which result in death are caused by cumulative developmental stresses, with adulthood health influenced by circumstances in earlier life. The life course approach to health can also be viewed as the intersection of socio-historical and cultural factors, with personal biological development. Elder (1994, p. 5) states: 'The life course can be viewed as a multilevel phenomen[on], ranging from structured pathways through social institutions and organisations to the social trajectories of individuals and their developmental pathways'. Elder's definition is the original formulation of the idea. Yet theory, like language, is dynamic; it is ever-developing. Elder's definition is still relevant: the life course perspective can be applied to areas beyond physical and emotional health. The life course perspective, in accordance with its multi-disciplinary origins, has been applied to other areas in the human services such as individuals, families, groups and organisations. Hutchison (2005, p. 144) suggests the life course approach could be viewed from micro and macro advantage points. It has been studied from the perspective of the individual as *event history*, that is, the sequence of events, experiences and transitions in a person's life from birth to death. It has also been studied from the perspective of the family, in terms of how family lives are synchronised across time. The life course has been studied as a property of cultures and social institutions that shape the pattern of individual and family lives. Some life course scholars have also conceptualised small groups, communities, formal organisations and social movements as having life courses marked by both continuity and change.

Hutchison's definition gives the approach broader perspective and greater application beyond traditional ideas of health. In general, the life course is affected by historical, social and cultural factors, the cumulative effects of circumstances and how these affect later events or outcomes. The approach can be applied to individuals, groups, communities and organisations. In regard to health, the approach challenges the dominance of adult risk factors as causes of adult diseases.

Stop and Think

- The life course approach can be applied to more than individuals. Using your family as an example, how have earlier events affected later events in your family?
- Try the same exercise with an organisation (e.g. an AFL team) or a social group (e.g. LGBTIQ Australians, or an ethnic group).

Life course approach: basic concepts

Cohorts

Cohort
A group who share the same experiences, in the same time, in the same sequence.

Cohorts are groups of people who share the same time together in the same time period. A cohort could also be a group of people born in the same (historical) time, in the same culture, and who experience the same social changes in the same order (Hutchison 2005). For example, Elder's data analysis of people born in the US during the Great Depression was the cohort he was studying when he noticed the effects of earlier life events on later life experiences (Elder 1974). Cohorts of people do not need to be born at the same time, in the case of an organisation or group. In such an instance, the cohort may be the people on a sporting team between 2008 and 2011. As a cohort on a sporting team, they share the same experiences in the same order with that team. A cohort could also be conceived as families whose first child was born in 1990. Cohorts can differ in size but face challenges in similar ways. For example, it is suggested that the baby boomer cohort faced the challenges of their demographic bubble by delaying marriage and childbirth, and having fewer children (Hutchison 2010).

Stop and Think

- People generally think of themselves as belonging to a birth cohort (e.g. Gen X, Gen Y, Gen Z, baby boomers), but we can also belong to other cohorts. Make a list of cohorts to which you belong. What experiences, in what time-frame and in what sequence, help define these cohorts?

Transitions

Transitions can be viewed as stage changes in life. Transitions are often culturally bound, yet at a macro level may be similar to other groups of transitions. Transitions can be thought of as markers in life as we transit from one state (childhood) to another (adolescence). Transitions can revolve around family life: birth, marriage, divorce, death (Hutchison 2005). They are about changes, exits and entrances. In the workplace, transitions may be marked by the change of managers in a job, or the start of a new group of graduates in an organisation.

Transition
Moving from one life stage to another, or from one life event to another.

Case Example 10.1

Micro transitions and macro transitions: markers of adulthood

The markers of entry into adulthood have changed, yet have not changed, since Dickens was chronicling life in the mid-1800s. Although on a micro level there are profound differences between Dickensian England and Australia in the 2010s, there are similarities on a macro level. Dickens describes some of his period's marks of transition from childhood to adulthood: the cultural idea of adolescence is very different now.

Adolescence is marked as the transition from childhood to adulthood. It is referred to as a liminal state—not quite one state (childhood) and not quite the other (adult). Biologically, it is defined by the development of secondary sex characteristics. Socio-culturally, it is marked by different experiences in different times and cultures. In contemporary Anglo-Australian culture, adolescence is (culturally) defined as the teenage years, when individuals experiment with adult identities and behaviours. Adolescence for most Australians begins at 13 and ends around 19. If we were to use biological markers for adolescence, it would begin somewhere around nine or 10 years for girls, and 11 to 13 years for boys; it would end at around 17 years for girls and 20 years for boys.

One of the markers of entering adulthood in Anglo-Australian society is finishing school and beginning employment. Another is moving out of home (although 'Dependults'—young people remaining in the family home until well into their 20s—challenge this notion) or getting married.

If we take the cultural definition of adolescence as the liminal state between childhood and adulthood, in Dickensian England the period lasted only two to three years. Childhood ended, as chronicled by Dickens, at around the age of 12 as many young people entered employment in their early teenage years. In some cases, young people moved out of home to take up service (in the case of girls) or an apprenticeship (in the case of boys). If the same markers of entry into adulthood were applied in Dickensian England, then adulthood would have begun around the age of 14. Society in mid-1800s England managed this transition by delaying the onset of adulthood until the young person had completed their service or apprenticeship and could function as an independent person.

So, on a micro level the transitions are quite different, yet on a macro level there are similarities. The markers of entry into adulthood are about independence in both cases. This is how transitions can be similar and different at the same time.

Case Example 10.2

Life transitions

One of the key issues in working with transitions is how we define them. One model is proposed by Bartley and colleagues (1997). Another possible way of looking at critical transition periods is to use Erik Erikson's Psychosocial Stages of Development (1968). Erikson argues that at critical times in our lives we need to resolve a conflict in order to progress positively through life. It is not so much the 'conflict' to be resolved that this model offers; rather, the age range represents critical periods of transitions. Erikson's model, like that of Bartley and colleagues, covers the life-span.

Bartley and colleagues (1997)

- transition from primary to secondary school
- school examinations
- entry to the labour market
- leaving parental home
- transition to parenthood
- job insecurity, change or loss
- onset of chronic illness
- exit from the labour market (retirement)

Erikson's Stages of Psychosocial Development (1968)

- infants, 0–1 year = hope: trust vs mistrust
- toddlers, 2–3 years = autonomy vs shame and doubt
- preschool, 3–5 years = purpose: initiative vs guilt
- childhood, 6–11 years = competence: industry vs inferiority
- adolescents, 12–19 years = fidelity: identity vs role confusion
- young adults, 20–40 years = love: intimacy vs isolation
- middle adulthood, 45–65 years = care: generativity vs stagnation
- seniors, 65+ years = wisdom: ego integrity vs despair

Stop and Think

- Bartley and colleagues (1997) and Erikson (1968) provide two potential lists of key transition periods in life. What would you list as key transitions in life?
- What do you consider to be key transitions you have experienced in your life? It might be turning 13, or starting secondary school or university.
- Draw two columns. On one side, write the transitions you have experienced. In the other column, write the effects these had on you at the time.

Transitions and **trajectories** are two key concepts in understanding life course determinants (Elder 1985). Where transitions are transitory, or moments in time, trajectories are more stable and follow a path towards a 'life destination' (Wheaton & Gotlieb 1997). Trajectories can consist of a number of transitions (Elder 1985; Macmillan & Elliason 2004). They can influence and be influenced by other trajectories. A change in trajectory results in a new 'life destination' (Wheaton & Gotlieb 1997). Trajectories, or 'careers', are multi-dimensional and interdependent (Elder 1985). Elder classes work, marriage and parenthood as trajectories a person might face in life. These trajectories are interdependent or interrelated. Macmillan and Elliason (2004, p. 2) define trajectories as the 'stable component of a direction toward a life destination [which] is given by the probability of occurrence'.

Trajectory
A stable path towards a life destination.

Life events

Life events can be defined as unexpected and sudden with an outcome markedly different from what was previously expected (Settersten Mayer 1997; Wheaton Gotlieb 1997). Life events require the individual to change and can result in experiences of great stress (Hutchison 2005). Some events in our lives are expected; for example, marriage after an extended period of dating. If one of these events happens out of normative sequence and results in significant change—marriage at a young age because of an unplanned pregnancy and so not completing university—then this is a life event. The change is unexpected and significant, and has consequences for our trajectory.

Life event
Abrupt and sudden change in life resulting in significant change in trajectory and stress.

Turning points

Turning points are classed as significant changes or change of direction in life (Rutter 1996) and result in crucially important moments in life (Wheaton Gotlieb 1997). A turning point may not be apparent at the time. To identify turning points we need a baseline that is stable over time. Turning points, unlike life events, may not be abrupt single events, unusual events or anything dramatic (Wheaton

Turning point
A crucial point in time that leads to significant change of direction.

Gotlieb 1997). Rutter (1996) identifies three types of life events that can also be turning points:

- an opportunity is closed off or opened up
- a change in an individual's personal environment (e.g. marriage) results in a change in social networks
- changes in an individual's self-concept, beliefs, values and views.

Trajectories are made up of transitions and life events. A change of trajectory results from a turning point in an individual's life. Turning points are not mere detours but result in a significant change of direction.

Stop and Think

- You have thought about the cohorts you belong to and transitions you have experienced. Now consider what trajectories you have been on in your life. What life events have resulted in detours? When did the trajectories change? What turning points caused the change in trajectory?
- What impacts may these phenomena have on your later life?

Elder's four themes of the life course

Elder (1994) posits four central themes in the life course approach that account for the interaction between the social and developmental trajectories. He argues that the link between our lives and historical events (times) accounts for some dynamic features of the life course, while the timing of events, the interdependence of our lives (with others) and our agency are all avenues that influence the paths we take (Elder 1994). Below is a summary of each of the four central themes.

Lives and historical times

Life and historical times
A way of accounting for cohort effects and how they affect the individual now and in the future.

Elder's phrase '**life and historical times**' refers to the intersection of our lives with the (historical) events that occur around us—for example, a cohort affected by the Vietnam War. Different birth cohorts experience different social worlds. Elder (1994) suggests that historical effects are cohort effects that not only affect us when they occur, but will affect our future and therefore indirectly affect the next generation. When applying a life course approach, we need to consider how the historical event, its effects and how we embody these effects become part of our life course. For example, does the event result in a transition, a life event or a turning point? Does the historical event effect a change in trajectories? Victorians in 2009 were impacted by the Black Saturday bushfires, and Queenslanders were hit by floods or cyclones in late 2010 and early 2011. How did these historical events affect their lives and how did they embody the changes? What will be the outcome on their health at the time, 15 years later and in another 10 or 15 years after that? A life course approach can help answer such questions.

Stop and Think

- In developing the map of your life course, what significant historical events have occurred in your life? Are these events unique to you or your family? If so, maybe these are life events or turning points. Remember, we are talking about events that affect cohorts.
- Make a list of historical events and describe how they affected your cohort.

The timing of lives

In developed nations, especially, there are parallels between chronological and social ageing (Elder 1994). In other words, the social events and transitions associated with marking periods of life are prescribed for individuals according to their chronological age. Adulthood in Australia is marked by an 18th birthday party, the social marker of the legal definition of adulthood. Social timing is the defining of values and beliefs about a role, alongside the incidence, duration and sequence of roles (Elder 1994). So, a childbirth in a marriage at a 'planned stage' has minimal impact, yet parenthood in adolescence is costly. The importance of **timing of lives** is that the impact of an event is moderated by where the person is in their life stage. Elder (1994) explored the service of men in the Second World War: men who entered service young with no family had minimal social disruption, while men in later life with families felt the full brunt of social disruption.

Timing of lives
Accounts for the age-graded perspective of social markers, roles and events.

Case Example 10.3

Understanding age: how old are you?

Age is not universally defined. It is a dynamic concept. I can recall working with a colleague, who was an anthropologist, on a survey. I wanted to ask respondents, 'How old are you?' The anthropologist informed me that the question had different meanings to different people—how age is defined is culturally bound. I needed to ask, 'In what year were you born?' in order to calculate the age.

Think of how we have described our age. When we were children, we might have said, 'I am nearly four' when in fact we had not long turned three. During late adolescence, when trying to convince parents we were old enough to make a decision, we might have said, 'I am nearly an adult', or might have believed that we looked adult enough to purchase alcohol. We hear older people say, 'I'm only 40'. All of these statements mark age differently. Earlier, we looked at the markers of childhood, adulthood and adolescence. Now we can consider the different ways we can define age.

Chronological age is age according to our birth year. This is how many of us think of age. If an individual was born in 1998, then in 2019 they will be 21 years old. Hutchison (2010) argues that chronological age is not the only aspect in the timing of our lives. Differences in roles and behaviours also result from biological, social and psychological processes. For example, being able to drive is a widely recognised marker of adulthood in many societies. Permission to engage in this adult behaviour is arbitrarily given by law in various localities at the age of 15, 16, 17 or 18, depending largely on social need and perception of the biological and psychological state of young people.

Biological age involves using biological development as an indicator of age, for example, when a paediatrician uses the Tanner Stages of Puberty (Marshall & Tanner 1969, 1970) to define a person's stage of physical development. Biological age can also be defined according to our health and how well our organs function.

Psychological age depends on the stages of psychological and cognitive development, for example, where an individual's cognitive or motor skills are in the developmental stages, or how well an individual copes with certain life crises (e.g. Erikson's Stages of Psychosocial Development).

Social age involves expected age-graded role and behaviours. For example, a society may have expectations of when it is acceptable for young people to begin romantic lives, or for children to begin household chores. Social age is often defined by markers and events. It could also be defined by asking 'How old do you feel?' Our perception of age is often based on social markers, or engagement with age-grade roles or behaviours.

Stop and Think

- Since age is dynamic and fluid, use the four examples of defining age and write down how you fit into each category. Is there a difference in how you could perceive your age?

Linked lives

Linked lives
The interdependence with others in our social networks and relationships and how these affect our life course.

Linked lives is Elder's (1994) recognition of the interdependence of our lives. We are all embedded in social relationships and networks. We are interdependent. We live in a family network with multiple social relationships. We study or work in a network with multiple social relationships. Sometimes our networks overlap. The life course approach recognises that relationships and networks are structures of socialisation and management, and also provide us with necessary interaction. These relationships and networks influence our decisions and therefore our transitions, life events and turning points—if not directly, then in reaction to them, which is of equal importance. Our parents can influence our immediate world and can also affect us in our later life. For example, parental socio-economic level can have an impact on infancy and childhood health and can also impact on health in later life.

Elder's (1974) work on the longitudinal data of the Great Depression children highlights the interdependence between parents and children over the life course. The parents expressed high levels of stress, depression and marital discord which in turn affected their ability to care for and nurture their children. This was to have an effect on the children's later lives. Linked lives are the interaction of our social worlds over the duration of our life (Elder 1994).

Stop and Think

- How is your life linked?
- On a large piece of paper, draw the networks of which you are a member. What networks are interdependent? How are these networks part of the multiple trajectories along which you might be travelling?
- Consider the role of these networks in your life and what impact they might have in the future.

Human agency

Human agency refers to our free will, or our ability to act independently of social constraints or structures (Abercrombie et al. 1994). In the life course approach, human agency is how we as actors in our social world make choices in relation to the world and events around us (Elder 1994). Elder believes that although we are influenced by the social structures around us, we can make decisions within and around the influences of the social structures. Human agency can account for some individual differences identified through the life course approach to exploring health issues.

Human agency
Our ability to negotiate the social structures and a way to account for individual differences in the life course.

Agency can also impact on our experiences of life and historical times (discussed earlier). We need to consider the individual's agency: what they contribute, how significant the event is to them, and the subsequent impact (Elder 1994). The impact of technological growth on young people is minimal and they have the skills to cope with a technological change in the workplace, whereas an older person might not have the skills and could therefore experience greater impact from the change. The lack of skills may result in a perceived lack of ability to engage with new technology and therefore have greater significance.

Social structures, on the other hand, can be conceived of as key institutions in society. These institutions can be constituted (e.g. school and education, the justice system) or more symbolic (e.g. gender, age, sexuality). Social theorists such as Durkheim and Marx argued that our lives are governed by social structures, while others, such as Weber and Habermas, suggested that life is about agency. A third school of thought argues that our lives are influenced by our agency engaging with social structures (e.g. Bourdieu). For example, social structures can be used to account for successes in life. Children from high socio-economic groups are more likely to succeed at school and more likely to have professional jobs with higher salaries, therefore better superannuation savings, resulting in a better quality of old age than someone of low socio-economic status (Blane 2006; see also Chapters 1 & 7).

Models of the life course approach

The key concepts described above can be applied in different ways in a life course approach. Three models used to explain the role of life course determinants on people's health are the critical period model, the accumulation model and the pathway model. Each model applies life course determinants in a slightly different way. I will explore each model and its utility.

The critical period model is based on the assumption that life outcomes result from events at critical periods in earlier life (Heikkinen 2011; Kendig & Nazroo 2016). Intrauterine events can influence health in adult life (Heikkinen 2011). Similarly, the change in activity patterns of children and young people have resulted in higher levels of later life obesity (Dietz 2001).

Kendig and Nazroo (2016) offer a number of critiques of this model, particularly as it applies to health of ageing populations. The critical period model has the potential to focus policy intervention on early life, and the focus on childhood does not account for the impact of agency or other events. They cite the influence of Michael Marmot's review on health inequalities and the role of early life, which does not take into account other influences which may mitigate (or exacerbate) life outcomes. This critique is addressed in the following two models.

As the name suggests, the accumulation model is based on the cumulative effect of life course events on later life outcomes (Ben-Shlomo & Kuh 2002; Kuh et al. 2003; Blane et al. 2007; Kendig & Nazroo 2016). Heikkinen (2011) suggests the accumulation model has 'good predictive power' and is applicable in understanding a variety of health issues. For example, financial insecurity in older age may result from a low socio-economic upbringing, where a child is not provided with educational opportunities, which in turn can influence job outcomes (lower-skilled jobs), higher occupational risks (e.g. impact of manual labour on physical well-being) and less superannuation in retirement (Blane et al. 1997). The more time a person is exposed to disadvantage, the greater the impact on their life outcomes. For example, in older age people who spent much of their life in manual labour experienced greater chronic health conditions, poorer self-rated health and higher rates of mortality (Blane et al. 2007).

The accumulation model is critiqued for not considering the timing of the events and how these impact on life outcomes, or the impact of moderation (where the dis/advantage is moderated, or widens, over time) (Kendig & Nazroo 2016). The role of **social mobility** also needs to be taken into account, as a protective factor, in the accumulation model.

The pathways model explores how the role of events at one point in life influences inequalities in later life. Events which occur at one point may have an indirect influence at another point—a pathway between events/factors. The role of **mediating factors** on the relationship between the earlier and later events needs to be considered (Kendig & Nazroo 2016). The pathway model can be used to explain how early disadvantage sets a pathway to later disadvantage. Ben-Shlomo and Kuh (2002) propose four potential pathways to explain the early–later inequalities pathway:

- a biological pathway, for example, the impact of foetal development on later life health
- a social pathway, for example, the impact of lower socio-economic disadvantage on healthy retirement
- a socio-biological pathway, that is, how the socio-economic position in childhood influences later life immunity
- a bio-social pathway, for example, repeated childhood infections influencing educational attainment and socio-economic status in later life (Ben-Shlomo & Kuh 2002).

Social mobility

The movement of individuals or groups (e.g. families, social groups) within or between the social strata; or a relative change in an individual's or group's social status.

Mediating factors

Factors which explain the relationship between two other factors or variables (events).

Health effects and the life course

Hertzman (2000) sees life course effects as a gradient that increases in time and with age. These gradual effects provide one way for us to understand how life course events affect our health. According to Hertzman, there are three types of outcome effects in the life course approach when looking at health: latent effects, pathway effects and cumulative effects. *Latent effects* are biologically or developmentally based and result in effects in later life, regardless of future experiences. They result from events occurring during foetal and infant development stages which program organ systems—for example, low birthweight and the increased likelihood of coronary heart disease (Delisle 2002). *Pathway effects* result from experiences which set us on particular trajectories that can later influence our health or well-being. Limited exposure to literacy in early childhood can lead to poor reading in early schooling (Baydar et al. 1993), in turn affecting educational outcomes and therefore later life experiences. Hertzman and Power (2004) suggest that children who are not prepared for school (emotionally, cognitively and behaviourally) are more likely to experience 'education failure', and people with poor educational outcomes are less likely to engage in health-enhancing behaviours. *Cumulative effects* are a combination of latent and pathway effects (Hertzman 2000) and can refer to an accumulation of either disadvantage or advantage. Hertzman argues that these effects could be risks or protective factors. He cites the study by Power and colleagues (1999) of the effect of socio-economic class on adult health, where low socio-economics status in early life may lead to cumulative effects on health outcomes in later adulthood. Cumulative effects are also affected by the social gradient.

Social gradient and the life course

Social gradient
Differences in social status that lead to different health outcomes. Individuals at the lower end of the ladder of social hierarchy tend to have worse health outcomes than those located at higher social levels.

When we consider the effects thesis put forward by Hertzman (2000), we can also discuss the effects of the life course in terms of the social gradient. When we apply the **social gradient** to life course determinants and health, we note that the health of people is better towards the top of the gradient (Oldroyd 2019). Most diseases, especially chronic diseases, are concentrated at the bottom of the gradient and at earlier stages (see Chapters 1, 2, 8 & 14).

Case Example 10.4

The social gradient and mortality

As we have just seen, people at the lower end of the socio-economic status (SES) scale have on average poorer health for a longer time than do people at the upper end of the scale. These differences affect not only when but also where people die.

The social gradient in health was first recognised through the relationship between age of death and social class: the lower people's SES, the lower their average age of death in comparison with that of higher SES groups. Further, people with lower SES have a higher average number of years of disability before their earlier deaths (Marmot 2010).

The most detailed studies of causes and place of death as a function of deprivation have been carried out in the UK (NAO 2008; NELIN 2010). These show higher rates of death from cancer and respiratory diseases, and more deaths in hospital, in more deprived (lower SES) groups. The available Australian data is consistent with this. For example, male mortality in Victoria occurs at a lower age than average in most rural areas and the western suburbs (DHS 1999; Draper et al. 2004). Tobacco- and alcohol-related diseases contribute more to deaths in lower SES groups, while accidents and suicide further reduce the average age of death for men in rural areas.

Surveys consistently show that the majority of people would prefer not to die in hospital but, as indicated above, people with lower SES are more likely to do so. The reasons for this are not clearly established. It has been shown that a combination of informal care (from family and friends) with formal care in the community significantly increases the odds that a person will be able to die at home. A study in Western Australia found that people who accessed community-based specialist palliative care had a seven times higher chance of dying in their usual place of residence (McNamara & Rosenwax 2007). Studies in Australia and overseas show that many people die in hospital when there is no clinical reason for them to be there. Not only is this contrary to their wishes in many cases, it also contributes to increased healthcare expenditure in the last days of life. Governments have endorsed Advance Care Planning as a means by which people can document their wishes about end-of-life care, but evidence to date indicates that the available options may not be able to deliver people's choices. The National Health and Hospitals Reform Commission even suggested that Advance Care Planning could become a consumer tool for shaping end-of-life services, but these services are inextricably linked with health service provision in general.

The policy implication seems clear. Providing more community services that are more accessible—that is, shaped by local needs and demand—should both meet people's expressed wishes to die at home (or in a 'home-like' environment such as a residential aged care facility) and reduce demand for expensive acute hospital services. It is clear that in the coming decades Australia will need to accommodate a large increase of ageing and deaths. A health service focus on providing primary care services that allow not only ageing in place, but also dying in place, is imperative.

This case study is contributed by Bruce Rumbold

According to Blane (2006), dis/advantage accumulates cross-sectionally and longitudinally, with dis/advantage in one stage of life affecting other phases of life. To accommodate this idea of accumulation of positive or negative impacts, Blane uses three processes: social accumulation, social mobility and social protection. *Social accumulation* is used to explain the continuity of parental socio-economic status to conditions throughout the life course (infancy, childhood, adolescence, adulthood) (Blane 2006). It also accounts for the intersection between biological programming and social conditions of life. Two possible disruptions to the cumulative role of social disadvantage are when a person shifts social class and when a socio-economic system evolves or changes. For example, Australia has moved from a production economy to a service economy. A similar effect is felt when economic events like the global financial crisis occur.

Social mobility accounts for the accumulation of health and social factors that can lead to better or poorer health in later stages of life (Blane 2006). Parental socio-economic status can influence whether their offspring move up the social ladder, down the social ladder, or remain in the same position. If a person moves up the social ladder (i.e. increases in status), they will add 'advantage' to their life course; they will have less advantage than those of already equal footing, but more advantage than those left behind. The corollary is also true. Downward mobility adds disadvantage, with the individual experiencing less advantage than those left behind but more advantage than those they have joined (Blane 2006).

Social protection
Factors which protect an individual or group from further disadvantage. It can include government policies aimed to reduce poverty.

Social protection explores the interaction between health and life course events. It moderates the experience of impact of new disadvantage (Blane 2006). New disadvantage has minimal impact on previous advantage—this is positive social protection. A new disadvantage, however, will have an increased impact on previous disadvantage. Blane (2006) explains the idea of social protection through examples from the Analysis of General Household Survey in the UK (Bartley & Owen 1996). Working men with a restrictive chronic illness were more likely to be unemployed than men who reported good health. Blane argues that people of low socio-economic status with a chronic illness were more likely to experience disadvantage from the chronic illness, as it affects life choices like employment, whereas people of high socio-economic status are likely to be protected from further disadvantage.

Case Example 10.5

Ageing and life course determinants

Ageing is a key focus area of health and well-being in the 21st century. Developed nations are impacted by the baby-boomer population bulge, and the phenomenon of an ageing population will continue for another three generations at least. Understanding how life course determinants impact ageing contributes to better planning and policy development.

Kendig and colleagues (2016) explored the impact of childhood and adulthood SES on subjective well-being in older Australians. They conclude the relationship between childhood SES and later life well-being is mediated by adult SES and other health factors (which may also be influenced by earlier life course determinants). The authors also conclude that early SES and health exposures impacted on mid-life achievements in education, social class and health, and later life well-being.

Kendig et al.'s (2016) study applied three models in the exploration of life course determinants on subjective well-being in later life. Support was reported for the accumulation model, with the number of negative SES and health exposures accumulating and effecting poorer well-being in later life. The critical period model was used to demonstrate the role of more recent adult life events impacting on later life well-being, rather than earlier (childhood) life events. The childhood events were reported to have an indirect impact on later well-being. Childhood life course influencers were found to have mediated adult exposures, with adult life course events mediating later life well-being.

Vanhoutte and Nazroo (2016) explored the pathways to later life well-being through an SES lens in the US and England. Early life SES was assessed using parental class (manual labour/service labour/professional labour) in the English cohort and, in the US cohort, parental education (low [0–8]/middle [8.5–11]/high [12+]). The authors included early adulthood occupational level and late mid-life occupational class. They applied a critical period approach, an accumulation approach and a social mobility approach to their analyses.

Socio-economic status was reported to be an influence as a proximal event (adult life), more than as a distal (childhood) event and a major influence on later life well-being (Vanhoutte & Nazroo 2016). Advantage/disadvantage accumulation had strong support in the study, with life satisfaction being associated with less accumulation (of disadvantage). Social mobility could also explain subjective well-being in later life. Downward social mobility during adulthood (from childhood status) was found to negatively impact on subjective well-being and those with an upward trajectory reported higher subjective well-being.

These two studies highlight the utility of life course determinants in understanding health in ageing populations. They also demonstrate the applicability of different models in exploring the impact of life course determinants on population health.

Reflection Exercise

Applying a life course approach to a health issue: addictions

A life course approach to understanding health requires consideration of past events and transitions in determining current experiences. Current health promotion campaigns to address addictions, whether smoking, gambling, or alcohol or other substances, focus on the individual to make a choice. Choose one form of addiction and apply a life course determinants approach to understanding addiction. Consider the following questions.

- What interventions would be required?
- At what point in life would the intervention need to take place?
- What are the implications of your suggested interventions?

Applying a life course approach to a health issue: developing policy

Little research has been undertaken in Australia in using life course determinants as a basis for social and economic policy. The UK government included life course determinants in social and economic policy development, with the establishment of an interdepartmental working group (Dorozynski 1994; Bartley et al. 1997). One of its first acts was to set a research agenda which explored factors that accumulate over the life course (Bartley et al. 1997). The Queensland government acknowledged the significance of life course determinants in health (Queensland Health 2001), yet to date this has not been explicitly articulated in policy development.

Bartley et al. (1997, p. 1194) recommend that policy development focus on key transitional periods in life which could have material and psychosocial effects, 'preventing dramatic falls in living standards and by a wider effect on the degree to which citizens experience a sense of control over their lives'. Policy that builds resilience will strengthen individual and community health and well-being (Queensland Health n.d.).

Based on a life course approach to policy development, consider the following questions.

- Identify key issues which impact on the well-being of your community. How are these issues determined through a life course approach?
- Identify key transitional periods in life which could be the focus of policy.
- Identify interventions which develop and/or strengthen resilience of individuals and/or the community, and address the life course determinants to the issues you identified above.

Summary

Points in the life course are social determinants of health and well-being. When we consider the causes of illness and disease, we need to look beyond the individual and explore their history (and possibly that of their families and communities) to gain a better understanding of the effects of their past. We know that effects accumulate over the life course and, when combined with the social gradient, have greater impact. The utility of life course determinants has moved beyond health and can be used in other areas of well-being, such as families (Hutchison 2005).

Although the early history of life course determinants focuses on foetal and early childhood development, researchers have acknowledged that events at any time in our lives can have an impact (Lynch & Smith 2005). The challenge for us as health and well-being practitioners is to advocate for acknowledgment of life course determinants and to advocate for policy change that addresses these determinants in the policy response.

Tutorial exercises

1. Throughout this chapter you have undertaken a number of exercises. Bring this information together and explore how your life course is affecting or could affect your health.
2. Many people confuse life course determinants with the life-span approach to development. How is each of these terms defined? How can life-span approaches be integrated into life course approaches?
3. What is the role of life course determinants in young women living with HIV in sub-Saharan Africa?
4. What policy action could we take to address the issues of life course determinants in the experiences of women living with HIV in sub-Saharan Africa?
5. Which critical periods in life would impact on domestic violence? How can we address this issue at those critical periods?

Acknowledgment

I would like to thank Dr Bruce Rumbold for his assistance in writing the first version of this chapter and for providing the text on which Case Example 10.4, 'The social gradient and mortality' is based.

Further reading

Ben-Shlomo Y., & Kuh, D (2002). A life course approach to chronic disease epidemiology: conceptual models, empirical challenges and interdisciplinary perspectives. *International Journal of Epidemiology*, 33, 285–293.

Blane, D. (2006). The life course, social gradient and health. In M. Marmot & R.G. Wilkinson (Eds), *Social Determinants of Health* (pp. 64–80). Oxford: Oxford University Press.

Blane, D., Netuveli, G., & Stone, J. (2007). The development of life course epidemiology. *Epidemiology and Public Health*, 55, 31–38.

Elder, G.J. (1994). Time, human agency, and social change: perspectives on the life course. *Social Psychology Quarterly*, 57(1), 4–15.

Hutchison, E. (2010). A life course perspective. In E. Hutchison (Ed.), *Dimensions of Human Behavior: The Changing Life Course* (pp. 3–38). London: Sage.

Kendig, H., Loh, V., O'Loughlin, K. et al. (2016). Pathways to well-being in later life: socioeconomic and health determinants across the life course of Australian baby boomers. *Population Ageing*, 9, 49. https://doi-org.ezproxy1.library.usyd.edu.au/10.1007/s12062-015-9132-0

Kuh, D., Ben-Shlomo, Y., Lynch, J., Hallqvist, J., & Power, C. (2003). Life course epidemiology. *Journal of Epidemiology and Community Health*, 57, 778–783.

Mayer, K.U. (2009). New directions in life course research. *Annual Review of Sociology*, 35, 413–433.

Mortimer, J.T., & Shanahan, M.J. (2004). *Handbook of the Life Course*. New York: Springer.

Websites

www.who.int/social_determinants/en

This is the website of the WHO Commission on Social Determinants of Health. It is a good source of discussions on social determinants and provides crucial background papers and reports as well as examples of actions in relation to social determinants.

http://aging.utoronto.ca

The Institute for Life Course and Aging is based at the University of Toronto. It focuses on ageing research from a life course perspective.

www.sfb186.uni-bremen.de/frames/main.htm

The Special Collaborative Centre 186: Status Passages and Risks in the Life Course is a research centre based at the University of Bremen. The website provides a link to an extensive bibliography and links to other organisations.

www.lebenslaufarchiv.uni-bremen.de/index.php?id=567&no_cache=1&L=

The Archive for Life Course Research is an archive for qualitative social science research and is available to life course researchers.

www.ucl.ac.uk/icls

The International Centre for Life Course Studies in Society and Health is a UK-based centre with a focus on UK birth cohort studies. The centre is under the directorship of Mel Bartley and David Blane, two leading researchers in life course determinants.

http://caepr.anu.edu.au/population/lectures2011.php

The Centre for Aboriginal Economic Policy and Research at the Australian National University, 2011 Online Lecture Series is on 'Measures of Indigenous well-being and their determinants across the life course'. There are 14 lectures, each with a transcript, a copy of the presentation and an audio file.

References

Abercrombie, N., Hill, S., & Turner, B.S. (1994). *The Penguin Dictionary of Sociology*. London: Penguin.

Bartley, M., Blane, D., & Montgomery, S. (1997). Socioeconomic determinants of health: health and the life course—why safety nets matter. *British Medical Journal*, 314, 1194–1195.

Bartley, M., & Owen, C. (1996). Relation between socioeconomic status, employment and health during economic change 1973–93. *British Medical Journal*, 313, 445–449.

Baydar, N., Brooks-Gunn, J., & Furstenberg, F.F. (1993). Early warning signs of functional illiteracy: predictors in childhood and adolescence. *Child Development*, 64(3), 815–829.

Ben-Shlomo, Y., & Kuh, D. (2002). A life course approach to chronic disease epidemiology: conceptual models, empirical challenges and interdisciplinary perspectives. *International Journal of Epidemiology*, 33, 285–293.

Blane, D. (2006). The life course, social gradient and health. In M. Marmot & R.G. Wilkinson (Eds), *Social Determinants of Health* (pp. 64–80). Oxford: Oxford University Press.

Blane, D., Netuveli, G., & Stone, J. (2007). The development of life course epidemiology. *Epidemiology and Public Health*, 55, 31–38.

Delisle, H. (2002). *Programming of Chronic Disease by Impaired Foetal Nutrition: Evidence and Implications for Policy and Intervention Strategies*. Geneva: World Health Organization.

DHS (Department of Human Services) (1999). *The Victorian Burden of Disease Study: Mortality*. Melbourne: Victorian Department of Human Services.

Dietz, W.H. (2001). The obesity epidemic in young children. *British Medical Journal*, 322, 313–314.

Dorozynski, A. (1994). British government looks at effects of wealth on health. *British Medical Journal*, 308, 1257–1258.

Draper, G., Turrell, G., & Oldenburg, B. (2004). *Health Inequalities in Australia: Mortality. Health Inequalities Monitoring Series No. 1.* Cat. No. PHE 55. Canberra: Queensland University of Technology & Australian Institute of Health and Welfare.

Elder, G.J. (1974). *Children of the Great Depression*. Chicago: University of Chicago Press.

Elder, G.J. (1985). *Life Course Dynamics: Trajectories and Transitions, 1968–1980*. Ithaca, NY: Cornell University Press.

Elder, G.J. (1994). Time, human agency, and social change: perspectives on the life course. *Social Psychology Quarterly*, 57(1), 4–15.

Erikson, E. (1968). *Identity: Youth and Crisis*. New York: Norton.

Heikkinen, E. (2011). A life course approach: research orientations and future challenges. *European Review of Aging and Physical Activity*, 8, 7–12. https://doi.org/10.1007/s11556-010-0069-2

Hertzman, C. (2000). The case for an early childhood development strategy. *Isuma: Canadian Journal of Policy Research*, 1(4), 10–18.

Hertzman, C., & Power, C. (2004). Child development as a determinant of health across the life course. *Current Paediatrics*, 14(5), 438–443.

Hutchison, E. (2005). The life course perspective: a promising approach for bridging the micro and macro worlds for social workers. *Families in Society*, 86(1), 143–152.

Hutchison, E. (2010). A life course perspective. In E. Hutchison (Ed.), *Dimensions of Human Behavior: The Changing Life Course* (pp. 3–38). London: Sage.

Kendig, H., Loh, V., O'Loughlin, K. et al. (2016). Pathways to well-being in later life: socioeconomic and health determinants across the life course of Australian baby boomers. *Population Ageing*, 9, 49. https://doi-org.ezproxy1.library.usyd.edu.au/10.1007/s12062-015-9132-0

Kendig, H., & Nazroo, J. (2016). Life course influences on inequalities in later life: comparative perspectives. *Population Ageing*, 9, 1–7. https://doi.org/10.1007/s12062-015-9138-7

Kuh, D., Ben-Shlomo, Y., Lynch, J., Hallqvist, J., & Power, C. (2003). Life course epidemiology. *Journal of Epidemiology and Community Health*, 57, 778–783.

Lynch, J., & Smith, G.D. (2005). A life course approach to chronic disease epidemiology. *Annual Review of Public Health*, 26, 1–35.

Macmillan, R., & Elliason, S.R. (2004). Characterising the life course as role configurations and pathways: a latent structure approach. In J.T. Mortimer & M.J. Shanahan (Eds), *Handbook of the Life Course* (pp. 529–554). New York: Springer.

Marmot, M. (2010). *Fair Society, Healthy Lives: The Marmot Review.* London: University College London.

Marshall, W.A., & Tanner, J.M. (1969). Variations in pattern of pubertal changes in girls. *Archives of Diseases in Childhood*, 44(235), 291–303.

Marshall, W.A., & Tanner, J.M. (1970). Variations in the pattern of pubertal changes in boys. *Archives of Diseases in Childhood*, 45(239), 13–23.

McNamara, B., & Rosenwax, L. (2007). The mismanagement of dying. *Health Sociology Review*, 16(5), 373–383.

NAO (National Audit Office) (2008). *End of Life: Report by the Comptroller and Auditor-General.* London: The Stationery Office.

NELIN (National End of Life Intelligence Network) (2010). *Variations in Place of Death in England: Inequalities or Appropriate Consequence of Age, Gender and Cause of Death?* www.endoflifecare-intelligence.org.uk/resources/publications.aspx#neolcin.

Oldroyd, J. (2019). Social determinants and public health. In P. Liamputtong (Ed.), *Public Health: Local and Global Perspectives*, 2nd edn (Chapter 6). Melbourne: Cambridge University Press.

Power, C., Manor, O., & Matthews, S. (1999). The duration and timing of exposure: effects of socio-economic environment on adult health. *American Journal of Public Health*, 89(7), 1059–1066.

Queensland Health (n.d.). *Social Determinants of Health: Life Course Fact Sheet.* Brisbane: Public Health Services.

Queensland Health (2001). *Social Determinants of Health: The Role of the Public Health Services Act.* Brisbane: Queensland Government.

Rutter, N. (1996). Transitions and turning points in developmental psychopathology: as applied to the age span between childhood and mid adulthood. *International Journal of Behavioral Development*, 6(3), 603–626.

Settersten, R.A.J., & Mayer, K.U. (1997). The measurement of age, age structuring and the life course. *Annual Review of Sociology*, 23, 233–261.

Vanhoutte, B., & Nazroo, J. (2016). Life course pathways to later life wellbeing: a comparative study of the role of socio-economic position in England and the U.S. *Population Ageing*, 9, 157. https://doi-org.ezproxy1.library.usyd.edu.au/10.1007/s12062-015-9127-x

Wheaton, B., & Gotlieb, I.H. (1997). Trajectories and turning points over the life course: concepts and themes. In I.H. Gotlieb & B. Wheaton (Eds), *Stress and Adversity over the Life Course* (pp. 1–28). Cambridge: Cambridge University Press.

Willis, E. (2004). *The Sociological Quest: An Introduction to the Study of Social Life*, 4th edn. Sydney: Allen & Unwin.

Chapter 11

Health and the Living Environment

Liz Hanna

Topics covered

This chapter covers the following topics:

- human dependence upon health environments
- living sustainably by caring for the environmental determinants of health
- the nine planetary boundaries
- urban environments: bringing it all together
- failures, consequences and challenges
- solutions

Key terms

Anthropocene
climate change
ecosystem services
environmental determinants of health
Planetary Boundary Framework
planetary health
Precautionary Principle
sustainability

Introduction

> Planetary Health is described by the Lancet Commission as 'the achievement of the highest attainable standard of health, wellbeing, and equity worldwide through judicious attention to the human systems—political, economic, and social—that shape the future of humanity *and* the Earth's natural systems that define the safe environmental limits within which humanity can flourish. Put simply, planetary health is the health of human civilisation and the state of the natural systems on which it depends' (Horton & Lo 2015, p. 1921).

The World Health Organization estimates that 23 per cent of global deaths (and 26 per cent of deaths among children under five) are due to modifiable environmental factors (Prüss-Üstün et al. 2016). These deaths can be prevented. In this chapter, I provide an understanding of the deep relationship between humanity and the planet upon which we evolved, flourished and developed successful, complex human societies. Focusing on the second part of the above quote, I explore how the social determinants of health are intricately linked with **environmental determinants of health**. In keeping with the UN Sustainable Development Goals, I take a planetary view of the environment as this determines global health—wherever we live.

Environmental determinants of health
All external factors and conditions that affect people's lives and health. From a health perspective, the definition adopts a more restricted meaning of the chemical, biological and physical agents that impinge on health. Examples include pollution of the air, water or land, exposure to hazards such as noise, vibrations, heat or chemicals, as well as global hazards such as stratospheric ozone depletion and climate change.

The concept of environmental justice emerged in the 1980s, drawing attention to the unfair distribution of environmental benefits and burdens and incorporating interdisciplinary work to link theories of the environment and justice, environmental laws and their implementation, environmental policy and planning, governance for development and sustainability, and political ecology. However, inequities persist as governments continue to ignore the plight of the planet, which exposes the global poor to the double burden of both economic and environmental disadvantage. Instead, they prioritise economic gain for the privileged. This is a recipe for poor global health.

An understanding of the relationship between human health and well-being and the environment in which we live, work and play must first examine the basis for this relationship (see also Chapter 1). Our evolutionary history illustrates the determinants that set humanity upon a course of survival to adulthood, which heralded population explosion, innovation and technological success. It also explains why humans have degraded the planet to such an extent that our survival is threatened. A deep exploration of this is beyond the scope of this chapter; the 'Further reading' section offers more detailed works which readers should access.

In essence, the story is this. Humanity flourished upon a healthy planet (clean soils, clean rivers, clean air and a stable climate) when agriculture was mastered. But, like microbes in a petri dish, human overpopulation is utilising all the available resources and generating waste that is choking the very resources needed to survive. Not everyone consumes equally: the wealthy countries consume more resources and create more waste, whereas the global poor struggle to find sufficient food (see Chapter 14).

Although this is an environmental chapter, I focus on issues vital to human health and societal well-being, through exploring the critical role played by ecological services, such as provisioning access to healthy food, water and air. When people live in harmony with the planet, resources extraction is balanced with renewal. Loss of balance is hazardous to human health. Imbalance generates contamination of air, food and water and interruptions to the climate system.

The discussion of human-induced environmental degradation is viewed through a health lens. The folly of disregarding the significance of healthy environments in nurturing human health is illustrated via the global scale of interruptions to the major geophysical systems which are increasingly challenging human existence and human flourishing, most significantly among the world's most vulnerable populations. Changing climate, recognised as the greatest health threat facing humanity (Costello et al. 2009), provides a case study to illustrate the ramifications of ignoring the systems that nurture us.

Policy responses and regulatory frameworks are woven throughout the chapter to challenge readers to consider how collective action is necessary to achieve health for all. I close with strategies for the health sector to minimise health harm and boost resilience among the most vulnerable communities.

Stop and Think

Question to consider at the outset of this chapter

Has the human species (Homo sapiens) evolved into self-destructive 'Homo lemming'? Are we driving ourselves towards annihilation?

- Take a moment to consider your thoughts on this, drawing on your experiences in your own community, your understanding of the current state of the world and your learning to date.

Humanity's wilful self-destruction may appear a preposterous scenario, especially to those who are new to environmental and ecological considerations. However, by the end of this chapter, readers will be sufficiently informed to provide rational input into debate about humanity's future health security, its current trajectory, its options, and how to plan for a healthy future for all.

Human dependence on healthy environments

Our species, *Homo sapiens*, evolved on a planet that was predominantly several degrees cooler than it is today (Hanna & McIver 2018). Earth is undergoing the most rapid warming witnessed by humans, which, given the upper limitations to thermoregulatory capacity, poses significant risks to human movement, to work and to survival (Hanna & Tait 2015). Throughout the first several hundred thousand years, human population numbers remained small. In contrast, the Earth's resources and available space appeared boundless; the concept that humans could influence planetary ecosystems would have been unimaginable. Evidence to the contrary now abounds, yet many people remain wedded to this misconception.

After a long evolutionary history as hunter gatherers, human societal development leapt forward with the advent of agriculture about 12 000 years ago. Significantly, agriculture emerged almost simultaneously on four continents, using distinctive endemic food sources and divergent farming practices. Those communities were not connected, so the knowledge could not have been transferred and yet it is unlikely that human brain development snapped into action simultaneously in different places to recognise the benefits of securing a stable food source. This advance did not occur until Earth's climate settled to its present unusually warm and unusually stable level—a global average of 13.5°C (NOAA 2017). This epoch is known as the Holocene. The **Precautionary Principle** suggests that human societies would be unwise to drive Earth's climate system substantially away from Holocene climatic conditions (Steffen et al. 2015). It involves statements that:

Precautionary Principle
The principle originated as a tool to bridge uncertain scientific information and a political responsibility to act to prevent damage to human health and to ecosystems.

> in cases of serious or irreversible threats to the health of humans or ecosystems, acknowledged scientific uncertainty should not be used as a reason to postpone preventive measures. The principle originated as a tool to bridge uncertain scientific information and a political responsibility to act to prevent damage to human health and to ecosystems … When an activity raises threats of harm to human health or the environment, precautionary measures should be taken, even if some cause-and-effect relationships are not fully established scientifically (Rio Declaration from the 1992 UN Conference on Environment and Development, also known as Agenda 21).

The mechanism underpinning this unlikely synchrony among disparate communities remains a mystery, yet the significance of a stable climate within a perfect 'Goldilocks' (McMichael 2017) range cannot be overestimated. The global average climate warmed and stabilised to provide perfect ambient conditions for food production (Hanna & McIver 2018). Relatively steady temperature and rainfall patterns are critical to achieving reliable yields. Abundant soil nutrients, unpolluted river systems and clean air provided the additional necessary ingredients.

Access to sufficient nutritious food is fundamental to life. Hence, the development of agriculture is often viewed as the most profound cultural innovation in human history. Similarly, access to potable water for domestic purposes is a necessity. A person risks death if deprived of water for a few days (or less, in hot weather), and can survive only a few weeks if starved of food. Without air, irreparable brain damage occurs within minutes. Earth's planetary systems provide us with air, food and water.

As agricultural successes grew, allowing others to purchase food rather than generate their own, congregations of people grew into settlements supported by local farmers. These expanded into villages, towns and ultimately cities. Humanity now inhabits almost all of Earth's surface, and the population explosion is testimony to successful and resourceful innovation. Today's 'megacities', defined as those with more than 10 million inhabitants, are projected to increase from 33 in 2018 to 43 by 2030, most of them in developing regions (UN 2018a).

By most metrics, health is better today than at any time in history. The global average life expectancy has soared from 47 years in 1950–1955, to 69 years in 2005–2010. Death rates in children younger than five years of age worldwide decreased substantially from 214 per thousand live births in 1950–1955 to 59 in 2005–2010 (Whitmee et al. 2015). The total number of people living in extreme poverty has fallen by 0.7 billion over the past 30 years, despite an additional 2.7 billion people living today. These advances are attributable to public health programs, healthcare, better nutrition, education, human rights legislation and technological development. Yet it is not all good news. These benefits have been delivered inequitably across the globe (see Chapter 14). Furthermore, these gains in human health have come at a high price: excessive resource extraction has degraded nature's ecological systems on a scale never seen in human history (UNEP 2016), as I discuss further in the sections below.

A growing body of evidence shows that the health of humanity is intrinsically linked to the health of the environment, but the collective actions of the world's population now threatens to destabilise Earth's key life-support systems. Humanity's impact upon global planetary systems has reached such a level of intensity that we have left the Holocene and entered a new epoch, the **Anthropocene** (Steffen et al. 2007).

Understanding that environmental damage harms human health dates back 2500 years, to the writings of Hippocrates (1923–1995.). Yet somewhere amid the rise of biomedicine, this wisdom lost prominence in mainstream western health thinking, despite the efforts of a few forward thinkers such as Professor Tony McMichael (1993). In 2000, as evidence increasingly emerged that humanity's unthinking and relentless utilisation of Earth's limited natural resources was polluting the planet, the UN Secretary-General Kofi Annan called for a Millennium Ecosystem Assessment (MEA) to assess the consequences of ecosystem change for human well-being. The MEA established the scientific basis for actions needed to enhance the conservation and sustainable use of those systems, so that they can continue to supply the ecological services that underpin all aspects of human life, now and into the future (Corvalan et al. 2005). The MEA described the life-supporting **ecosystem services** (ES) provided by healthy ecosystems (Table 11.1).

Anthropocene
The current geological age during which the combined influence of one species—*Homo sapiens*—has acted with sufficient power and scale to change the Earth system, now viewed as the dominant influence on climate and the environment.

Ecosystem services (ES)
The benefits provided by ecosystems that contribute to making human life both possible and worth living. Examples include products such as food and clean water, regulation of the carbon cycle, or floods, soil erosion and disease outbreaks, and non-material benefits such as psychological, spiritual and recreational benefits.

Table 11.1 Typology of four ecosystem services, using a classification developed by the Millennium Ecosystem Assessment

Ecosystem service	Example
Provisioning	Food crops (e.g. wheat fields, rice paddies, market gardens) and fibre crops (cotton, bamboo), biofuels (e.g. from corn and sugarcane), animal products (e.g. sheep flocks, chicken farms), aquaculture ponds, fish stocks, fresh water, medicinal (e.g. codeine, pyrethrum), mangroves (fish nurseries)
Regulating	Forests on slopes that stabilise soil, lessening erosion, coastal protection from storms and (partially) tsunamis (carbon stabilisation), some cases of infectious disease limitation (e.g. Lyme disease, malaria in some cases, onchocerciasis)
Culturally enriching	Inspiration (charismatic landscapes and species, e.g. coral reefs, tiger reserves, old-growth forests), spiritual refreshment (sacred groves), religious observation, ancestral links, ceremonial decorations (red ochre, bird of paradise feathers)
Supporting	Soil fertility and nutrient recycling (micro-organisms, earthworms, fungi), pollinators (insects, birds, bats), insect control (birds), seed dispersers (bats, birds, apes, elephants), detoxification and nutrient recycling

Butler & Hanna (2013)

Living sustainably by caring for the environmental determinants of health

The intrinsic value of healthy ecosystems to human survival and flourishing is recognisable even without intellectual or scientific understanding of the mechanisms involved.

Stop and Think

> You must teach your children that the ground beneath their feet is the ashes of our grandfathers. So that they will respect the land, tell your children that the earth is rich with the lives of our kin. Teach your children what we have taught our children—that the earth is our mother. Whatever befalls the earth, befalls the sons of the earth. If men spit upon the ground, they spit upon themselves.
>
> This we know. The earth does not belong to man; man belongs to the earth. This we know. All things are connected like the blood which unites one family. All things are connected.
>
> Whatever befalls the earth befalls the sons of the earth. Man did not weave the web of life; he is merely a strand in it. Whatever he does to the web, he does to himself ...
>
> And of the ways of the white folk who landed on their shores from afar he spoke '... He treats his mother, the Earth, and his brother, the same, as things to be bought, plundered, sold like sheep or bright beads. His appetite will devour the Earth and leave behind only a desert.

Note: This 1854 text reflects the Native American relationship with Earth. Similar belief systems are held dearly by other First Nations, such as Australian Indigenous peoples. If written today, the wording would more likely be inclusive of females.

- Consider this quote from one of America's First Nation leaders, Chief Seattle, contrasting Native American lore with the culture of the colonising peoples. Do his words ring true to you? Do they reflect the teachings of your elders?

Urbanisation sets in place geographic, visual, psychological and cognitive barriers that separate urban dwellers from natural places, the source of our food and water. In 2018, 55 per cent of the world's population reside in urban areas (UN 2018a), deprived of seeing a full horizon, through clear skies, to a land of bounteous natural beauty. In modern societies, food is primarily sourced from supermarkets, water emanates from taps and energy is available at the flick of a switch. The importance of ecological services, ensured only by a healthy planet, such as clean air, clean food and clean water, is often forgotten. This divorce from nature produces a profound lack of understanding of the dynamic relationship between humans and the life-supporting role played by natural systems. It has resulted in an overly intensive and disruptive, not a **sustainable**, human interaction with the natural world.

Sustainability
The process of living within the limits of available physical, natural and social resources in ways that allow the living systems to thrive in perpetuity.

A human population of 7.1 billion, of which an estimated 24 per cent (WorldWatch Institute 2017) enjoy the benefits of highly developed life-styles, is evidently unsustainable. Earth Overshoot Day is the day each year by which the world's population has consumed the entire year's supply of renewable planetary resources. The date creeps forward every year as resource extraction and waste generation accelerate. In 2017, it was 2 August. If everyone on the planet lived the Australian life-style Earth Overshoot Day would occur on 12 March, and 5.2 Earths would be needed to supply the global population with sufficient resources—and to absorb the waste generated—for an entire year. Yet if all humanity adopted the average life-style consumption patterns of India, only 0.6 planets would be needed.

Those who are attuned to the empirical evidence of environmental degradation and its threats to global health are raising a call to action. The *Lancet,* one of the world's leading medical journals, established a series of commissions to explore and promulgate the evidence and risks to human health arising from environmental degradation. The aim is to raise awareness and influence the health sector and world leaders to place greater importance on protecting the life-supporting systems that form our natural ecosystems. The Commission on Pollution and Health identified pollution as the largest environmental cause of disease and premature death in the world today (Landrigan et al. 2017). Diseases caused by pollution were responsible for an estimated 9 million premature deaths in 2015, or 16 per cent of all deaths worldwide, and were responsible for more than one death in four in the most severely affected countries.

Planetary health
The achievement of the highest attainable standard of health, well-being and equity worldwide through judicious attention to the human systems—political, economic and social—that shape the future of humanity and the Earth's natural systems that define the safe environmental limits within which humanity can flourish.

The *Lancet* journal joined forces with the Rockefeller Foundation to develop a Commission on Planetary Health and create a new *Lancet* journal of the same name, and their definition of **planetary health** appears in the opening quote to this chapter. The movement is snowballing as many other groups have joined in an effort to protect humanity's future.

Planetary Boundary Framework
Considers planetary resources and defines a safe operating space for humanity, to map how far humanity has progressed towards irreparably damaging key aspects of Earth's biophysical processes and ecosystems

The collective damage is detectable in so many differing ecosystems that addressing the problem can appear overwhelming. Launched in 2009, the **Planetary Boundary Framework** breaks down the problem into nine planetary boundaries to provide information on how humanity can safely exist and flourish within each system (Rockström et al. 2009).

Transgressing one or more planetary boundaries may be deleterious or even catastrophic, due to the risk of crossing thresholds that will trigger non-linear, abrupt environmental change within continental- to planetary-scale systems (Rockström et al. 2009). The term 'tipping point' is widely used to describe a critical threshold beyond which rapid physical feedback mechanisms can drive the Earth system into a new state, that may present intolerable challenges to ecosystems.

The nine planetary boundaries are:

1. climate change
2. change in biosphere integrity (biodiversity loss and species extinction)
3. land-system change (agriculture)
4. freshwater use
5. biogeochemical flows (phosphorus and nitrogen cycles)
6. ocean acidification
7. atmospheric aerosol loading (microscopic particles in the atmosphere that affect climate and living organisms)

8. stratospheric ozone depletion
9. introduction of novel entities (e.g. organic pollutants, radioactive materials, nanomaterials and micro-plastics).

The Stockholm Environment Institute developed the Planetary Boundaries Framework as a basis for examining the areas where human activities are compromising major planetary systems (see Figure 11.1). Although the framework's strength lies in its focus on key threatened ecological systems, examining these through a health lens allows readers to fully appreciate the health implications that arise when key environmental health determinants are threatened.

Figure 11.1 Nine planetary boundaries. Credit: F. Pharand-Dschenes/Globaia

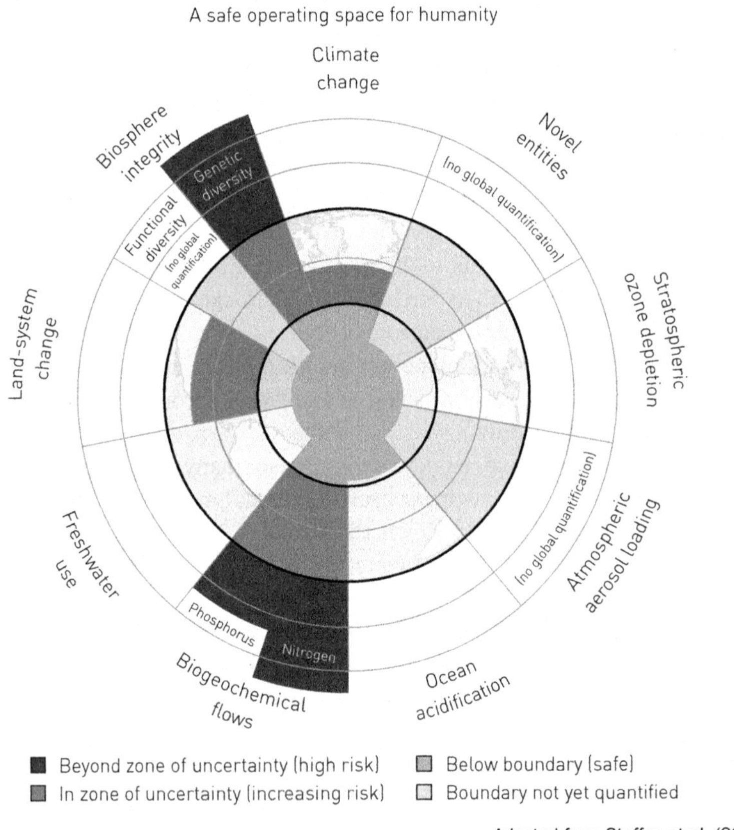

Adapted from Steffen et al. (2015)

Climate change

A change in the state of the climate, identified via statistical tests as changes in the mean and/or the variability of its properties that persist for an extended period, typically decades or longer.

Climate change

Climate change affects the social and environmental determinants of health, such as clean air, safe drinking water, sufficient food and secure shelter (WHO 2016b). Climate-related shocks and stresses, already a major obstacle to global poverty reduction, will worsen with climate change. The global poor are disproportionately affected—not only because they are often more exposed to the effects of climate extremes and are more vulnerable to climate-related shocks, but also because they have fewer resources and receive less material support from family, community, the financial system and even social safety nets to prevent, cope and adapt (Hallegatte et al. 2017). Climate change will worsen these shocks and stresses, contributing to a decoupling of economic growth and poverty reduction, thereby making it even harder to eradicate poverty in a sustainable manner. Climate change is making it harder for poor countries to achieve their Sustainable Development Goals (SDG), hence it was recognised by the *Lancet* journal as 'the biggest global health threat of the 21st century' (Costello et al. 2009, p. 1693). Between 2030 and 2050, climate change is expected to cause approximately 250 000 additional deaths per year, from malnutrition, malaria, diarrhoea and heat stress (WHO Director-General 2018).

Human health is negatively impacted by climate change via many direct and indirect pathways (Watts et al. 2017). In a warming world, heat exposure presents a dire threat to survival, to people's capacity to conduct their activities of daily living, and to work. Death rates increase in cold weather, but the rise in deaths in hot weather is more pronounced, as there is little escape from the heat (see Figure 11.2).

Figure 11.2 The exposure–response relationship for temperature-associated mortality

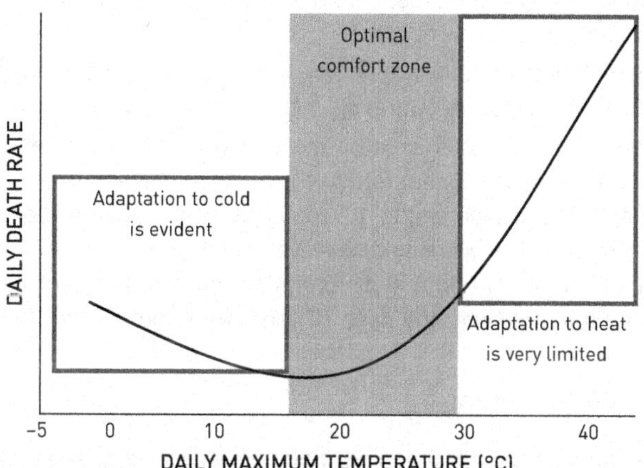

Hanna (2017)

Case Example 11.1

Climate change: ignoring the science

The known science (Hanna & McIver 2018).

- Throughout the past 2.6 million years, atmospheric carbon dioxide (CO_2) levels oscillated between 180 parts per million (ppm) (during ice ages) and 280 ppm (during warmer interglacial periods). In 2017, global atmospheric CO_2 levels peaked at 412 ppm).

- More than a century ago, scientists understood the relationship between CO_2 levels and the greenhouse effect which could change the global climate.
- Global warming was observed in the 1930s.
- Burning of fossil fuels has contributed to 75 per cent of the observed 1°C rise in global temperatures since the start of the industrial era (c.1750).

This elevation in atmospheric CO_2 forebodes more global warming. Today's CO_2 levels transgress safe planetary boundary thresholds.

Climate change effects

- All years since 2014 (up to mid 2018, the time of writing) have broken heat records by significant margins.
- Antarctic ice volume has decreased by more than 300 km^3/yr since 1994 (Shepherd et al. 2018), and this rate has tripled since 2012 (Cole & Buis 2018) to 219 billion metric tonnes.
- Antarctic ice loss could raise global sea levels by 58 m.
- Anthropogenic emissions from burning fossil fuels have released sufficient carbon into the global atmosphere that the loss of summer Arctic sea-ice is already considered irreversible.
- White ice reflects the sun's radiation, whereas dark oceans absorb heat which further accelerates warming, thus ice loss accelerates warming.
- In the first half of the 20th century, the average global sea level rose by about 1.4 mm/yr. Since 1993, that rate has more than doubled to 3.2 mm/yr. And since 2012, it's jumped to 4.5 mm/yr and is accelerating at 0.084 ± 0.025 mm/yr, which will double sea-level rise by 2100 (Nerem et al. 2018).
- The annual number of natural disasters attributable to the climate has increased threefold over the past 35 years (Hoeppe 2016).

Impact upon humanity

- Rapid economic growth, urban development and migration are expected to increase the number of people living in the low-elevation coastal zone to 1.4 billion by 2060 (Neumann et al. 2015).
- Low-lying areas along coastlines, in delta regions and atoll nations will be submerged sooner.
- Even with aggressive mitigation, sea-level rise will continue to 2300 (Brown et al. 2018).
- Currently, 30 per cent of the world's population is exposed to lethal heat thresholds for at least 20 days a year (Mora et al. 2017).
- By 2100, this proportion will increase to between 48 per cent and 74 per cent, depending on the rate at which CO_2 emissions grow.
- Heat exposure is a rapidly rising threat to those working outdoors, especially in humid zones (Hanna et al. 2011).

- Flood hazards from increased rainfall intensities are being observed across the world, and projected to increase in more than half the world's regions (World Bank Group 2016).
- The number of people at risk from floods is projected to rise from 1.2 billion today to around 1.6 billion in 2050 (nearly 20 per cent of the world's population).
- An estimated 1.8 billion people are currently affected by land degradation/desertification and drought.
- Climate change triggers cascading disasters with far-reaching effects, as demonstrated by the Syrian conflict which was precipitated by a profound drought. The Arab Spring, subsequent mass migration and rise of the far-right anti-migration political movement across Europe can be traced back to the global food crisis of 2008–10 (Werrell & Femia 2013).

Global response

- The UN Framework Convention on Climate Change was established in 1992. The Kyoto Protocol, adopted in 1997, represents the world's first international agreement on international emission reduction targets. The Paris Agreement (2015) set pledges to accelerate and intensify nations' emission reduction targets and timelines, and investments needed for a sustainable low-carbon future.
- The Paris Agreement Intended Nationally Determined Contributions (INDCs) were voluntary, not binding. There is a 50 per cent chance of keeping warming to 2°C if all countries adhere to their stated pledges. Yet the stated policies to achieve the targets fell short, resulting in a 99.5 per cent chance of exceeding 2°C, and only a 50 per cent chance of staying under 3.6°C.
- To date (2018), international agreements fail to protect human health by keeping global warming within safe limits.
- The delayed response to climate change over the past 25 years has jeopardised human life and livelihoods (Watts et al. 2017).

Agriculture presents a major global challenge. The sector is directly affected by climate change, yet agriculture, forestry and other land use changes are responsible for almost a quarter of anthropogenic greenhouse gas (GHG) emissions (van Meijl et al. 2018). Among crop species, rice is the primary food source for more than 2 billion people (Zhu et al. 2018). Rice and wheat provide two out every five calories that humans consume, and these are produced from photosynthesis from atmospheric CO_2 (Zhao et al. 2017). The increase in atmospheric CO_2 since the Industrial Revolution is thought to have increased the production of sugars and other carbohydrates in plants by up to 46 per cent, and these will continue to rise in the coming decades. Conversely, higher concentrations of CO_2 lead to lower levels of proteins, nitrogen, zinc, magnesium, potassium, calcium and iron in plants (Loladze

2014), as well as vitamins B1, B2, B5 and B9 (Zhu et al. 2018). The impact of a continued increase in foodstuff ratio of starch to micronutrient could be profound, notably among the poor whose diets consist of proportionally more rice or wheat and less vegetable, meat and fish than do the diets of rich nations.

Insufficient intake of micronutrients, protein and vitamins, and bouts of diarrhoea, contribute to nutritional deficiencies among 2 billion people in developing and developed countries (Zhu et al. 2018). These deficiencies can directly (cognitive development, metabolism, immune system) and indirectly (obesity, type 2 diabetes mellitus) affect human health on a panoptic scale (Stein 2009).

Loss of biosphere integrity (biodiversity loss and extinctions)

The Millennium Ecosystem Assessment of 2005 concluded that changes to ecosystems due to human activities were more rapid in the past 50 years than at any time in human history, increasing the risk of abrupt and irreversible changes. The world's growing population demands for food, water and natural resources are the major drivers of severe biodiversity loss and are eroding the health of life-giving ES (Haines et al. 2018). Damage is escalating yet, globally, insufficient commitment means there is insufficient global action to halt that harm. By ignoring environmental impacts, humanity's blinkered approach to producing food en masse has inadvertently reduced the planet's food-producing capacity. The ES concept shows that environmental impact plays an important role in agriculture (Danckaert & Gijseghem 2013). To produce the provisioning services (food, feed, fibre, fuel) and other cultural services such as an aesthetic landscape, agriculture needs ES such as regulation (pollination, natural pest control, water and atmospheric regulation) and supporting services (soil structure, nutrient cycling, genetic biodiversity) (Butler & Hanna 2013). Using those regulating and supporting services correctly—thereby minimising disservices such as habitat loss, nutrient runoff and pesticide use—comes close to the concept of sustainable agriculture. The ES concept makes non-productive services more visible, as these need to be included in full accounting processes.

It has been estimated that the production of 84 per cent of crop species cultivated in Europe depends directly on insect pollination, especially by bees, and 70 per cent of the 124 staple food crops in the world require pollinators (Carreck 2016). These percentages vary dramatically among crops, with the highest level of pollinator dependence found predominantly in fruits, vegetables and nuts. The total economic value of insect pollination worldwide has been estimated at over $162 billion. Many wild bee species are declining rapidly across North America and Europe, a potential consequence of land-use change driven by agricultural intensification and urbanisation (Vaidya et al. 2018) The collapse of pollinators presents a catastrophic loss to global nutrition, and the economic collapse of many farming communities (Bauer & Sue Wing 2016). Lower food yields would elevate prices, making nutritious food prohibitively expensive for those on lower incomes.

Flying insect biomass has declined 82 per cent in the past 27 years (Hallmann et al. 2017), raising concerns for cascading effects on food webs and jeopardised ES. Agricultural crops are necessary to feed human populations, and livestock provide human protein. It is estimated that approximately 75 per cent of the globally produced food crops rely on pollinating insects, among which honeybees are economically most important. Approximately 30 per cent of the 2.8 million tons of pesticides applied annually worldwide are insecticides, which kill the pollinators needed in the production of crops.

Pesticides are biocidal—designed specifically to kill life-forms by interrupting biological processes, many of which are shared with humans. Pesticide-related diseases have burgeoned over recent decades (Hanna 2005). Such perverse outcomes result from linear thinking, but the biology of life is a food web. Everything is connected. Interference in one system has impacts on many, if not all, others.

Land system change

Land is converted to human use all over the planet, predominantly for agriculture, forestry of wood products, and covering the land with urban settlements—often on the best prime farming land next to the best water sources, and the oceans. Urban expansion is creeping over agricultural land, especially in coastal and riverine regions. In 2009, only 9 per cent of Earth's landmass showed no sign of human footprint, and most of that land was in places that are unsuited to agriculture or cities, such as the Sahara, Gobi and Australian deserts, the most remote portions of tropical rainforests in the Amazon and Congo, and the tundra (Venter et al. 2016). There is little arable land that is not already farmed.

This land-use change is driving serious reductions in biodiversity, and interfering with water flows and the biogeochemical cycling of carbon, nitrogen and phosphorus and other important elements. A key factor, often overlooked, is that while each incident of land cover change occurs on a local scale, the aggregated impacts can have consequences for Earth system processes on a global scale. This collective destruction is known as the Tragedy of the Commons (Hardin 1968). Modern examples are where broad-scale farming patterns interrupt balanced ecosystems by replacing biodiversity with mono-species. Large volumes of foodstuffs ripening at once provide a food boom for pests, attracting them in high concentrations. Farmers respond with pesticides, which alter the local, nearby and downstream ecosystems and waterways.

Pesticides and artificial fertilisers run off into rivers and streams. Downstream organisms are exposed and die, and the enriched chemical nutrient load creates eutrophication, which generates algal blooms that can make the water hypoxic, and toxic for human and agricultural use. The combined effect drives environmental degradation and diminished food yields, which further motivates farmers towards heavier application of chemicals.

Forests hold soil and support diverse ecosystems as well as induce rain (Syktus & McAlpine 2016), such that cleared land receives less rainfall while providing fewer niches for wildlife, including natural controllers of pests. Mechanical tilling of the soil weakens the soil structure, thus facilitating dust storms and loss of top soil. Global annual dust emissions have increased by 25 per cent to 50 per cent over the last century due to a combination of land-use change and climate change involving increased droughts (UNEP et al. 2016).

Despite decades of increases in agricultural yields and progress towards achieving SDG 2, 'End hunger, achieve food security and improved nutrition', global numbers of chronically undernourished people are increasing—815 million people in 2016, up from 777 million in 2015 (FAO et al. 2017). The world is well short of achieving SDG 2 targets, and climate change and other anthropogenic degradation of ecosystems is escalating the challenge. Furthermore, meeting the global food demand of roughly 10 billion people by the middle of this century will become increasingly challenging as Earth's climate continues to warm, and previous measures (land-clearing, irrigation and chemicals) are no longer available.

Global warming and increased rain variability are anticipated to outstrip any potential gains in additional CO_2, or modest yield gains in the higher-latitude regions (Myers et al. 2017). For every degree increase in global mean temperature, yields are projected to decrease, on average, by 7.4 per cent for maize, 6 per cent for wheat, 3.2 per cent for rice and 3.1 per cent for soybean (Zhao et al. 2017). Warming and rainfall variability have amplified global cereal production yields and price volatility—where prices can surge 300 per cent—that creates uncertainty for the entire agribusiness sector and the ~800 million people living in extreme poverty who are most vulnerable to food price spikes (Tigchelaar et al. 2018). Back-to-back droughts have left at least 8.5 million people in Ethiopia in need of food aid. In the Somali region, rains failed for four consecutive years, causing a breakdown in pastoral livelihoods (FAO 2017). By the end of 2017, 866 000 people were in need of emergency food supplies.

The food system is responsible for more than a quarter of all greenhouse gas emissions, and current unhealthy diets of high intakes of meat, fats, salt and sugar cause obesity and a range of disorders which are the greatest contributors to premature mortality in the developed world. Agriculture also places great strain on biodiversity, soils, water and the atmosphere, and these strains will be exacerbated if the current trends in population growth, meat and energy consumption, and food waste continue.

Thus, farming systems that are highly productive yet minimise environmental harms are critically needed, while diets need to be considered for their environmental footprints. Transitioning toward more plant-based diets in line with standard dietary guidelines could reduce global mortality by 6–10 per cent and food-related greenhouse gas emissions by 29–70 per cent compared with today. Monetising the improvements in health could even exceed the value of the environmental benefits, at US$1–31 trillion, equivalent to 0.4–13 per cent of global gross domestic product in 2050 (Springmann et al. 2016).

The resurgence in organic farming that attempts to improve soil quality is showing benefits, and the food yields are little short of conventional (chemical) farming practice yet come without the price tag of degraded soils (Ponisio et al. 2015). Long-term accounting leaves 'healthy farming' practices ahead of highly mechanised farming systems.

Freshwater consumption and the global hydrological cycle

Whereas a healthy well-nourished human can survive up to three weeks without food, most would die within about a week without water, and within days if exercising or in a hot climate. Water is abundant on Earth. Yet although 71 per cent of the planet is water-covered, 96.5 per cent of it is saline (oceanic) (USGS 2018). Most human water resources are derived from rivers and lakes, which comprise a mere 0.0072 per cent of total planetary water. Freshwater is thus a very precious resource. Since the 1990s, water pollution has worsened in almost all rivers in Africa, Asia and Latin America (WWAP 2018). Water shortages are trending, notably where ice sheets or glaciers are diminishing in response to climate change and where groundwater is being withdrawn at an unsustainable rate. Groundwater meets the domestic needs of roughly half of the world's population and boosts food supply by providing for 38 per cent of global consumptive irrigation water demand (Rodell et al. 2018).

Climate change-induced drought frequency and intensity has risen measurably and is projected to further increase, leading to longer and slower recovery and more time spent in drought (Schwalm et al. 2017). Droughts are a leading cause of famine and disease (Oxfam 2017), and conflict (UNHCR 2017). Climate refugees flee when they have no other feasible option; poverty increases vulnerability and minimises adaptation and options. Climate change is another tragic example of the poor suffering disproportionately from the actions of the wealthy.

Around 2 billion people, or almost one-fifth of the world's population, live in areas of water scarcity, and two-thirds of the world's population (4 billion people) currently live in areas that experience water scarcity for at least one month a year (Mekonnen & Hoekstra 2016; UN Water n.d.). By 2025, half of the world's population will be living in water-stressed areas (WHO 2017b), and by 2050, 4.8–5.7 billion are likely to be living in water stress.

Nitrogen and phosphorus flows to the biosphere and oceans

Continuing the interconnectedness theme, land-use change drives the serious reductions in biodiversity, and interferes with water flows and the biogeochemical cycling of carbon, nitrogen, phosphorus and other important elements.

Nitrogen and phosphorus are essential elements for plant growth, but heavy fertiliser production and agricultural application have depleted this natural resource. Rather than being taken up by crops, a more reactive form of artificially produced nitrogen is emitted to the atmosphere, so that runoff after rain pollutes waterways and coastal zones. Similarly, much of the phosphorus mobilised by humans ends up in aquatic systems and ultimately the sea, causing algal blooms which consume the available oxygen and can suffocate marine creatures, to form ocean 'dead zones' (Van Meter et al. 2018). For example, the Mississippi River carries agricultural runoff into the Gulf of Mexico and creates an ever-increasing dead zone. The largest to date was in 2017 at 22 729 km^2, and it will require decades of determined action to reverse current agricultural practices and return the ocean to a healthy status that would again support fish stocks (Van Meter et al. 2018). Human efforts to produce food supplies can destroy other food sources, if environmental considerations are ignored.

Ocean acidification

Around a quarter of the CO_2 emitted into the atmosphere dissolves in the oceans to form carbonic acid, which lowers the pH of the surface water (from 8.1 to 8.0), and has to date increased ocean acidity by 30 per cent (USGCRP et al. 2017). The associated loss of available carbonate ions presents a critical barrier to the formation of calcium carbonate exoskeletons of marine shellfish (mussels, prawns, krill) and coral. Plankton and krill form the basis of the marine food web; their numbers are declining and shells are thinning (ACCSP 2015). Increasing ocean temperatures, loss of chlorophyll and increasing acidification may also place marine larvae into suboptimal conditions, close to the limits of their physiological tolerance (Piñones & Fedorov 2016). Their loss could herald collapse of the entire marine food web and wreak devastating impacts on fisheries and the nutritional status of the 3.1 billion people who derive at least 20 per cent of their dietary protein from marine sources (FAO 2016). Significant nutritional deficits could arise from marine fisheries stock losses when acidification and warming sea temperatures compound existing threats from overfishing (Hanna & McIver 2018).

Atmospheric aerosol loading

Air quality can deteriorate from human and natural causes. Clearing and burning of forests release dust and smoke into the air. Industrial activities and fossil-fuelled transport systems release a toxic chemical mix, particulates and greenhouse gases. The increased combustion of fossil fuels in the last century is the primary culprit in the progressive change in the atmospheric composition. Air pollutants, such as carbon monoxide (CO), sulphur dioxide (SO_2), nitrogen oxides (NOx), volatile organic compounds (VOCs), ozone (O_3), heavy metals and respirable particulate matter (PM2.5 and PM10), differ in their chemical composition, reaction properties, emission, time of disintegration and ability to travel long or short distances airborne (WHO 2014). Polluted air crosses international borders with impunity, which decouples the benefit–cost matrix as those forced to breathe polluted air are frequently not those who burned the fossil fuels.

The World Health Organization (2018) reports that nine out of 10 people across the world breathe polluted air, and that one in nine dies as a result. Global distribution of air pollution is uneven, as high levels of local emissions affect local residents, then distant peoples as the winds disperse to neighbouring regions. Atmospheric pollutant concentrations depend upon modes of transport, household fuels and industrial activities, fossil fuel reliance and emissions, along with the existence of and compliance with government policies to protect air quality. Effects on human health depend on exposure concentrations and duration, the mix of air toxics, general health status and vulnerability. There are increasing rates of stroke, heart disease, lung cancer and chronic and acute respiratory diseases. Air pollution disproportionately affects populations in countries undergoing rapid industrialisation, population growth, urbanisation and motorisation (Alexandra et al. 2018).

Global annual mortality from ambient (outdoor) air pollution exceeds 4.2 million, with 91 per cent of these deaths reported in low- and middle-income countries (WHO 2018). Most sources of outdoor air pollution are well beyond the control of individuals and demand concerted action by local, national and regional level policy-makers working across sectors (transport, energy, waste management, urban planning and agriculture). Wealthy countries have regulatory frameworks to outlaw polluting practices and protect the air.

The high morbidity and mortality in low- and middle-income countries, two-thirds of which occur in cities in WHO's south-east Asia and western Pacific regions (WHO 2016a), result from weak regulation. In China, the density of urban air pollution reached concentrations levels high enough to interrupt sunlight, photosynthesis and plant growth (Chen 2014), and halt solar voltaic energy production (Li et al. 2017). China's response was to become the world leader in investment in renewable energy sources (IRENA 2018b), which provides employment (IRENA 2018a).

The transition away from burning fossil fuel delivers multiple benefits: climate change mitigation, clean jobs and substantial global health benefits.

Stratospheric ozone depletion

The stratospheric ozone layer protects against skin cancer by filtering out ultraviolet radiation from the sun. Since about the 1970s, anthropogenic emissions of ozone-depleting gases depleted the protective layer of ozone, and a hole in the ozone layer over Antarctica was detected in 1987 (Thompson et al. 2011). A multilateral agreement known as the Montreal Protocol aimed to reduce and ultimately ban the global use of chlorofluorocarbons and halons frequently used as refrigerant gases. The 2016 Kigali Amendment added hydrofluorocarbons. This international treaty stands as testament to coordinated global action to cooperate to protect human health and reduce environmental damage—the ozone hole over Antarctica is notably reducing (UNEP 2017) (see Figure 11.3).

Chemical pollution and the release of novel entities

Pollution is not merely an environmental issue, it is also an equity issue. Nearly 92 per cent of pollution-related deaths occur in low- and middle-income countries. In wealthier countries, disease caused by pollution is most prevalent among minorities and the marginalised (Landrigan et al. 2017). Children are at high risk of pollution-related disease. Even extremely low-dose exposures to pollutants during windows of vulnerability in utero and early infancy can result in disease, disability across the life-span, and premature death. Globally, pollution causes three times more deaths than AIDS, tuberculosis and malaria combined and 15 times more than those caused by wars and other forms of violence (Landrigan et al. 2017).

Due to large-scale global application, bioaccumulation and persistence, pesticides are now ubiquitous throughout global ecosystems, including the Arctic (Hung et al. 2016). Emissions of toxic and long-lived substances such as synthetic organic pollutants, heavy metal compounds and radioactive materials represent some of the key human-driven changes to the planetary environment. These compounds can have potentially irreversible effects on living organisms and the physical environment (by affecting atmospheric processes and climate). For example, approximately 800 chemicals have been classified as known or suspected endocrine disruptors and are known to cause a range of serious health problems, yet they appear in common everyday products such as metal food cans, pesticides, food and cosmetics (WHO 2017a).

Stop and Think

Return to the quote from Chief Seattle, specifically the section 'Whatever he does to the web (of life), he does to himself'.

- What is your view about humanity destroying the ecoservices that support human life and societal flourishing? Do you think people are doing this by intent, or through ignorance/disbelief, or lack of care about the welfare of themselves, their children or other people?

Urban environments: bringing it all together

Environmental challenges often concentrate in cities. Case Example 11.2 illustrates some of the key problems, and the global responses to protect urban health.

Case Example 11.2

Urban environments and urban renewal

SDG 11: 'Making cities and human settlements inclusive, safe, resilient and sustainable'.

Over 55 per cent of the world's population live in cities and by 2050 this is projected to increase to 68 per cent, with another 2.5 billion people living in urban environments. Close to 90 per cent of this increase will take place in Asia and Africa (UN 2018b). Cities are engines of innovation and wealth creation but are also sources of environmental stress, pollution and disease.

Extreme weather conditions, displacement from disasters, heat stress, unsafe water and inadequate sanitation, water- and food-borne diseases, mosquito- and tick-borne diseases, food insecurity and air pollution—all converge in the urban setting. Urban slum-dwellers are especially vulnerable. In developing countries, rapid increases in urban population and demand for services, a lack of funding, inadequate planning and pre-existing patterns of social marginalisation mean that large sections of the urban population are lacking in economic power and political voice (Hanna et al. in press). Such a scenario can result in slow alleviation of their unhealthy environments. It has prompted a rise in global philanthropy and development aid, such as the following groups that focus on rapidly urbanising regions.

International Healthy Cities celebrated its 30th year in 2018 with the theme 'Healthy people and healthy places: participation and prosperity for a healthy and peaceful planet' for its annual conference. The Rockefeller Foundation launched a 100 Resilient Cities (100RC) campaign in December 2013 with an initial group of 32 cities (Kernaghan & da Silva 2014). The 100RC aims not only to help individual cities become more resilient, but to facilitate the building of a global practice of resilience among governments, NGOs, the private sector and individual citizens.

Local Governments for Sustainability is a world-leading network of over 1000 cities that aims to help its members make their cities and regions sustainable, low-carbon, resilient, eco-mobile, biodiverse, resource-efficient and productive, healthy and happy, with a green economy and smart infrastructure. These projects have facilitated south–south transfer of good practices between cities.

The Making Cities Resilient Campaign, which was launched by the UN International Strategy for Disaster Reduction in 2010, has acted as a vehicle for local governments to give more attention to disaster risk reduction and to develop partnerships with key stakeholders, including civil society, the private sector and academics. More than 1400 local governments signed up to the campaign and adopted the 10 Essentials for Making Cities Resilient (UNISDR 2013). These ground-level projects provide opportunities for environmental and health promotion practitioners and professionals to jointly develop actions with a health focus.

Care and sensitivity are required. The World Bank 2016 report *Regenerating Urban Land* documents eight cities that underwent successful regeneration (Amirtahmasebi et al. 2016). Inner urban areas with poor education levels, environmental issues, low standard housing and high crime rates were refashioned to return enterprise, green spaces and public access. The report identifies the main objective of urban regeneration projects as local economic development, and lists a range of social benefits that follow regeneration. Gentrification is listed as an 'unintended consequence' of urban regeneration, although it is difficult to imagine planners finding it a surprising outcome. Bulldozing existing dwellings and shops forces residents from their homes, followed by a protracted building phase. Post rejuvenation, higher property values drive the shift towards wealthier residents and businesses, which precludes the return of former residents, who lose their neighbourhoods and networks and suffer significant loss of social capital. The report does not expand on relocation strategies for the poor residents nor how their needs are met.

Failures, consequences and challenges

In 1992, the Union of Concerned Scientists, along with over 1700 scientists from around the world (this author included), including 99 of the 196 then-living Nobel laureates in the sciences, drafted and signed the first World Scientists' Warning to Humanity. They came together again in 2017 to release a Second Warning, this time signed by 20000 scientists, which illustrated the collective damage humanity is inflicting upon planetary resources (Ripple et al. 2017).

Figure 11.3 provides clear evidence that substantial and continuing environmental degradation is occurring across the world's landmasses, the global freshwater sources, the oceans, the air and climate. Humanity's stance as 'guardian of the planet' has unquestionably failed. The current trajectory is a dangerous one. First to suffer have been the disadvantaged but gradually, as degradation deepens, the quality of life all people living on this planet will suffer. Refusal to recognise the impending peril will inevitably threaten survival of the human and other species.

Solutions

Humanity is facing many challenges. But the knowledge is available, and the solutions are known. What is lacking is the collective will to make the transformations to sustainable living. It is not the poor who are leading us down this perilous path.

Figure 11.3 Trends over time in nine key environmental parameters, showing pre (grey line) and post (black line) the release of the first Scientists' Warning

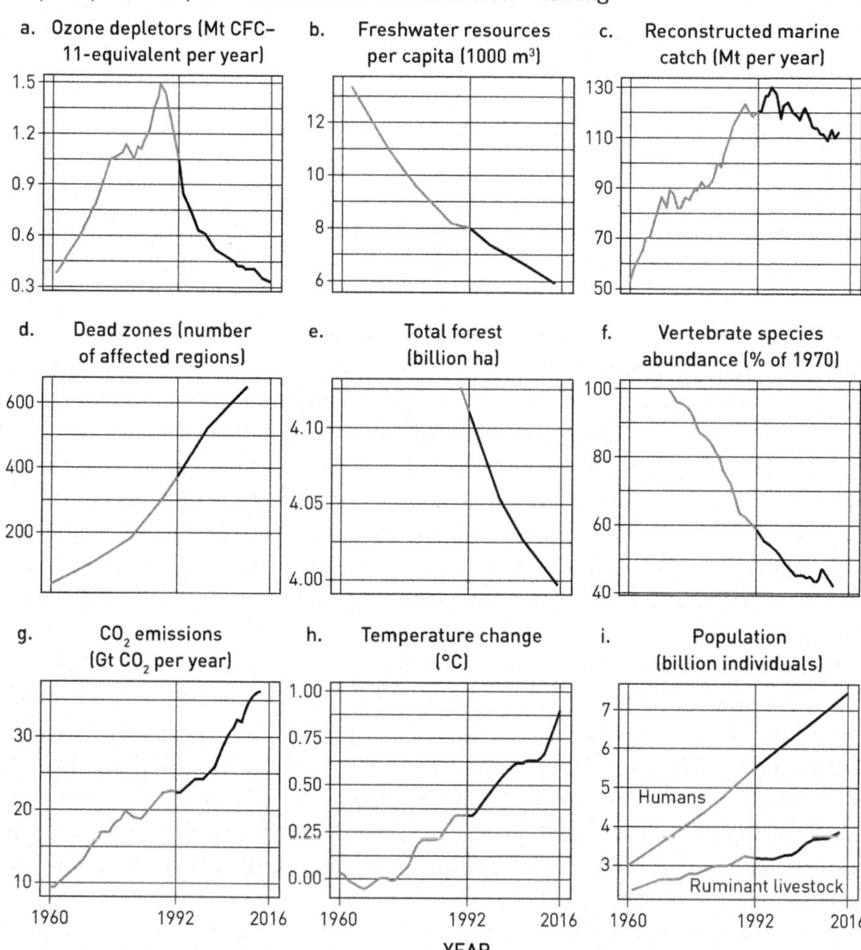

It is the high end and middle consumer class. It is vital to debunk the myth that purchasing more 'stuff' is the answer to happiness and well-being.

The first step towards solving problems is recognising that a problem exists. The second key step involves gaining an understanding of the nature of the problem: its depth and breadth; who is affected, and in what ways; its causes; and its trajectory if left unaddressed. Next, a detailed understanding of what exacerbates the problem and what might alleviate it is required. Such deep understanding does not emerge without effort, and is a critical step towards developing the most appropriate responses. Lastly, given the seriousness of environmental degradation for all nations, all people need to firmly commit to pursuing solutions, unwaveringly and with vigour.

The good news is that in the field of environmental health, this endeavour is well advanced. The UN spearheaded the pathway with the first Earth Summit in 1972 in

Stockholm, which produced the Report of the World Commission on Environment and Development: Our Common Future. The second meeting was held in Nairobi in 1982, the third in 1992 in Rio de Janeiro. It was there that the ground-breaking Rio Declaration and Agenda 21 were born (UNCED 1992).

Johannesburg hosted the fourth Earth Summit in 2002 and in 2012, Rio de Janeiro hosted the fifth, Rio+20. The significance of these Summits cannot be overstated, as they represent a global multilateral response to a global problem. They set the mould for future international agreements to identify and agree to find solutions to reduce and reverse harm. The UN summits led the most far-reaching agreement to date. The Sustainable Development Goals brought international attention to the urgent need for new paradigms for sustainable development. A high level of commonality exists between the SDGs and improvements (Donkin et al. 2018).

When countries abide by an international treaty success is achievable, as can be seen in graph (a) of Figure 11.3, through the Montreal Protocol on Substances that Deplete the Ozone Layer. Another intergovernmental body established under UN auspices is the Intergovernmental Panel on Climate Change. This recruits the world's best climate scientists, researchers, adaptation experts and policy-makers to collate and review all the current knowledge on climate change, its causes, its development, its effects, who is vulnerable and how, and options for mitigation. Reports are released every seven years, after they have been vetted and approved by all governments.

Many other organisations are also working to improve sustainability and protect the planet, humans and ecosystems. The Stockholm Institute's Planetary Boundaries, the Lancet's *Planetary Health* journal and various commissions have been discussed. There are many other groups. Health Care without Harm involves the world's health sectors working together to prevent environmental degradation. It supports the Global Green and Healthy Hospitals Network, which facilitates health organisations across the community and acute sectors to reduce their environmental and carbon footprint (HCWH 2018).

Often, cities and subnational governments are taking action even when their national governments are refraining. Hundreds of cities have created climate change adaptation plans and strategies during the last decade (Sanchez Rodriguez et al. 2018).

There is hope. Seventy years after the Universal Declaration of Human Rights and 50 years after UN Covenants on civil and political rights and on economic, social and cultural rights were proclaimed, the environment is now to receive legal protection. On 10 May 2018, the UN General Assembly adopted a resolution that paved the way for negotiations on a Global Pact for the Environment. This international treaty is intended to enshrine the rights and duties of states, public and private entities and individuals relating to the conservation, protection and restoration of the environment (100 Jurists 2018). The UN started the formal process in January 2019 with the first Conference, entitled 'Towards a Global Pact for the Environment'. Granting legal status to the environment represents a major step forward in protecting human health and well-being for future generations.

Case Example 11.3

Climate change = global inequity writ large

Climate change exemplifies the inequitable situation that lies at the core of environmental injustice.

The wealthy consume planetary resources at a rate that far exceeds consumption by the global poor. Only the wealthy have access to large amounts of space, food, water and the capacity to burn fossil fuels for heating and cooling, and transport. These public goods are used to advance the health of themselves and their family and associates, to advance their education and business interests and as recreational pursuits. The consequence is resource utilisation and waste generation. The global poor have minimal access to all of these. Yet the poor often live in areas exposed to high-level pollution, with minimal social and national infrastructure.

The environmental and health consequences of climate change, which disproportionately affect low-income countries and poor people in high-income countries, have profound effects on human rights and social justice.

Climate change presents within-country and between-countries inequalities. The relationship is characterised as a vicious cycle, whereby initial inequality causes the disadvantaged groups to suffer disproportionately from the adverse effects of climate change, resulting in greater subsequent inequality (Islam & Winkel 2017).

Climate change thus flouts human rights and social justice, by threatening rights embodied in the Universal Declaration of Human Rights (see Chapter 5). These include the right to security and the right to a standard of living adequate for health and well-being, including food, clothing, housing, medical care and necessary social services. Climate change threatens civil and political rights, such as the inherent right to life, and rights related to culture, religion and language, as people are forced to flee their lands and nations to become refugees. Climate change threatens economic, social and cultural rights, including the right of self-determination. High fossil fuel emissions unarguably sentence young people to a massive, implausible clean-up or to growing deleterious climate impacts—or both. Environmental degradation and climate change are grievous examples of intergenerational inequity.

Reflective Exercise

The mantra of the health sector derives from a quote by Hippocrates 2500 years ago: 'First—do no harm'. The health sectors in the US and UK realised that healthcare services were contributing substantially to environmental degradation and global warming, thus contravening their core mission.

Through the Global Green and Healthy Hospitals Network, Health Care without Harm runs the Health Care Climate Challenge. It pledges to meet the challenge posed by climate change—a test perhaps as great as human civilisation has ever known—by taking the following steps.

1. Reducing climate footprint: our collective vision is to reduce our healthcare systems' emissions, moving toward low carbon, and ultimately, carbon neutral healthcare. We will measure and report on our progress, including financial savings related to these actions.
2. Preparing for climate impacts: in order to serve our communities, hospitals and health centres need to remain operational during and after an extreme weather event. We need to understand, anticipate and be equipped to manage the health needs of our immediate community and prepare for shifting disease patterns.
3. Leading the way to a low-carbon future: as healthcare providers respected by local communities, government and business, we commit to provide leadership in our societies for a healthy climate.

The full text of this can be found at https://www.greenhospitals.net/join-climate-challenge/

- Consider your own workplace. What changes might you be able to institute, including enlisting others, to 'Do no harm' to the health of humanity?

Summary

After a long evolutionary history as hunter gatherers, human societal development accelerated with the advent of agriculture during the Holocene. The success brought about by agriculture delivered a range of benefits in health, power and trade. Agriculture gave sustenance and allowed humans to flourish, but we have steadfastly destroyed Earth's life-giving capacity, polluted the waterways and the air we breathe, and disrupted global climate systems. We'd best tend Mother Earth, for without her well-being, we will surely die.

I have described multiple ways in which we risk our health and the survival of our species by damaging various aspects of the environment. Climate change is one of many areas in which human activity is altering planetary forces, and not for the better. Unless every person alive considers their ecological footprint and their carbon emissions, our future is one of reduced food supplies, reduced water availability, polluted air and intensifying climatic extremes, such as unbearable heat, fires, storms, floods, droughts and incursions of rising seas. Resource shortages will drive competition, widen the disadvantage gap and generate unheralded interpersonal and international conflict. The disruption to human society and health will be unimaginable.

We must ask ourselves, would an intelligent species be the architect of their own annihilation? We should join forces with those who are trying to protect our planet and protect our children's future.

Tutorial exercises

1. Consider Case Example 11.1. Discuss in groups why the world is so reluctant to fully commit to the task of mitigating climate change.
2. We produce more than enough food to feed everyone, yet 815 million people go hungry. As reflected in SDG 2, one of the greatest challenges is how to ensure that a growing global population—projected to rise to around 10 billion by 2050—has enough food to meet its nutritional needs. To feed another 2 billion people in 2050, food production will need to increase by 50 per cent globally. Food security is a complex condition requiring a holistic approach to all forms of malnutrition, the productivity and incomes of small-scale food producers, the resilience of food production systems and the sustainable use of biodiversity and genetic resources (FAO et al. 2017).

   Discuss what strategies might serve to reduce wastage and reduce ecosystem damage, while ensuring everyone has sufficient nutritious food.
3. Planetary health situates human health within human systems and ecosystems. It has been said that the threats we face are not restricted to physical risks, such as disease, climate change, ocean acidification and chemical pollution. The risks we face lie within ourselves and the societies we have created (Horton & Lo 2015).

   Discuss how could we change the mindset of humanity to recognise that every person alive affects the planet and that, to ensure health for all, we must tread lightly and equitably share Earth's resources.
4. This chapter described multiple ways in which we risk our own health and survival of our species by damaging various aspects of the environment that supports us.

   Discuss some implications of the issues raised in the chapter, in relation to how you might alter your work practices.
5. Climate change is a result of anthropogenic emission, primarily from the burning of fossil fuels.

   Consider Case Example 11.2. Discuss how climate change presents a glaring example of environmental inequity, social inequity and intergenerational inequity.

Further reading

Hanna, E.G., & McIver, L.J. (2018). Climate change: a brief overview of the science and health impacts for Australia. *Medical Journal of Australia*, 208(7), 311–315.

Hanna, E.G., & Tait, P.W. (2015). Limitations to thermoregulation and acclimatisation challenges human adaptation to global warming. *International Journal of Environmental Research and Public Health*, 12(7), 8034–8074.

Islam, S.N., & Winkel, J. (2017). *Climate Change and Social Inequality*. DESA Working Paper No. 152. UN Department of Economic & Social Affairs. Retrieved from http://www.un.org/esa/desa/papers/2017/wp152_2017.pdf

Kampa, M., & Castanas, E. (2008). Human health effects of air pollution. *Environmental Pollution*, 151(2), 362–367.

Levy, B.S., & Patz, J.A. (2015). Climate change, human rights, and social justice. *Annals of Global Health,* 81(3), 310–322.

McMichael, A.J. (1993). *Planetary Overload: Global Environmental Change and the Health of the Human Species*. Cambridge: Cambridge University Press.

McMichael, A.J. (2017). *Climate Change and the Health of Nations: Famines, Fevers, and the Fate of Populations*. Oxford: Oxford University Press.

Tait, P.W., McMichael, A.J., & Hanna, E.G. (2014). Determinants of health: the contribution of the natural environment. *Australia and New Zealand Journal of Public Health*, 38(2), 104–107.

WHO (World Health Organization) (2017). *Don't Pollute my Future! The Impact of the Environment on Children's Health*. Retrieved from http://apps.who.int/iris/bitstream/10665/254678/1/WHO-FWC-IHE-17.01-eng.pdf?ua=1

WHO (World Health Organization) (2017). *Preventing Noncommunicable Diseases (NCDs) by Reducing Environmental Risk Factors*. Retrieved from http://apps.who.int/iris/bitstream/10665/258796/1/WHO-FWC-EPE-17.01-eng.pdf?ua=1

Websites

https://sustainabledevelopment.un.org/outcomedocuments/agenda21

Agenda 21 was a special product of the 1992 Earth Summit. It is a vast work program for the 21st century, approved by consensus among the world leaders in Rio de Janeiro, representing over 98 per cent of the world's population. It aims at optimising human health without creating environmental harm.

https://www.un.org/sustainabledevelopment/sustainable-development-goals/

In January 2016, 193 countries adopted the 17 UN Sustainable Development Goals—SDGs that call for action by all countries, poor, rich and middle-income, to promote prosperity while protecting the planet. This link opens to the UN Sustainable Development Goals homepage, showing all 17 SDGs.

http://www.who.int/phe/en/

This link takes you to the World Health Organization page for public health, environmental and social determinants of health. From there you can search specific topics.

https://www.unenvironment.org/

This links to the UN Environment Program. While it does not have a dedicated health focus, it links to UN programs that deal with environmental determinants of health.

http://www.ipcc.ch/

This is the home page for the Intergovernmental Panel on Climate Change, the UN body for assessing the science related to climate change. It links to all the IPCC reports, including special reportsand the five Assessment Reports.

http://www.ipcc.ch/report/ar5/wg2/

This links to the IPCC Working Group II report for the latest Assessment Report, AR5. It includes adaptation, a chapter on human health, and regional chapters.

https://www.uclg.org/sites/default/files/the_sdgs_what_localgov_need_to_know_0.pdf

This links to the UN SDGs, focusing on what local governments need to know (United Cities and Local Governments, 2015).

http://unsdsn.org/wp-content/uploads/2016/07/9.1.8.-Cities-SDG-Guide.pdf

Getting Started with the SDGs in Cities (Sustainable Development Solutions Network and German Cooperation, 2016).

https://www.greenhospitals.net/ and **https://noharm.org/**

These two sites take you to the Global Green and Healthy Hospitals, and Health Care Without Harm. The GGHH Network provides a free service to assist organisations reduce their environmental impact, managed by HCWH.

References

100 Jurists (2018). *100 Jurists Call for Action for the Adoption of a Global Pact for the Environment.* Paris: UN General Assembly. Retrieved from http://pactenvironment.emediaweb.fr/wp-content/uploads/2018/10/Appel-EN-1.pdf

ACCSP (Australian Climate Change Science Programme) (2015). *What is Ocean Acidification and How Will it Impact on Marine Life?* Retrieved from http://www.cawcr.gov.au/projects/climatechange/docs/OA_paper_v4.pdf

Alexandra, K., Tracey, H., Patrick, L.K., Arlene, M.F., Ruth, D., Gregor, K., & Chris, H. (2018). Urban versus rural health impacts attributable to PM 2.5 and O_3 in northern India. *Environmental Research Letters*, 13(6), 064010.

Amirtahmasebi, R., Orloff, M., Wahba, W., & Altman, A. (2016). *Regenerating Urban Land: A Practitioner's Guide to Leveraging Private Investment.* Urban Development Series. Retrieved from http://documents.worldbank.org/curated/en/979091467993467764/pdf/106149-PUB-ADD-DOI-ISBN-SERIES-AUTHORS-OUO-9.pdf

Bauer, D.M., & Sue Wing, I. (2016). The macroeconomic cost of catastrophic pollinator declines. *Ecological Economics*, 126(June), 1–13. doi:https://doi.org/10.1016/j.ecolecon.2016.01.011

Brown, S., Nicholls, R.J., Goodwin, P., Haigh, I.D., Lincke, D., Vafeidis, A.T., & Hinkel, J. (2018). Quantifying land and people exposed to sea-level rise with no mitigation and 1.5°C and 2.0°C rise in global temperatures to year 2300. *Earth's Future*, 6(3), 583–600. doi:10.1002/2017EF000738

Butler, C.D., & Hanna, E.G. (2013). Ecosystems, biodiversity, climate, and health. In J. Adegoke & C. Wright (Eds), *Climate Vulnerability: Understanding and Addressing Threats to Essential Resources. Vol. 1. Health* (pp. 69–78). Amsterdam: Academic Press.

Carreck, N. (2016). Decline of bees and other pollinators. In J.F. Schroder (Ed.), *Biological and Environmental Hazards, Risks, and Disasters.* https://doi.org/10.1016/B978-0-12-394847-2.01001-9, pp. 109-117). Boston: Elsevier.

Chen, S. (2014). Agriculture feels the choke as China smog starts to foster disastrous conditions. Pollution is blocking natural light and threatening agriculture, say experts. *South China Morning Post.* Tuesday, 25 February. Retrieved from http://www.scmp.com/news/china/article/1434700/china-smog-threatens-agriculture-nuclear-fallout-conditions-warn

Cole, S., & Buis, A. (2018). *Ramp-up in Antarctic Ice Loss Speeds Sea Level Rise.* NASA Media Release 18-053. Retrieved from https://www.nasa.gov/press-release/ramp-up-in-antarctic-ice-loss-speeds-sea-level-rise

Corvalan, C., Hales, S., & McMichael, A. (2005). *Ecosystems and Human Well-being: Health Synthesis. A Report of the Millennium Ecosystem Assessment.* Retrieved from http://www.millenniumassessment.org/documents/document.357.aspx.pdf

Costello, A., Abbas, M., Allen, A., Ball, S., Bell, S., Bellamy, R., & Friel, S. (2009). Managing the health effects of climate change. *Lancet*, 373 (9676), 1693–1733.

Danckaert, S., & Gijseghem, D.V. (2013). Obstacles to use an ecosystem services concept in agriculture A2—Jacobs, Sander. In N. Dendoncker & H. Keune (Eds), *Ecosystem Services* (pp. 377–379). Boston: Elsevier.

Donkin, A., Goldblatt, P., Allen, J., Nathanson, V., & Marmot, M. (2018). Global action on the social determinants of health. *BMJ Global Health*, 3(Suppl.1), e000603. doi:10.1136/bmjgh-2017-000603

FAO (Food and Agriculture Organization) (2016). *The State of World Fisheries and Aquaculture 2016: Contributing to Food Security and Nutrition for All.* Retrieved from http://www.fao.org/3/a-i5555e.pdf

FAO (Food and Agriculture Organization) (2017). Hunger crises will escalate unless we invest more in addressing root causes, say UN food agency chiefs on visit to drought-hit Ethiopia. Addis Ababa: UN Food and Agriculture Organization.

FAO, IFAD, UNICEF, WFP, & WHO (2017). *The State of Food Security and Nutrition in the World 2017: Building Resilience for Peace and Food Security.* Rome: UN Food and Agriculture Organization.

Haines, A., Hanson, C., & Ranganathan, J. (2018). Planetary Health Watch: integrated monitoring in the Anthropocene epoch. *Lancet Planetary Health*, 2(4), e141–e143. doi:10.1016/S2542-5196(18)30047-0

Hallegatte, S., Bangalore, M., Bonzanigo, L., Fay, M., Kane, T., Narloch, U. … Vogt-Schilb, A. (2017). *Shock Waves: Managing the Impacts of Climate Change on Poverty.* Climate Change and Development Series. Retrieved from https://openknowledge.worldbank.org/bitstream/handle/10986/22787/9781464806735.pdf

Hallmann, C.A., Sorg, M., Jongejans, E., Siepel, H., Hofland, N., Schwan, H. … de Kroon, H. (2017). More than 75 percent decline over 27 years in total flying insect biomass in protected areas. *PLOS ONE*, 12(10), e0185809. doi:10.1371/journal.pone.0185809

Hanna, E.G. (2005). Environmental health and primary health care: towards a new workforce model. PhD thesis. La Trobe University, Melbourne. Retrieved from http://arrow.latrobe.edu.au:8080/vital/access/services/Download/latrobe:19661/SOURCE1 (Open Access Theses and Dissertations. No. 235990)

Hanna, E.G., Kjellstrom, T., Bennett, C., & Dear, K. (2011). Climate change and rising heat: population health implications for working people in Australia. *Asia Pacific Journal of Public Health*, 23(2 Suppl.), 14S–26S. doi:10.1177/1010539510391457

Hanna, E.G., & McIver, L.J. (2018). Climate change: a brief overview of the science and health impacts for Australia. *Medical Journal of Australia*, 208(7), 311–315. doi:10.5694/mja17.00640

Hanna, E.G., Mercado, S.P., & de Pinho-Campos, K. (in press). Urban climate change resilience: a desired health promotion outcome for the 21st century. In V. Lin, S. Fawkes, K. Englehart & S.P. Mercado (Eds), *Health Promotion Systems and Strategies in Asia: Preparing for the Asia Century*. New York: Springer.

Hanna, E.G., & Tait, P.W. (2015). Limitations to thermoregulation and acclimatisation challenges human adaptation to global warming. *International Journal of Environmental Research and Public Health*, 12(7), 8034–8074. doi:10.3390/ijerph120708034

Hanna, L. (2017). *Climate Change: A Risk to Workers? Heat: An Underestimated Threat*. Paper presented at the Justice and Community Safety Directorate, Canberra.

Hardin, G. (1968). The tragedy of the commons. *Science*, 162(3859), 1243–1248. doi:10.1126/science.162.3859.1243

HCWH (Health Care without Harm) (2018). *Leading the Global Movement for Environmentally Responsible Healthcare*. Retrieved from https://noharm.org/ and https://www.greenhospitals.net/join-climate-challenge/

Hippocrates (1923–1995). *Selected Works*. Loeb Series. Cambridge, MA: Harvard University Press.

Hoeppe, P. (2016). Trends in weather related disasters: consequences for insurers and society. *Weather and Climate Extremes*, 11, 70–79. doi:http://dx.doi.org/10.1016/j.wace.2015.10.002

Horton, R., & Lo, S. (2015). Planetary health: a new science for exceptional action. *Lancet*, 386(10007), 1921–1922.

Hung, H., Katsoyiannis, A.A., Brorström-Lundén, E., Olafsdottir, K., Aas, W., Breivik, K. ... Wilson, S. (2016). Temporal trends of persistent organic pollutants (POPs) in arctic air: 20 years of monitoring under the Arctic Monitoring and Assessment Programme (AMAP). *Environmental Pollution*, 217, 52–61. doi:https://doi.org/10.1016/j.envpol.2016.01.079

IRENA (2018a). *Renewable Energy Benefits: Leveraging Local Capacity for Offshore Wind*. Retrieved from http://www.irena.org/-/media/Files/IRENA/Agency/Publication/2018/May/IRENA_Leveraging_for_Offshore_Wind_2018.pdf

IRENA (2018b). *Renewable Capacity Statistics 2018*. Retrieved from http://www.irena.org/-/media/Files/IRENA/Agency/Publication/2018/Mar/IRENA_RE_Capacity_Statistics_2018.pdf

Islam, S.N., & Winkel, J. (2017). *Climate Change and Social Inequality*. DESA Working Paper No. 152. Retrieved from http://www.un.org/esa/desa/papers/2017/wp152_2017.pdf

Kernaghan, S., & da Silva, J. (2014). Initiating and sustaining action: experiences building resilience to climate change in Asian cities. *Urban Climate*, *7*(0), 47–63. doi:http://dx.doi.org/10.1016/j.uclim.2013.10.008

Landrigan, P.J., Fuller, R., Acosta, N.J.R., Adeyi, O., Arnold, R., Basu, N. ... Patrick, N., & Breysse, T. (2017). The Lancet Commission on pollution and health. *Lancet*, 391(10119), 462–512.

Li, X., Wagner, F., Peng, W., Yang, J., & Mauzerall, D.L. (2017). Reduction of solar photovoltaic resources due to air pollution in China. *Proceedings of the National Academy of Sciences*. doi:10.1073/pnas.1711462114

Loladze, I. (2014). Hidden shift of the ionome of plants exposed to elevated CO2 depletes minerals at the base of human nutrition. *eLife*, 3, e02245. doi:10.7554/eLife.02245

McMichael, A.J. (1993). *Planetary Overload: Global Environmental Change and the Health of the Human Species*. Cambridge: Cambridge University Press.

McMichael, A.J. (2017). *Climate Change and the Health of Nations: Famines, Fevers, and the Fate of Populations*. Oxford: Oxford University Press.

Mekonnen, M.M., & Hoekstra, A.Y. (2016). Four billion people facing severe water scarcity. *Science Advances*, 2(2). doi:10.1126/sciadv.1500323

Mora, C., Dousset, B., Caldwell, I.R., Powell, F.E., Geronimo, R.C., Bielecki, C.R. ... Trauernicht, C. (2017). Global risk of deadly heat. *Nature Climate Change*, 7, 501–506. doi:10.1038/nclimate3322

Myers, S.S., Smith, M.R., Guth, S., Golden, C.D., Vaitla, B., Mueller, N.D. ... Huybers, P. (2017). Climate change and global food systems: potential impacts on food security and undernutrition. *Annual Review of Public Health*, 38, 259–277. doi:10.1146/annurev-publhealth-031816-044356

Nerem, R.S., Beckley, B.D., Fasullo, J.T., Hamlington, B.D., Masters, D., & Mitchum, G.T. (2018). Climate-change driven accelerated sea-level rise detected in the altimeter era. *Proceedings of the National Academy of Sciences*, 115(9), 2022–2025. doi:10.1073/pnas.1717312115

Neumann, B., Vafeidis, A.T., Zimmermann, J., & Nicholls, R.J. (2015). Future coastal population growth and exposure to sea-level rise and coastal flooding: a global assessment. *PLOS ONE*, 10(3), e0118571. doi:10.1371/journal.pone.0118571

NOAA National Centers for Environmental Information (2017). *Global Analysis: State of the Climate, June 2017*. Retrieved from https://www.ncdc.noaa.gov/sotc/global/201706

Oxfam (2017). *A Climate in Crisis: How Climate Change is making Drought and Humanitarian Disaster Worse in East Africa*. Retrieved from https://d1tn3vj7xz9fdh.cloudfront.net/s3fs-public/mb-climate-crisis-east-africa-drought-270417-en.pdf

Piñones, A., & Fedorov, A.V. (2016). Projected changes of Antarctic krill habitat by the end of the 21st century. *Geophysical Research Letters*, 43(16), 8580–8589. doi:10.1002/2016GL069656

Ponisio, L.C., M'Gonigle, L.K., Mace, K.C., Palomino, J., de Valpine, P., & Kremen, C. (2015). Diversification practices reduce organic to conventional yield gap. *Proceedings of the Royal Society B: Biological Sciences*, 282(1799). doi:10.1098/rspb.2014.1396

Prüss-Üstün, A., Corvalán, C., Bos, R., & Neira, M. (2016). *Preventing Disease through Healthy Environments: A Global Assessment of the Burden of Disease from Environmental Risks*. Retrieved from http://apps.who.int/iris/bitstream/10665/204585/1/9789241565196_eng.pdf?ua=1

Ripple, W.J., Wolf, C., Newsome, T.M., Galetti, M., Alamgir, M., Crist, E. … & 15 625 other scientists (2017). *Scientists' Warning: 2nd Notice.* Retrieved from http://www.scientistswarning.org/

Rockström, J., Steffen, W., Noone, K., Persson, A., Chapin, F.S., Lambin, E.F. et al. (2009). Planetary boundaries: exploring the safe operating space for humanity. *Ecology and Society*, 14(2), 32.

Rodell, M., Famiglietti, J.S., Wiese, D.N., Reager, J.T., Beaudoing, H.K., Landerer, F.W., & Lo, M.H. (2018). Emerging trends in global freshwater availability. *Nature*, 557(7707), 651–659. doi:10.1038/s41586-018-0123-1

Sanchez Rodriguez, R., Ürge-Vorsatz, D., & Barau, A.S. (2018). Sustainable Development Goals and climate change adaptation in cities. *Nature Climate Change*, 8(3), 181–183. doi:10.1038/s41558-018-0098-9

Schwalm, C.R., Anderegg, W.R.L., Michalak, A.M., Fisher, J.B., Biondi, F., Koch, G. … & Tian, H. (2017). Global patterns of drought recovery. *Nature*, 548(7666), 202–205. doi:10.1038/nature23021

Shepherd, A., Fricker, H.A., & Farrell, S.L. (2018). Trends and connections across the Antarctic cryosphere. *Nature*, 558(7709), 223–232. doi:10.1038/s41586-018-0171-6

Springmann, M., Godfray, H.C.J., Rayner, M., & Scarborough, P. (2016). Analysis and valuation of the health and climate change cobenefits of dietary change. *Proceedings of the National Academy of Sciences*, 113(15), 4146–4151. doi:10.1073/pnas.1523119113

Steffen, W., Crutzen, P.J., & McNeill, J.R. (2007). The Anthropocene: are humans now overwhelming the great forces of nature? *Ambio*, 36(8), 614–211.

Steffen, W., Richardson, K., Rockström, J., Cornell, S.E., Fetzer, I., Bennet, E.M. … & Sörlin, S. (2015). Planetary boundaries: guiding human development on a changing planet. *Science*, 347(6223), 736–747. doi:10.1126/science.1259855

Stein, A.J. (2009). Global impacts of human mineral malnutrition. *Plant and Soil*, 335(1–2), 133–154. doi:http://dx.doi.org/10.1016/j.gfs.2014.09.003

Syktus, J.I., & McAlpine, C.A. (2016). More than carbon sequestration: biophysical climate benefits of restored savanna woodlands. *Scientific Reports*, 6, 29194. doi:10.1038/srep29194

Thompson, D.W.J., Solomon, S., Kushner, P.J., England, M.H., Grise, K.M., & Karoly, D.J. (2011). Signatures of the Antarctic ozone hole in Southern Hemisphere surface climate change. *Nature Geoscience*, 4(11), 741–749.

Tigchelaar, M., Battisti, D.S., Naylor, R.L., & Ray, D.K. (2018). Future warming increases probability of globally synchronized maize production shocks. *Proceedings of the National Academy of Sciences*, 115(26), 6644–6649. doi:10.1073/pnas.1718031115

UN (2018a). *World Urbanization Prospects 2018: More Megacities in the Future.* Retrieved from https://www.un.org/development/desa/publications/graphic/world-urbanization-prospects-2018-more-megacities-in-the-future

UN (2018b). *World Urbanization Prospects: The 2018 Revision*. Retrieved from https://esa.un.org/unpd/wup/

UN Water (n.d.). *Water and Climate Change*. Retrieved from http://www.unwater.org/water-facts/climate-change/

UNCED (1992). *Rio Declaration on Environment and Development. The Earth Summit and Agenda 21* (A/CONF.151/26). Retrieved from http://www.unesco.org/education/pdf/RIO_E.PDF

UNEP (2016). *Rate of Environmental Damage Increasing Across the Planet but There is Still Time to Reverse Worst Impacts if Governments Act Now, UNEP Assessment Says.* Retrieved from http://www.unep.org/NEWSCENTRE/default.aspx?DocumentId=27074&ArticleId=36180#sthash.mT6IbL1O.dpuf

UNEP (2017). *The Emissions Gap Report 2017.* A UN Environment Synthesis Report. Retrieved from https://wedocs.unep.org/bitstream/handle/20.500.11822/22070/EGR_2017.pdf?sequence=1&isAllowed=y

UNEP, WMO & UNCCD (2016). *Global Assessment of Sand and Dust Storms.* UN Environment Programme, Nairobi. Retrieved from http://library.wmo.int/opac/doc_num.php?explnum_id=3083

UNHCR (2017). *Climate Change, Disaster and Displacement in the Global Compacts: UNHCR's Perspectives*. Retrieved from www.who.int/social_determinants/SDH-Brochure-May2017.pdf

UNISDR (2013). *Making Cities Resilient: Summary for Policymakers. A Global Snapshot of how Local Governments Reduce Disaster Risk—April 2013*. Retrieved from http://www.unisdr.org/files/33059_33059finalprinterversionexecutivesu.pdf

USGCRP, Wuebbles, D.J., Fahey, D.W., Hibbard, K.A., Dokken, D.J., Stewart, B.C., & Maycock, T.K. (Eds) (2017). *Climate Science Special Report: Fourth National Climate Assessment, Vol. I*. Washington, DC: US Global Change Research Program.

USGS (2018). *How much Water is There on, in, and above the Earth?* Retrieved from https://water.usgs.gov/edu/earthhowmuch.html

Vaidya, C., Fisher, K., & Vandermeer, J. (2018). Colony development and reproductive success of bumblebees in an urban gradient. *Sustainability*, 10(6), 1936.

van Meijl, H., Havlik, P., Lotze-Campen, H., Stehfest, E., Witzke, P., Domínguez, I.P. … & Willem-Jan van, Z. (2018). Comparing impacts of climate change and mitigation on global agriculture by 2050. *Environmental Research Letters*, 13(6), 064021.

Van Meter, K.J., Van Cappellen, P., & Basu, N.B. (2018). Legacy nitrogen may prevent achievement of water quality goals in the Gulf of Mexico. *Science*, 360, 427–430. doi:10.1126/science.aar4462

Venter, O., Sanderson, E.W., Magrach, A., Allan, J.R., Beher, J., Jones, K.R. … & Watson, J.E.M. (2016). Global terrestrial human footprint maps for 1993 and 2009. *Scientific Data*, 3, 160067. doi:10.1038/sdata.2016.67

Watts, N., Amann, M., Ayeb-Karlsson, S., Belesova, K., Bouley, T., Boykoff, M. … & Costello, A. (2017). The Lancet Countdown on health and climate change: from 25 years of inaction to a global transformation for public health. *Lancet*, 30 October. http://dx.doi.org/10.1016/S0140-6736(17)32464-9), 1–50. doi:10.1016/S0140-6736(17)32464-9

Werrell, C.E., & Femia, F. (Eds) (2013). *The Arab Spring and Climate Change: A Climate and Security Correlations Series*. Center for Climate and Security. Retrieved from https://climateandsecurity.files.wordpress.com/2017/12/climatechangearabspring-ccs-cap-stimson.pdf

Whitmee, S., Haines, A., Beyre, C., Boltz, F., Capon, A.G., de Souza Dias, B.F. … & Yach, D. (2015). Safeguarding human health in the Anthropocene epoch: report of the Rockefeller Foundation–Lancet Commission on planetary health. *Lancet*, 386(10007), 1973–2028. doi:10.1016/S0140-6736(15)60901-1

WHO (World Health Organization) (2014). *Ambient (Outdoor) Air Quality and Health.* Fact Sheet No. 313. Retrieved from http://www.who.int/mediacentre/factsheets/fs313/en/

WHO (World Health Organization) (2016a). *Ambient Air Pollution: A Global Assessment of Exposure and Burden of Disease*. Retrieved from http://www.who.int/iris/bitstream/10665/250141/1/9789241511353-eng.pdf?ua=1

WHO (World Health Organization) (2016b). *Climate Change and Health.* Fact Sheet. Retrieved from http://www.who.int/mediacentre/factsheets/fs266/en/

WHO (World Health Organization) (2017a). *Don't Pollute my Future! The Impact of the Environment on Children's Health*. Retrieved from http://apps.who.int/iris/bitstream/10665/254678/1/WHO-FWC-IHE-17.01-eng.pdf?ua=1

WHO (World Health Organization) (2017b). *Drinking Water.* Fact Sheet. Retrieved from http://www.who.int/mediacentre/factsheets/fs391/en/

WHO (World Health Organization) (2018). *Air Pollution.* Fact Sheet. Retrieved from http://www.who.int/airpollution/en/

WHO (World Health Organization) Director-General (2018). *Health, Environment and Climate Change. 71st World Health Assembly Provisional Agenda Item 11.4.* Report No. A71/10. Retrieved from http://apps.who.int/gb/ebwha/pdf_files/WHA71/A71_10-en.pdf?ua=1

World Bank Group (2016). *High and Dry: Climate Change, Water, and the Economy*. Retrieved from https://openknowledge.worldbank.org/bitstream/handle/10986/23665/K8517.pdf?sequence=11&isAllowed=y

WorldWatch Institute (2017). *The State of Consumption Today*. Retrieved from http://www.worldwatch.org/node/810

WWAP (World Water Assessment Programme) (2018). *The United Nations World Water Development Report 2018: Nature-Based Solutions for Water*. Retrieved from http://unesdoc.unesco.org/images/0026/002614/261424e.pdf

Zhao, C., Liu, B., Piao, S., Wang, X., Lobell, D.B., Huang, Y. … & Asseng, S. (2017). Temperature increase reduces global yields of major crops in four independent estimates. *Proceedings of the National Academy of Sciences*, 114(35), 9326–9331. doi:10.1073/pnas.1701762114

Zhu, C., Kobayashi, K., Loladze, I., Zhu, J., Jiang, Q., Xu, X. … & Ziska, L.H. (2018). Carbon dioxide (CO_2) levels this century will alter the protein, micronutrients, and vitamin content of rice grains with potential health consequences for the poorest rice-dependent countries. *Science Advances*, 4(5). doi:10.1126/sciadv.aaq1012

Chapter 12

Health and the Media

Linda Portsmouth

Topics covered

This chapter covers the following topics:

- impact of the mass media on public health
- utilising the mass media to promote public health
- developing media materials to communicate health messages

Key terms

entertainment-education
health literacy
marketing
mass media
media advocacy
public health communication
semiotics
social marketing

Introduction

The mass media is a social determinant of health. The media plays an important role in the human social landscape and thus forms part of the 'conditions in which people are born, grow, live, work and age' (WHO 2018, para. 1). It is one of the many features of a society that impact on people's knowledge, attitudes and beliefs about health—and thus on their health behaviours. The mass media that people are exposed to, and interact with, has a measurable impact on their health choices and outcomes. Many people gain much of their understanding of health from what they see and hear on television, the internet, radio, social media, newspapers and magazines. The mass media is pervasive and persuasive, reaching population-wide with health information in a way that promotes and normalises the health concepts portrayed. The mass media plays a part in the socialisation of children and adolescents—influencing them as to what to expect and what is expected of them in their society.

The US Institute of Medicine (IoM 2003) identified the mass media as a 'key partner' in 'assuring the conditions for public health' (p. 30) as it 'plays a central role in people's lives' because 'a growing proportion of "life experience" is mediated through communication technologies instead of being directly experienced or witnessed' (p. 307). Dugassa (2016) highlighted this relationship in the context of the politically driven denial of free mass media for the people of Oromia in Ethiopia. The author confirmed that mass media enables a population to build and communicate public health knowledge and take control over their own health: 'inequalities in the distribution of access to information and knowledge are directly linked to inequality in health' with an 'independent media critical to the social transformation of a society and to the betterment of public health conditions' (pp. 66–67). It was proposed that the long-standing lack of mass media developed for Oromo people by Oromo people in the Oromo language from the Omoro point of view is a social justice issue which has contributed to poorer health for the already marginalised Oromo people.

In this chapter, I will discuss the impact of the mass media on health, and how it can be used to promote health. News and current affairs, entertainment, the internet, social media—and the advertising that pays for most of it—often contain messages of public health significance. Public health practitioners seek to explore the impact of the mass media, aiming to describe, quantify and counter any negative influence on population health. We study the effective techniques used by media practitioners and how to work in partnership with them. This enables us as public health practitioners to successfully communicate health messages via the mass media in a way that promotes population health. We seek to influence news and current affairs content to increase people's awareness of health issues, often advocating for a change in policy or legislation. We seek to influence existing entertainment programming and develop entertainment-education media. We have successfully developed social marketing campaigns that include the use of media advertising (among other activities) to promote health.

In the chapter, I will also outline the process by which successful media materials and campaigns can be developed. Working closely with members of population groups at risk allows us to develop concepts, messages and media materials that will communicate most effectively with that particular group—and thus have a greater impact on their health.

Mass media

Mass media
The means by which messages are communicated throughout a society, transmitting the same message to large numbers of people over a large geographical area at the same time—for example via television, cinema, radio, the internet, social media, newspapers and magazines.

Media means 'middle' in Latin and the media lies in the middle of the communication process—between the people who send messages and the people who receive them (O'Shaughnessy & Stadler 2016). The media is the means by which we 'transmit information and entertainment across time and space', with **mass media** enabling mass communication to a large audience (p. 3). The mass media is usually run for financial profit and requires technology and electricity to produce; some mass media also requires technology and electricity to consume at the other end. Mass media is an important mode of communication between the members of a society.

Mass media can be contrasted with 'limited-reach' media, which communicates with individuals or smaller groups of people within a limited geographical area. Limited-reach media includes items such as pamphlets, DVDs, posters, T-shirts, drink bottles, stickers and fridge magnets. Mass media can also be contrasted with 'folk media' or 'popular media'—the traditional media that humans used to communicate long before we could read and write. People everywhere enjoy music, song, theatre, puppetry and dance as forms of entertaining communication. Public health practitioners use folk media when this is the best way to communicate their health message; it might be the most culturally appropriate form of communication for the health issue and the target audience. Folk media may also be valuable if the target audience has low literacy levels and/or limited access to forms of mass media that require technology and electricity.

The traditional dividing line between mass media and both limited-reach and folk media has become blurred over the past 20 years. Limited-reach media such as pamphlets is now routinely put up on websites and gains frequent hits as people search for health information using web browsers. Videos of folk media performances can be seen on YouTube by people all over the world. Some may argue that social media is limited-reach media as people need to sign up to access other members—but how many hundreds of millions of members are needed before Facebook can be considered a mass media tool in its own right? Some commentators refer to social media as 'masspersonal' communication (Johnston 2013). Perhaps a more useful way of categorising mass media is to consider it in terms of its level of interactivity. 'Active' media platforms such as social media and the internet involve users exchanging, sharing and creating content, in contrast to 'passive' media platforms where users have little or no influence, such as watching television (Sterin & Winston 2018).

The mass media constitutes a powerful, far-reaching social influence—particularly with the impact of globalisation of media and the internet over the past couple of decades. Never before, in the history of the planet, has such a large proportion of the population been exposed to the same messages at the same time.

O'Shaughnessy and Stadler (2016, p. 35) argued that media 'shows us what the world is like; it makes sense of the world for us' as it represents, interprets and evaluates the world, noting that many media products 'do not show or present the real world; they construct and re-present reality' (p. 36). However, they acknowledged that media is 'not the only social force to make sense of the world for us, nor does it have total control over how we see and think about the world' (p. 36), noting the influence of, for example, family, religion and education.

Mass media impact on health

Health literacy

People increasingly choose to seek health information via the internet ('Internet self-diagnosis increasing' 2016) and are consistently exposed to health content in the entertainment, news or social media they access. The impact of these mass media messages on people's health is mediated by their level of **health literacy**.

Health literacy
An individual's ability to successfully seek, identify, interpret and act on health information so as to protect and improve their health.

Health literacy was initially conceptualised as people's ability to understand medical information impacting on their treatment outcomes, such as compliance with prescribed medication or appropriate management of their disease or condition (Van den Broucke 2014). More recently, public health practitioners have recognised that people with lower levels of health literacy are less likely to engage in prevention and protection, including adopting healthy behaviours and participating in screening programs (Van den Broucke 2014). The following definition was proposed by Sørensen et al. (2012) and adopted by the World Health Organization (Kickbusch et al. 2013). **Health literacy** 'entails people's knowledge, motivation and competences to access, understand, appraise and apply health information in order to make judgements and take decisions in everyday life concerning healthcare, disease prevention and health promotion to maintain or improve quality of life during the life course' (Sørensen et al. 2012, p. 3; Kickbusch et al. 2013, p. 4). The WHO views health literacy as a 'key determinant of health' (p. 2) and noted that it includes the ability to assess whether health information presented in the mass media is reliable (Kickbusch et al. 2013).

Health literacy levels in Australia are lower than expected of a high-income country with free government-provided education. The 2006 Adult Literacy and Life Skills Survey (ALLS) measured the health literacy of almost 9000 Australians aged 15–74 years (ABS 2008). Less than half (41 per cent) of those assessed were considered to have adequate or better health literacy skills. Health literacy is related to, but not the same as literacy. People can have high educational levels with a well-developed ability to read and write, yet not have highly developed health literacy, and vice versa. However, the 2006 ALLS survey found that health literacy is lower among people on low incomes, older people and those who speak English as a second language and it is higher among those with a university degree and on a higher income (ABS 2008). The WHO recommends that public health practitioners develop 'plain language' communications to enable people to understand health information the first time they are exposed to it (Kickbusch et al. 2013).

Mass media representation of health

The knowledge, attitudes, beliefs and behaviours of many people are influenced by the health messages they are exposed to via mass media. The health issues reported in the newspaper, explored on a television current affairs program, shared by celebrities on the front cover of a magazine displayed at the supermarket checkout, and experienced by characters on television dramas or in movies enter the public consciousness. People are stimulated to think about the particular health issue and, unless they have firsthand experience of it, will tend to think of it in the way it has been presented by the media.

It is important to consider how the mass media can impact on the health of some of society's most vulnerable members: children and adolescents. Strasburger et al. (2014) discussed extensive research which concluded, for example, that aggression is a behaviour learnt from witnessing media violence and that while media violence is not the major cause of violence, it is a 'socially significant … part of a complex web of cultural and environmental factors that can teach and reinforce aggression as a way of solving problems' (p. 193). Strasburger and colleagues also reviewed the literature regarding children's and adolescents' frequent exposure to sexual material via mass media. They argued that most of this material is either suggestive or explicit, with few messages about safer sex and sexual responsibility. The authors noted that several studies reveal that the media is an important source of information about sex for teenagers. They discussed several studies which concluded that teenagers who are exposed to a high level of media are more likely to overestimate the number of their peers who are engaged in sexual activity, and feel pressure from the media to begin having sex; this increases the likelihood of earlier sexual activity.

Stop and Think

Karl is 18 and is planning to go to a bar with a group of friends on Friday night. He wants to have fun and meet new women. He is a bit shy and worries that he will say the wrong thing and not look or act 'cool'. In movies, he has noticed that the main male characters often seem to be having a drink while romantic things happen to them. A TV ad he has found amusing shows sporty guys having a great time drinking beer together and getting the attention of beautiful women by offering them a drink. Karl decides that he will have a few drinks to relax and feel more confident.

- What could be the adverse health outcomes of his night out?
- How do you think his attitudes and behaviours are influenced by the media?

Jasmine is 13. She loves social media and has Instagram and Snapchat accounts. She logs on to her accounts more than 10 times per day. Her parents have never accessed these platforms and do not know how they work or who she is in contact with. She met a friend online two months ago. He says he is a 14-year-old boy who lives a couple of suburbs away. They have been getting closer and he has started to ask about her body and if she has ever had sex. She has not told her parents about this boy because she thinks they would stop her talking to him if they knew she planned to meet him in the local park next weekend.

- What could be the adverse health outcomes of this social media contact?
- How do you think Jasmine's attitudes and behaviours are influenced by the nature of the media she is using?

The relationship between mass media and mental health is another important example of mass media impact. In a review of two decades of research, Klin and Lemish (2008) concluded that the mass media has perpetuated misconceptions and stigma about people with mental illness due to 'inaccuracies, exaggeration, or misinformation' (p. 434). They argued that the mass media tends to portray people with mental illness as male, violent and unpredictable. They noted that through news coverage, entertainment and advertising the mass media has shaped community attitudes towards people with mental illness, and that this acts as a barrier to people seeking assistance. Pirkis and Francis (2012, p. 3) reviewed news reporting of mental illness and revealed that while it often presents a 'distorted and inaccurate' view of mental illness, it is nevertheless ranked as a highly influential information source for both the community and people with mental illness. The authors noted that its promotion of myths and stigma can result in the belief that people with mental illness are dangerous and to be avoided.

There is also a clear link between mass media and suicide. Stack (2003) discussed the 'copycat effect'—that suicides reported in the media trigger people to emulate what they have seen reported. News reporting of real suicides (4.03 times) and suicides of celebrities (14.3 times) are more likely to trigger suicides than fictional suicides in the entertainment media (Stack 2003). Sudak and Sudak (2005) pointed to more suicides resulting from media reports that 'romanticize or dramatise the description of suicidal deaths' (p. 495). An Australian study supported these findings, reporting that 39 per cent of media items resulted in increased male suicide and 31 per cent resulted in increased female suicide (Pirkis et al. 2006). The effect noted by the researchers was more likely if there were several media reports, it was reported on television, and the suicides were completed rather than attempted. Recommendations for media reporting were made by all the above authors and the Australian Press Council introduced standards for suicide reporting in 2011 (see the weblink at the end of the chapter to online information provided by Mindframe National Media Initiative). However, the internet and social media do not have the same editorial control as the traditional mass media. Growing attention has been paid to the negative role of the internet and social media in informing and encouraging suicide, as well as its positive role in tracking the possibility or probability of suicides via the use of key words, and providing suicide prevention information and interventions (Oritz & Khin 2018; Robinson et al. 2016).

Marketing
The strategies used by commercial or non-profit enterprises—including the use of persuasive media communications such as advertising—that aim to change attitudes so that the consumer feels positive towards, and decides to buy or use, the advertised product or service.

Marketing was defined by Armstrong et al. (2017, p. 4) as 'the process by which marketing organisations engage customers, build strong customer relationships and create customer value in order to capture value from customers in return'. Marketing is often thought of as just selling and advertising, but Armstrong et al. (p. 4) described these activities as 'the tip of the marketing iceberg'. Marketing discovers and meets the customer's needs, building an ongoing relationship that leads to profit. Marketers aim to provide the right product, at the right price, in the right place, at the right time—and advertising is one method used to promote this to customers. Advertising has an enormous impact on purchasing behaviours—this is why companies have advertising budgets worth millions of dollars.

Stop and Think

Public health practitioners are concerned when a product or service being marketed has a negative impact on health. Tobacco advertising is an important example. Tobacco was advertised in Australia—and still is in many places in the world—despite clear evidence that it damages health. How do tobacco companies advertise their product? Australians only see tobacco advertising when they travel, or if the tobacco product is promoted by placement in media such as movies or television dramas. Exploration of tobacco advertising gives an interesting insight into how advertising is crafted to be so persuasive. Link to these two websites to see some tobacco advertising posters—but do not be too influenced by them!

http://wellmedicated.com/lists/40-gorgeous-vintage-tobacco-advertisements
http://tobacco.stanford.edu/tobacco_main/index.php

Semiotics
The study of the meaning of signs and symbols (e.g. images and colours) within a particular culture, how they communicate specific information and influence the interpretation of messages.

Semiotics is the study of sign systems and the meanings (feelings, beliefs, ideas) that people within a culture attach to them (O'Shaughnessy & Stadler 2016). Signs and symbols include language, colours, objects, facial expressions, clothing and hairstyles. Note the images and words that were used in the advertisements in the above two internet links. What were the advertisers promising when they placed the words and images alongside the cigarettes they were trying to sell? Analyse the semiotics. The people in the images are attractive and many of them are having a wonderful time with other attractive people. They are shown enjoying a golden and wealthy, carefree and relaxing, or highly romantic life-style. They are having fun, are proud of their choice or are quietly satisfied by their success. There are celebrities or trusted community members (e.g. doctors) promoting tobacco. The Virginia Slims advertisements promise a voice and freedom for women. The Marlboro advertisements link tobacco with a rugged outdoors cowboy life-style for men. Many of the advertisements suggest that sexual success is associated with tobacco. Advertising often presents stereotypes of what is generally agreed as something we should aspire to be, do or have in order to be successful. Stereotypes enable customers to quickly see that desirable people are connected to this product—thus the product must be desirable too. Tobacco advertising offers a wonderful life if we choose to smoke cigarettes.

Case Example 12.1

Television food advertising and children

The levels of childhood obesity are increasing globally, and overweight and obese children are more likely to become overweight adults who are at higher risk of health problems such as cardiovascular disease, diabetes and some cancers (WHO 2010). Using BMI measurements, it has been estimated that between 1985 and 1995 the proportion of Australian children who were overweight rapidly increased by 60–70 per cent and the proportion of Australian children who were obese more than tripled (Magarey et al. 2001; Booth et al. 2003). The 2014–2015 Australian Health Survey indicated that 27.4 per cent of children aged five to 17 years are overweight or obese and that levels have started to plateau in recent years (ABS 2017).

Public health practitioners looked for the reason for this sudden rise in childhood obesity. While it was recognised that there was a genetic predisposition to obesity (Wardle et al. 2008), this did not explain the rapid increase from the 1980s. The 2007 Australian National Children's Nutrition and Physical Activity Survey (CoA 2008) revealed that 26.2 per cent of children did not meet the recommended 60 minutes of moderate to vigorous physical activity per day and 66.6 per cent of children exceeded the recommended two hours of screen time per day. A link was discovered between the amount of television watched and childhood obesity (Wake et al. 2003; Salmon et al. 2006). Public health practitioners wondered if the time spent watching television rather than participating in physical activity had contributed to the development of obesity. The link between physical activity levels and obesity was explored and it was concluded that the obesity caused the lack of physical activity, rather than the other way around (Metcalf et al. 2010).

The Australian National Children's Nutrition and Physical Activity Survey (CoA 2008) also discovered that Australian children's diets were higher in saturated fat, sugar, and salt—and lower in fruit and vegetables—than recommended by the Australian National Dietary Guidelines. Several Australian and international studies demonstrated that children's television viewing was associated with a higher consumption of fatty foods, soft drinks and sweet and salty snacks, and a lower consumption of fruit and vegetables (Woodward et al. 1997; Coon et al. 2001; Coon & Tucker 2002; Lowry et al. 2002; Boynton-Jarrett et al. 2003; Giammattei et al. 2003; Zuppa et al. 2003). Children from families that routinely watched television during meal-times were found to consume fewer fruits and vegetables and more fast foods than children whose families did not (Coon et al. 2001).

During the rapid rise in their level of overweight and obesity, Australian children were estimated to watch an average of 23 hours of television per week (just over three hours per day) (Woodward et al. 1997; Story 2003), with an average of eight food ads per hour. They were estimated to be exposed to over 10 000 food advertisements every year (Story 2003). Almost 80 per cent of the food ads were for non-core foods and approximately 50 per cent were for fast foods, chocolate and confectionery (Zuppa et al. 2003; Neville et al. 2005; Chapman et al. 2006). Children of all ages who watched more television were consistently found to desire more advertised products than children who watched less television. Children asked for and ate the foods that they saw advertised and ate more of them after seeing television advertisements. This particularly applied to obese children (Halford et al. 2007). Giveaways such as toys, and messages promoting taste or fun, were the commonest marketing strategies aimed at Australian children. The most frequently used features were cartoons and scenes of people eating the food in a social setting. Goris et al. (2010) attributed 10–28 per cent of Australia's childhood obesity to television food advertising.

There was a resulting international call to ban television food advertising to children (WHO 2010); this has been put into effect in several countries. Australian parents were concerned about the amount of advertising their children were exposed to and supported tighter restrictions on television food advertising (Morley et al. 2008). The Australian Communications and Media Authority produced the Children's Television Standards 2009: https://www.acma.gov.au/theacma/childrens-television-standards-2009-childrens-tv-i-acma. The standards stipulate that popular characters cannot be used to promote foods during children's viewing times, pressure cannot be put on children to ask parents to purchase, children who have the food cannot be shown as superior, and those who buy the food cannot be implied to be more generous. Recent studies have concluded that the subsequent industry self-regulatory pledges have not reduced children's exposure to television advertising for unhealthy foods and that breaches of the regulations are frequent (King et al. 2012; Roberts et al. 2013; Watson et al. 2017).

Advocacy groups (discussed below) are lobbying for the Australian government to ban advertising of unhealthy food to children, but this has not yet occurred. Some influential advocacy and information-sharing groups include the Public Health Association of Australia, which has written a policy document, www.phaa.net.au; the Australian Council on Children and the Media, https://childrenandmedia.org.au/; Obesity Policy Coalition, http://www.opc.org.au/; and The Parent's Voice, https://parentsvoice.org.au.

Utilising mass media for health promotion

Public health communication
A variety of carefully developed communication strategies aimed at improving or maintaining the health of a population.

Health communication is the 'study and use of communication strategies to inform and influence individual and community decisions that enhance health' (NCI 2002, p. 2). **Public health communication** can be seen as a subset of health communication that 'focuses more on the health of communities and populations', being 'inherently interventionist, seeking to promote and protect health through change at all levels of influence' (Bernhardt 2004, p. 2052). The major mass media communication strategies used in public health communication are discussed in the sections below: social marketing, media advocacy and entertainment-education. Public health communication aims to change knowledge, attitudes, beliefs and, ultimately, behaviours (including behaviours that relate to policy change). The term 'behaviour change communication' is often used, particularly in low- and middle-income countries, to refer to communication programs that aim for behaviour change. In high-income countries, 'social marketing' is more commonly used to refer to such programs.

Social marketing

The most commonly cited definition for **social marketing** is that of Andreasen (1995, p. 7), who explains it as 'the application of commercial marketing technologies to the analysis, planning, execution, and evaluation of programmes designed to influence the voluntary behaviour of target audiences in order to improve their personal welfare and that of society'. Social marketers can be seen as 'selling' health and social development. The advertising on television and radio and in newspapers—urging the community to quit smoking, drive within the speed limit, watch their waistline or increase their physical activity levels—are very visible examples of this conceptualisation of social marketing.

Social marketing
The application of commercial marketing techniques (including media communications) to the promotion of health and other socially desirable outcomes.

Social marketing campaigns have successfully influenced population-wide changes in knowledge, attitudes, beliefs and behaviours of relevance to public health (see also Chapter 6). Campaigns have targeted a range of public health issues (see the list of websites at the end of this chapter regarding current Australian campaign messages, materials and evaluations). Social marketing is suitable for communicating simple messages about public health issues that affect a large proportion of the general population. Current mass media campaigns aim to reduce people's sugar intake and increase their social activity within their community, for example, but there isn't a mass media campaign that promotes safer injecting techniques aimed at people who inject drugs (that very important public health message is best communicated in a trusted face-to-face setting). Messages and images that may offend sections of the community are usually avoided. While there are occasional safe sex campaigns in the mass media, for example, the messages and materials are less explicit than in the limited-reach media developed for specific target groups. Most of the links at the end of the chapter relate to physical health, but the last link—the innovative Western Australian 'Act, Belong, Commit'—is the first population-wide attempt to promote mental health.

Social marketing campaigns are most effective if the mass media campaign is coordinated with limited-reach media and activities within the community that support and extend the reach of the 'brand' and the message (Donovan & Henley 2010). A successful, comprehensive and evaluated Australian social marketing strategy was the 'Go for 2 & 5®' campaign promoting increased consumption of fruit and vegetables (see Case Example 12.2).

Donovan and Henley (2010, p. 1) take a wider view of social marketing, arguing that it is 'the one discipline to embody, within one framework, most of the principles, concepts and tools necessary for the development and implementation of effective social change campaigns'. They believe that Andreasen's definition needs to be extended to include involuntary behaviours—we now know that behaviours are influenced by environment and are thus not entirely under an individual's control. Social marketing, they state, also needs to target policy-makers in order to create supportive environments. They propose that social marketing needs to enable individuals to reach their potential by seeking to change social structures and influence the social determinants of health. Donovan and Henley would thus argue that both media advocacy and entertainment-education (discussed in the following sections) are actually social marketing activities.

Case Example 12.2

The 'Go for 2 & 5®' Campaign

www.livelighter.com.au

www.crunch&sip.com.au

The 'Go for 2 & 5®' Campaign was a national campaign involving mass media (television, radio, newspaper, magazines and the internet). It ran in Western Australia from 2002 to 2012 and was adopted by other Australia states once its success was evident. This campaign developed paid advertising, gained publicity via public relations events, and launched excellent websites. It led to the development of many limited-reach media (e.g. cookbooks, pamphlets, posters, billboards, signs on taxis), point-of-sale marketing (e.g. signs on supermarket trolleys, cooking demonstrations) and school-based activities (e.g. 'Crunch & Sip®', a program involving a break in the school day during which children drink water and eat fruit or vegetables).

Australians do not eat the amount of fruit and vegetables recommended for good health and the prevention of many chronic diseases such as cardiovascular disease and some cancers. The 'Go for 2 & 5®' campaign, as summarised by Pollard et al. (2008a, 2009a), was first run by the Department of Health in Western Australia from March 2002 to June 2005. Research revealed that people knew fruit and vegetables were 'good for them' but they did not know the recommended level of intake and thought that they were already eating enough. Research also uncovered that people did not believe they had enough time or the skills to prepare vegetables. The campaign aimed to increase Western Australian adults' knowledge about the required number of serves, inform them as to what constitutes a serve, increase their perceived need to eat more (especially vegetables), and persuade them that vegetables were easy to prepare and eat. The main target group was the family meal preparer and grocery shopper. All of the campaign materials were strongly branded with the registered, colourful, memorable logo and attention-grabbing vegetable characters based on the celebrities who provided their voices (search YouTube to view many of the television ads). The first message was: 'It is easy to get an extra serving of vegies into your day.' In 2003, a question was added to encourage honest self-assessment: 'How many servings of vegies did you really eat today?'

Pollard et al. (2008a, 2009a) detailed how telephone surveys tracked the responses of thousands of Western Australian adults over time—before, during and after the campaign. These surveys discovered that 90 per cent of adults in the Perth metropolitan area were aware of the campaign, mainly via the television advertising. The surveys revealed that the campaign successfully increased awareness of the recommended servings and improved attitudes towards eating more fruit and vegetables, and that consumption rose as a result. From 2002 to 2005 there was an increase from 1.6 to 1.8 serves of fruit, and vegetable intake rose from 2.6 to 3.2. The proportion of the adult population who reported eating the recommended two or more serves of fruit a day and five or more serves of vegetables rose from 7 per cent in 2001 to 13.4 per cent in 2005. Pollard et al. (2009b) noted the direct link between increased knowledge and behaviour change—people who knew what a correct serving size was, were more likely to eat more fruit and vegetables. Australian states that did not run the campaign did not show any behaviour changes and had consumption levels similar to those in Western Australia before the campaign (Pollard et al. 2008a). The increases were so impressive that the campaign has been implemented by all other Australian states and territories.

This success was not just due to the visible campaign. 'Go for 2 & 5®' also demonstrated the successful impact of the wider view of social marketing (Donovan & Henley 2010). Partnerships were developed between government organisations, non-government organisations and industry to increase the availability of affordable, high-quality fruit and vegetables and to increase opportunities for the consumption of fruit and vegetables within different community settings (Pollard et al. 2008b). The authors listed some achievements that targeted the environmental and social determinants of fruit and vegetable consumption. Examples included the development of nutrition policies for schools and childcare centres, award schemes that rewarded the food industry, promotion of the correct storage, handling and preparation of fruit and vegetables, and supporting welfare agencies in the provision of fruit and vegetables.

Note: Crunch & Sip® is now managed in Western Australia by Cancer Council Western Australia and in New South Wales by the Healthy Kids Association. Aspects of the original Go for 2 & 5® campaign now form part of the wider Live Lighter® campaign which is run in several Australian states by branches of the Cancer Council and/or Heart Foundation.

Media advocacy

'Advocate' comes from the Latin word meaning 'to be called to stand beside' (PHAI WA 2013) and advocacy is 'the pursuit of influencing outcomes—including public policy and resource allocation decisions within political, economic, and social systems and institutions—that directly affect people's lives' (Cohen 2001, p. 7). According to Chapman (2004, p. 361), **media advocacy** aims to 'develop and shape ... news stories in ways that build support for public policies and ultimately influence those who have the power to change or preserve laws, enact policies, and fund interventions that can influence whole populations'. While some advocacy is more behind-the-scenes, such as meetings with politicians or policy-makers, traditional media advocacy involves public health practitioners carefully planning and telling their 'story' so that it is reported in the mass media in a way that can bring about the desired changes in society. Increasingly, media advocacy involves practitioners' strategic use of social media platforms to reach the large segment of the population who access them.

Media advocacy
Using mass media to stimulate public support and obtain the attention and sympathy of policy-makers and legislators, in order to gain changes in law and policy which have a positive impact on public health.

Gaining this kind of publicity for a health issue can be cost-free—unlike the high cost of a large social marketing campaign, for example—but it is less within the control of public health practitioners when the established news media is involved. Journalists and news editors decide what will be reported, as well as how, when and where it will be reported. As Johnston (2013, p. 71) said, 'News doesn't just happen—it is created from the vast amount of daily activity on the planet, chosen by the newsmakers'.

Public health practitioners working in media advocacy need to develop good working relationships with journalists. They need to know what journalists consider 'newsworthy' or 'news value', as this will affect how health messages need to be 'framed' for maximum media interest. This in turn impacts on how journalists will 'frame' the event to make it understood (Johnston 2013). The major news values, according to Johnston (2013, p. 73), are those that have 'impact; conflict, timeliness, proximity, prominence, currency, human interest, the unusual/novelty' and 'money'. Public health practitioners are more likely to have their message communicated if they can provide memorable stories that will connect with people's emotions. They need, for example, to give local statistics; introduce local members of the target group who are willing to be photographed or filmed and tell their story; give a new angle to the issue such as recent and compelling evidence; suggest powerful images that can be photographed or filmed; and involve celebrities or high-profile spokespeople.

Public health practitioners working for large organisations usually have a public relations or media department to assist them, while those who work for small community-based organisations will need to develop media relations skills. After careful planning, the issue in question needs to be brought to the attention of journalists. Large organisations have the skills and resources to hold press conferences; this works well when the issue is of interest to journalists and you are sure they will attend. Many health organisations fax or email media releases (short written pieces summing up the main points about the issue) in order to interest the journalist, to invite contact or attendance at an event. Journalists are often open to clear, concise emails or clear telephone messages, particularly if they have worked with the public health practitioners before. Events can show that many and/or prominent people feel strongly about the issues. For example, a media release can invite journalists to a protest, a public meeting, the presentation of a petition to a politician or the launch of an intervention that is being attended by a politician or a concerned celebrity. Another effective, no-cost strategy is to write a letter to the editor of the newspaper. This way—should the letter be well written and topical enough to be chosen—a public health viewpoint can be put onto the public agenda quickly using a few words in an email. Once media interest is shown in their issue, public health practitioners need to plan for newspaper, television or radio interviews. They need to find and train articulate and credible spokespeople, while being aware that some interviews about urgent issues can happen with little warning!

Social and online media are an effective way to advocate with more control over the messages than that allowed in traditional media coverage. In addition to being the preferred communication tool for an increasing proportion of the population, they can draw the attention of traditional mass media which may report on social media content—particularly if the people involved are prominent. Online polling and petition sites can bring large numbers of people together to take a position on an issue in a way that is easily communicated to those who can create the desired change. For example, change.org is the world's largest online petition platform; it enables anyone to start a petition. There are successful examples of a change.org petition drawing attention to an issue and contributing to a change, with positive public health impact.

Advocacy in Action: A Toolkit for Public Health Professionals (PHAI WA 2013) is an excellent and easily accessible 'how to' guide for public health practitioners. This manual describes how public health practitioners can plan and implement media advocacy strategies—how to write media releases and letters to the editor, how to prepare for interviews, and how to influence journalists and politicians. Also included in the 'Further reading' list at the end of this chapter are two useful manuals advising on the use of social media, produced by the US Centers for Disease Control and Prevention.

Case Example 12.3

Anti-tobacco media advocacy

Australia is an international leader in the use of media advocacy to create supportive environments that encourage people to not start smoking and to assist smokers to quit. Australia has implemented a highly successful multi-faceted campaign encouraging and supporting people to quit smoking: www.quitnow.gov.au/.

Chapman and Wakefield (2001, p. 274), in their exploration of 30 years of tobacco control in Australia, cited tobacco company documents that stated that 'Australia has one of the best organised, best financed, most politically savvy and well-connected anti-smoking movements in the world. They are aggressive and have been able to use the levers of power very effectively to propose and pass draconian legislation ... Australia is a seed-bed for anti-smoking programs around the world'. They chronicled the achievements of tobacco control advocacy since 1970: harm reduction via reduction in the tar and nicotine levels in cigarettes; 'civil disobedience' as activists 'graffitied' tobacco advertising billboards with anti-tobacco messages; banning of tobacco advertising and sponsorship; tobacco taxes; replacement of tobacco sponsorship of sport and arts by using some of the tobacco tax income; warnings printed on cigarette packs; ban on the small packs popular with children; ban on smokeless tobacco; and bans on smoking in transport, workplaces and domestic environments. More recent advocacy action gained Australian government support for the world-first introduction of plain packaging for cigarettes, in 2012. Plain packaging has been found to decrease smoking appeal and increase intention to quit (Wakefield et al. 2013; Moodie et al. 2014).

Smoking rates in Australia have fallen from the peak levels of 72 per cent for adult males in 1945 and 31 per cent for adult females in 1983 (Chapman & Wakefield 2001) to some of the lowest in the world. The 2016 National Drug Strategy Survey estimated that 12.2 per cent of Australians aged 14 years or over are daily smokers, comprising 13.8 per cent of males and 10.7 per cent of females (AIHW 2017). It also revealed that 62 per cent of the Australian population has never smoked and 23 per cent of people are ex-smokers. Statistical projections estimate that if current trends continue, smoking will disappear in Australia by 2028 (Daube & Walker 2008).

Chapman and Wakefield (2001, p. 278) noted that media advocacy 'challenges radio and television audiences and newspaper readerships—including the politicians at whom it is often ultimately directed—to locate themselves in a moral debate'. Of course, we include internet and social media audiences in this discussion. The authors argued that casting the tobacco industry as a 'pariah' which requires heavy regulation was an essential part of this process, giving examples of how advocates framed tobacco as a series of newsworthy issues such as advertising that seduced vulnerable children, and revelation of the hidden and dangerous chemical additives in tobacco. Advocacy's role was to successfully frame the public health issue so it gained the support of the public and politicians, and to communicate problems which require solutions that politicians are usually responsible for finding (Chapman & Wakefield 2001).

Media advocacy in Australia was first undertaken by the advocacy group Australian Council on Smoking and Health (ACOSH), which was formed in 1967 out of frustration with the government response to calls for tobacco control (Daube & Walker 2008). ACOSH worked in partnership with government health departments and non-government organisations such as the Heart Foundation, Cancer Council and Australian Medical Association. Daube and Walker described

ACOSH's attention-getting media strategies which reduced the credibility of the tobacco industry, increased the sympathy of the media, and eventually gained the required legislation. The strategies included buying shares in tobacco companies so that ACOSH members could attend AGMs and ask questions holding a press conference to release a report on the number of body parts removed each year due to smoking; a 'death cards' campaign where doctors sent postcards to politicians when patients' deaths were smoking-related; a report for each MP showing the impact of smoking in their electorate; and presenting statistics in forms that could be easily understood and reported on, such as bookies' odds.

It is interesting to note that, after exploring the concepts of deviance and stigma in Chapter 4, 'smoking, smokers and the tobacco industry are today routinely depicted in everyday discourse and media representations in a variety of overwhelmingly negative ways' (Chapman & Freeman 2008, p. 25). Mass media advocacy and social marketing have been so successful in 'denormalising' smoking behaviour that this national 'culture change' may be impacting on the mental and social health of people who smoke. Smoking is now seen as dirty and smelly and smokers are publicly framed as selfish, undesirable, undereducated, lower-class or addicts who are a drain on health services and should not be employed (Chapman & Freeman 2008). A 2007 Western Australian survey revealed that smokers feel like 'social pariahs' and receive 'disdainful looks' and 'social verbal bashing' when they smoke in public—with many stating that they would consider quitting so that they could 'rejoin society' (Carter 2008, p. 28). This situation presents an ethical dilemma. Public health practitioners used effective media strategies that aimed to reduce the population level of smoking, placing the overall population health good above the mental and social health of the minority of people who smoke. Public health would normally seek to promote the health of all population groups—so this is a rare case where public health is culpable of a negative impact on the mental and social health of a particular group in society.

Entertainment-education

The terms **entertainment-education** and *edu-tainment* were used interchangeably in the past, but De Fossard (2008) noted that a clear difference between the two was becoming widely accepted, and described it. Edu-tainment is education made entertaining, for example by the use of a story, so that learners were emotionally engaged in the educational experience. Entertainment-education is an entertainment experience that is sought out and appreciated by a general audience who are emotionally involved with characters they identify with. Within this entertainment experience, the 'behavior change messages are woven and modeled gradually, naturally and subtly' (De Fossard 2008, p. 19). Entertainment-education connects with people in a unique way. It becomes a part of the social fabric of their lives, and thus a social influence on their health.

Entertainment-education
A mass media vehicle which is designed to entertain a wide general audience while changing societal attitudes and norms. It models and normalises behaviour change that promotes health and social development.

Interestingly, Singhal and Rogers (2004) pointed out that the first recognisable entertainment-education intervention was in Australia—in 1944 a radio series called *The Lawsons* encouraged farmers to adopt agricultural innovations. However, they also noted that, for a long period, the most common form of entertainment-education was donor-supported television and radio soap opera in low- and middle-income countries, which communicated health messages to audiences without much experience of mass media exposure. Barker (2005) described the successful serial drama formula pioneered by Miguel Sabido in the late 1970s and early 1980s, who made an enormous impact on family planning in Mexico using serial television dramas (*telenovelas*). The Sabido Methodology involves a serial drama that captures people's attention and emotions over several months or years. This allows the audience to increasingly identify with the main characters as they change their behaviour slowly, in a realistic way, in a realistic social context—various subplots enable the introduction of different issues in a believable way through different characters (Barker 2005). Techniques used to keep the audiences thinking and wondering about the storylines include mystery, suspense, dilemmas and cliffhangers at the end of episodes (Singhal & Rogers 2004). Piotrow and De Fossard (2004) pointed out that, when communicating health risks that are routine or longer-term, well-written drama scripts can make the health issue appear more important, urgent or dangerous. They mentioned examples such as contraceptive pills being angrily thrown into the fire, with the resulting panic to replace them before morning (highlighting that they need to be taken daily), and a fruit seller whose poor personal hygiene contaminates his fruit, resulting in a stampede of people to the village latrine. Singhal and Rogers (2004) noted that evaluation of this type of entertainment-education reveals that it is memorable—people can recall health messages years later—and has resulted in millions of people changing their health behaviours.

Entertainment-education is now widely applied and many forms of entertainment media are utilised. Some entertainment-education reaches a local audience, particularly when folk media such as theatre is used. Other media, such as comics and *fotonovelas* (stories told via photos with brief dialogue in 'bubble text'), reach an increasingly wider audience via the internet. The scope of mass media entertainment-education ranges from the placement of a few lines of dialogue into an existing mass media program (e.g. the Harvard Alcohol Project; see Case Example 12.4) to an ongoing multi-media TV, radio, internet and print program spanning several countries over several years (e.g. Soul City; see Case Example 12.5).

Case Example 12.4

The Harvard Alcohol Project

The Harvard Alcohol Project (Winsten 1994; Winsten & DeJong 2001) is the first, biggest and most famous example of public health working with existing commercial mass media to successfully promote a health message to an entire population. This project was launched across the US in 1988 and ran until 1992. It demonstrated how a new concept and new behaviour could be introduced and disseminated via entertainment programming to a whole society—and actually shift social norms (i.e. what is considered normal behaviour).

All of the major Hollywood studios and the ABC, CBS and NBC television networks worked with the Center for Health Communication at Harvard School of Public Health to promote the idea of the 'designated driver'—one person in a group who does not drink alcohol at a given event because their role on that occasion is to drive everyone home safely. It was intended, according to Winsten (1994), to give the non-drinker's role social legitimacy and to encourage people to plan for their transport if they intended to drink. The author met with more than 250 television producers and writers who agreed to insert drink-driving prevention messages, including mention of designated drivers, into scripts of top-rated television programs such as *Cheers*, *L.A. Law* and *The Cosby Show*. The characters acted as role models for safer behaviours. Over four years, more than 160 prime-time television programs, with audiences of up to 45 million, incorporated the health message. The networks also agreed to air frequent Public Service Announcements promoting the designated driver concept, a number of prominent individuals and organisations endorsed the message and the campaign was widely reported in the news media (Winsten 1994; Winsten & DeJong 2001).

The term 'designated driver' became a household phrase in the US, appearing in the 1991 edition of Webster's *College Dictionary* (Winsten 1994). Research revealed that, by 1998, 62 per cent of adults who were frequent drinkers had been a designated driver on various occasions or had been driven home by one (CHC 2011). The Center for Health Communication (2011) estimated that a 30 per cent reduction in alcohol-related traffic fatalities was gained over the six years following the launch of the campaign—compared with a reduction of 0 per cent in the three years preceding the campaign. This equated to 50 000 lives saved by the end of 1998.

Case Example 12.5

Soul City, South Africa

www.soulcity.org.za

Soul City: Institute for Health and Development Communication (since 2016, Soul City Institute for Social Justice) is a highly successful, health-promoting mass media entertainment-education organisation. It is a highly recognised and trusted source of health information in South Africa and was the first to address national health priorities with an ongoing, nationwide multi-media strategy.

Soul City was established in 1992 by two medical doctors, Garth Japhet and Shereen Usdin, who wanted to prevent the serious health and social issues that impacted on the lives of their patients. Dr Japhet had been writing a newspaper column but realised that he was only reaching people who were literate (UNAIDS 2005). He discovered that educational programs on South African television might reach an audience of 500 000 and that prime-time television drama would reach more than 7 million (UNAIDS 2005). Japhet and Usdin brought together government, donors and business to develop prime-time, health-promoting mass media that was entertaining and well made (Singhal & Rogers 2003; UNAIDS 2005).

Singhal and Rogers (2003), UNAIDS (2005) and Usdin et al. (2004) described the media materials produced by Soul City and how success is ensured by undertaking extensive research with audience groups to develop realistic scripts that resonate powerfully with the audience. Each year Soul City produces a 13-part one-hour television drama on the most popular television channel; 60 episodes of 15-minute prime-time radio drama (with different characters and storylines from the television series) in nine languages covering all regional stations on a daily basis; and three nationally distributed 36-page booklets which are designed around the television characters and serialised in 11 major newspapers. Soul City also has relationships with newspaper journalists who regularly publish features based on Soul City activities. In 2000, for children aged eight to 10, the organisation began 'Soul Buddyz'—a television series, radio series and print materials. More recently, Soul City has developed a significant social media presence via Facebook and Twitter.

Soul City reaches millions of people in South Africa and the neighbouring countries of Botswana, Zimbabwe, Lesotho, Swaziland, Namibia and Zambia. Series 7, which was broadcast in 2005 and 2006 and focused on HIV/AIDS, was very well evaluated (HDA 2007). Research revealed that 87 per cent of the total adult population of South Africa was exposed to at least one Soul City program component in 2006, with wide reach across rural and urban areas and all educational levels, particularly among black Africans; 76 per cent of women and 69 per cent of men watched Soul City on television in 2006, with 60 per cent of those watching nine or more episodes. The series had a measurable impact on HIV issues, including increased HIV testing, increased condom use and an increased willingness to accept and assist people living with HIV/AIDS. Soul City has been identified by the WHO as an example of best practice in the use of mass media to communicate about HIV/AIDS (UNAIDS 2005). This positive media impact has continued. Evaluation of Series 12 (which was broadcast in 2014–2015 and focused on primary healthcare for women and children), indicated that every episode reached over 6 million people and was one of the top four television shows in South Africa (SCI 2015). The evaluation report discussed the findings of qualitative research which indicated that Series 12 successfully raised awareness, stimulated communication, influenced attitudes and beliefs and facilitated behaviour change.

Soul City has also had an influence on knowledge, attitudes and behaviours relating to many other health and social issues. Usdin et al. (2004) detailed the now famous example of the impact that the 1999 Series 4 had on community practices relating to domestic violence. In one episode, people in a neighbourhood gathered around a house where a husband was beating his wife, loudly banging cooking pots and pans to show their disapproval. This newly suggested practice of pot beating, or making other loud banging noises, was reported to occur in response to domestic violence in several locations after the episode was broadcast and is now widely used across South Africa. The series also resulted in communities organising several protest marches to highlight violence against women. An evaluation of Series 4 reported that it stimulated public discussion of domestic violence; increased recognition of the abuse of women; increased knowledge and use of a telephone hotline; and that many viewers subsequently acted to stop domestic violence in their lives or in the lives of others. Interviews with viewers revealed that some women had invited their husbands to watch episodes so that they could recognise their perpetration of domestic violence, and that some men who saw the series recognised for the first time that violence against their wives was wrong.

Developing media materials to communicate health messages

The National Cancer Institute (2002) in the US has developed a useful way of conceptualising the process of developing health communication media materials (see Figure 12.1). Media materials are most successfully developed when public health practitioners and media professionals follow the four stages described below. This process can be used for the development of mass media, limited-reach media and folk media materials. The process is a cycle because, after evaluating the health communication program they have undertaken, public health practitioners are better informed when they plan for future communications.

Stage 1: planning and strategy development

Adequate time spent at this vital stage will ensure a greater chance of success at later stages, and for the health communication program's overall objectives. Some practitioners want to rush into developing media materials as the first stage of their intervention. However, this usually results in them developing materials that work for them, rather than materials that are effective for the target audience.

Figure 12.1 Stages in the health communication process

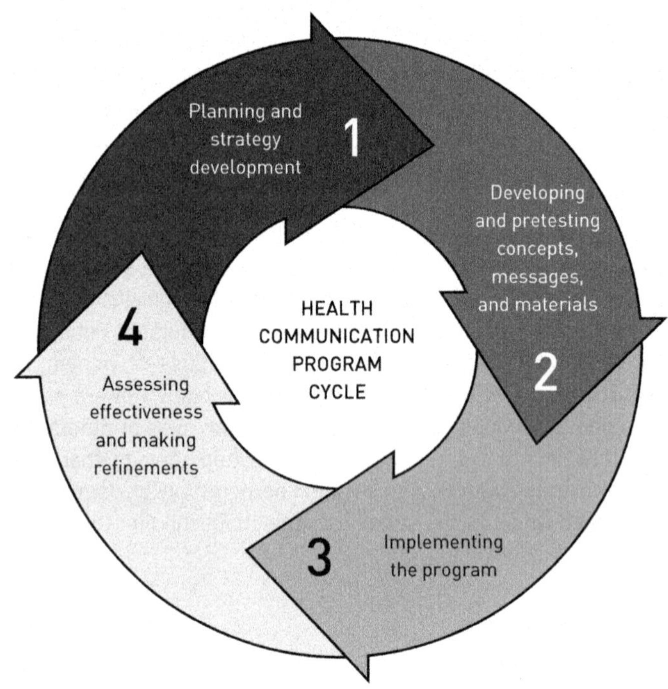

NCI (2002, p. 11)

Public health practitioners first need to assess the health issue and identify all parts of a possible solution. It could be that communication to the community via media materials is not the best plan of action—or that it is an excellent idea but needs to happen concurrently with communication with policy-makers about changes in policy or with healthcare providers about changes in health services. It could be that the communication needs to be accompanied by changes to the physical or social environment. It can be impossible for individuals to decide to change their behaviours if the required enablers of change are not available. We cannot, for example, produce a social marketing campaign encouraging women to go for breast screening if they are unable to access affordable, acceptable screening services close to where they live. It is difficult for people living in remote and rural areas of Australia to 'Go for 2 & 5®' when the local shops do not stock affordable, high-quality fresh fruit and vegetables.

Public health practitioners need to find out as much as possible about their intended audience. The target group may be of a different culture, language, religion, gender, age and educational level from the public health practitioners. Research will often reveal that the target group is made up of different audiences that require different media and messages. Surveys, interviews or focus groups can be used to ask members of the target group questions: What do you know about this issue? What are you doing now? What have you tried before? What happened then? What do you think about it? What do you believe has caused it or is making it worse? What would help you to change? What is stopping you from changing? What would be the benefit—or the cost—of change to you? Do you think it is worth changing? What media do you pay attention to? What media do you believe? What media would you trust communicating about this health issue? Where are you and what are you doing when you access this media? The answers to these sorts of questions are invaluable when developing communication objectives and planning for the communication program. If these questions are not asked, public health practitioners may develop media materials that make sense to them, not to a target group with a different understanding and lived experience of the particular health issue.

Stage 2: developing and pretesting concepts, messages and materials

The first thing public health practitioners need to do in this stage is to review existing media materials and discover if there are any that meet their needs or can be adapted to suit their target audience. If the decision is made that new materials need to be developed, it is useful to work with experienced media professionals who have expertise in research to ensure that the concepts, messages and materials are going to be the most effective for that particular target group. The concepts and messages need to be put together (in terms of words, images, colours and sounds) in a way that is understandable, believable, convincing and culturally appropriate. All of the information discovered in Stage 1 needs to be considered as this will shape the concept and the message. It is best practice to involve members of the target group in developing the concepts, messages and materials. It is essential to then test the materials with different members of the target group to check that they are having the intended effects.

Stage 3: implementing the program

The concepts, messages and materials implemented are as varied as the health issue and the target group. Mass media approaches can be expensive and may not be the correct approach for the issue and target group. Mass media campaigns have been found to work best when an appropriate range of limited-reach media and person-to-person approaches also form part of the plan of action. Public health practitioners can discover the kinds of messages and media that have worked for other people in similar projects, but must always be most influenced by what the target audience tells them. Members of the target audience are the experts on what will work for them, and it might not be what the public health practitioners expect. Public health practitioners may find that directly involving the target group in the program implementation (e.g. peer outreach and support) may enhance the impact of the media materials produced.

Stage 4: assessing effectiveness and making refinements

Public health practitioners need to ask such questions as: How appropriate was the message for the target audience? How effective were the media channels? How well did the message reach the target audience? What changes resulted? To what extent were the goals achieved? Were the benefits worth the cost? Evaluating the health communication program is not something that can be left until the end. Stage 1 activities include plans for evaluation. The program, methods and media materials need to be evaluated while they are being developed and used. Surveys, interviews and focus groups can assist in gaining the required information, but information can also be collected while the program is running. The people delivering the program can record useful information while they work (e.g. number of calls to the telephone information and support line, or hits on the website after advertising appears in print, television or radio).

Reflection Exercise

Consider whether you see the following as questionable.

- A young primary school-aged girl sits with her mother watching a reality television show in which overweight people are shamed and bullied to lose weight by thinner people.
- A group of older primary school girls dance to a music video on television and decide that they are fat because they don't look like the dancers.
- A young teenage girl explores an 'ana and mia' website where underweight female bodies are celebrated and advice is provided on how to prevent weight gain by induced vomiting and avoiding eating.
- An older teenage girl looks at her social media news feed and notices that her favourite celebrity is being widely critiqued for weight gain and there are many close-up photographs of her thighs and bottom, with commentary about her 'loss of control' and 'downward spiral'.
- A woman in her 20s is flicking through a fashion magazine enjoying the new season's colours, fabrics and styles but knows that the clothes only look good on individuals who are as thin as the models.
- A woman in her 30s sits with her male partner watching a movie and realises that the attractive, sophisticated and romantically successful female lead characters are underweight and that the one overweight and bumbling female character is consistently laughed at by the male characters as she attempts to gain their attention.
- A woman in her 40s is listening to the radio as she drives to work. She hears an advertisement encouraging her to join a dieting organisation as women her age always put on weight over winter and that she must lose this weight or be at risk of developing a terrible disease and die early.

- What do these situations say about the pervasive nature of many media messages in our society?
- How might these messages negatively impact on the physical health, mental health and social well-being of females?
- Why does society accept that these messages exist? Should vulnerable young girls be protected? How could they be protected?

We need to take time to analyse the media messages that surround us. We may not even notice what is being communicated—we have grown up with these messages being part of our society. We may even have internalised the messages so that we unquestioningly apply them to ourselves.

- Why is media content constructed as it is? Should there be a change? How could we achieve change? Is change even possible?

Summary

Mass media constitutes a powerful social determinant of health. Many people gain much of their understanding of health from messages in the mass media. This influences their health knowledge, attitudes, beliefs and behaviours.

Mass media can have a negative impact on health. Media representation and reporting of violence, sexuality, mental health and suicide, for example, have been implicated in poor health outcomes. The marketing of products and services detrimental to health (such as tobacco) are of public health concern. Public health practitioners need to recognise and study these negative impacts—then act to counter them.

Once the mass media impacts on health are understood, public health practitioners can use this knowledge to work in partnership with media professionals to utilise mass media to promote health. Social marketing, media advocacy and entertainment-education are the forms this activity usually takes—all have demonstrated a strong positive impact on public health.

Public health professionals need to carefully plan, implement and evaluate health communication programs. It is vital, at all stages of the health communication process, to work closely with members of the media audience (target group) in order to successfully develop media materials to communicate appropriate health messages.

Tutorial exercises

Watch the American documentary *Super Size Me*, which was nominated for the Academy Award for Best Documentary in 2005. It is available via many online video streaming services. The film documents one man's decision to consume McDonald's food and drink every meal for 30 days—and the impact on his physical and mental health. Note how the documentary was made.

1. What role do you think fast food marketing plays in the obesity epidemic?
2. What did the film-makers choose (in terms of words, vision, sound, music and graphics) to make the film more persuasive?

Watch a commercial television station during a timeslot for children's programs. Note the advertisements for food and drink. Choose one, record it and bring it to class.

3. What messages are being communicated by the advertisement?
4. What stereotypes, images, sounds, music and colours were brought together to make the advertisement more persuasive to children?
5. Do you think the advertisement adheres to the Australian Children's Television Standards?

Find an internet site that is potentially harmful to health. It may contain incorrect information, have information presented with bias (e.g. a commercial site selling 'cures'), or openly promote poor health choices (e.g. anorexia, suicide).

6. What are the main messages being communicated, and how were they communicated? What words, images, colours and sound were used—and what do those choices communicate?
7. Is the site presented as being more credible than it really is? Does it contain references for any scientific information? Does it contain advertising? What other sites does it link to?
8. Is it clear who wrote it and how you can contact them? How might it harm health?

Link to the examples of the Australian social marketing campaign websites listed below. Watch their television advertisements. For each advertisement, note the way it has been constructed and answer the following questions.

9. Who do you think the target group is?
10. What is the key message?
11. What do you think the initial research revealed about the target audience?

Further reading

CDCP (Centers for Disease Control and Prevention) (2011). *The Health Communicator's Social Media Toolkit*. Atlanta: CDC, US Department of Health and Human Services. Retrieved from www.cdc.gov/socialmedia/tools/guidelines/pdf/socialmediatoolkit_bm.pdf

CDCP (Centers for Disease Control and Prevention) (2012). *CDC's Guide to Writing for Social Media*. Atlanta: CDC, US Department of Health and Human Services. Retrieved from www.cdc.gov/socialmedia/Tools/guidelines/pdf/GuidetoWritingforSocialMedia.pdf

Donovan, R., & Henley, N. (2010). *Principles and Practice of Social Marketing: An International Perspective*, 2nd edn. Melbourne: IP Communications.

NCI (National Cancer Institute) (2002). *Making Health Communication Programs Work*. Bethesda, MD: National Institutes of Health, US Department of Health and Human Services. Retrieved from https://www.cancer.gov/publications/health-communication/pink-book.pdf

O'Shaughnessy, M., & Stadler, J.M. (2016). *Media and Society*, 6th edn. Melbourne: Oxford University Press.

PHAI WA (Public Health Advocacy Institute of Western Australia) (2013). *Advocacy in Action: A Toolkit for Public Health Professionals*, 3rd edn. Perth: Curtin University. www.phaiwa.org.au/wp-content/uploads/2015/12/PHAIWA-Advocacy-in-Action-3rd-Edition.pdf

Websites

www.comminit.com

The Communication Initiative Network connects people all over the world so they can share their work in media communication to promote health, peace and social development.

www.cdc.gov/healthcommunication

The Centers for Disease Control and Prevention's 'gateway' to many health communication and social marketing resources.

www.jhuccp.org

Center for Communication Programs, Johns Hopkins Bloomberg School of Public Health, promotes international public health through partnering organisations to assist in health communication. This website links to many resources such as downloadable publications/reports and examples of health communication materials.

www.populationmedia.org

The Population Media Center works to improve global health through the use of entertainment-education strategies. This website shares its current projects and links to many resources.

www.communicationforsocialchange.org

The Communication for Social Change Consortium is a non-profit organisation working globally to help people living in poor communities to communicate in such a way as to influence the change they need in their societies and in their lives.

http://www.mindframe-media.info/for-media/reporting-suicide

http://www.mindframe-media.info/for-media/reporting-mental-illness

Mindframe National Media Initiative provides guidelines for the reporting and portrayal of mental illness and suicide in Australia.

www.alcoholthinkagain.com.au

https://www.rsc.wa.gov.au/Your-Safety/Safety-Topics

https://campaigns.health.gov.au/drughelp/resources

https://playsafe.health.nsw.gov.au/

http://www.quitnow.gov.au/internet/quitnow/publishing.nsf/Content/campaigns

https://livelighter.com.au/

www.actbelongcommit.org.au

Interesting examples of Australian social marketing campaigns and health communication media materials.

www.phaiwa.org.au

The Public Health Advocacy Institute of Western Australia.

References

ABS (Australian Bureau of Statistics) (2008). *Health Literacy, Australia 2006*. Cat. No. 4233.0. Retrieved from http://www.abs.gov.au/ausstats/abs@.nsf/Latestproducts/4233.0Main%20Features22006

ABS (Australian Bureau of Statistics) (2017). *National Health Survey: First Results, 2014–15. Children's Risk Factors.* Cat. No. 4364.0.55.001. Retrieved from http://www.abs.gov.au/ausstats/abs@.nsf/Lookup/by%20Subject/4364.0.55.001~2014-15~Main%20Features~Children's%20risk%20factors~31

AIHW (Australian Institute of Health and Welfare) (2017). *National Drug Strategy Household Survey 2016: Detailed Findings.* Drug Statistics Series31. Cat. No. PHE 214. Retrieved from https://www.aihw.gov.au/getmedia/15db8c15-7062-4cde-bfa4-3c2079f30af3/21028a.pdf.aspx?inline=true

Andreasen, A. (1995). *Marketing Social Change: Changing Behaviour to Promote Health, Social Development, and the Environment*. San Francisco: Jossey-Bass.

Armstrong, G., Adam, S., Denize, S.M., Volkov, M., & Kotler, P. (2017). *Principles of Marketing*, 7th edn. Melbourne: Pearson Australia.

Barker, K. (2005). Sex, soap, and social change: the Sabido methodology. In M. Haider (Ed.), *Global Public Health Communication: Challenges, Perspectives, and strategies* (pp. 113–153). Subury, MA: Jones & Bartlett Publishers.

Bernhardt, J.M. (2004). Communication is at the core of effective public health. *American Journal of Public Health*, 94(12), 2051–2052.

Booth, M.L., Chey, T., Wake, M., Norton, K., Hesketh, K., Dollman, J., & Robertson, I. (2003). Change in the prevalence of overweight and obesity among young Australians, 1969–1997. *American Journal of Clinical Nutrition*, 77, 29–36.

Boynton, R., Thomas, T., Peterson, R., Wiecha, J., Sobol, A., & Gortmaker, S. (2003). Impact of television viewing patterns on fruit and vegetable consumption among children and adolescents. *Pediatrics*, 112(6), 1321–1326.

Carter, O. (2008). Changes in the attitudes and beliefs of West Australian smokers, 1984–2007. In Cancer Council Western Australia, The Progress of Tobacco Control in Western Australia: Achievements, Challenges and Hopes for the Future (pp. 23–29). Perth: Cancer Council Western Australia. Retrieved from http://www.cancerwa.asn.au/resources/2010-07-07-Tobacco-Control-Monograph.pdf

Chapman, K., Nicholas, P., & Supramaniam, R. (2006). How much food advertising is on the Australian television? *Health Promotion International*, 21(3), 172–180.

Chapman, S. (2004). Advocacy for public health: a primer. *Journal of Epidemiology and Community Health*, 58, 361–365.

Chapman, S., & Freeman, B. (2008). Markers of the denormalisation of smoking and the tobacco industry. *Tobacco Control*, 17(1), 25–31.

Chapman, S., & Wakefield, M. (2001). Tobacco control advocacy in Australia: reflections on 30 years of progress. *Health Education and Behavior*, 28(3), 274–289.

CHC (Center for Health Communication, Harvard School of Public Health) (2011). *Harvard Alcohol Project*. Retrieved from https://www.hsph.harvard.edu/chc/harvard-alcohol-project/

CoA (Commonwealth of Australia) (2008). *2007 Australian National Children's Nutrition and Physical Activity Survey: Main Findings*. Retrieved from www.health.gov.au/internet/main/publishing.nsf/Content/health-pubhlth-strateg-food-monitoring.htm#07survey

Cohen, D. (2001). Advocacy: its many faces and a common understanding. In D. Cohen, R. De la Vega & G. Watson. (Eds), *Advocacy for Social Justice: A Global Action and Reflection Guide*. Bloomfield, Conn.: Kumarian Press.

Coon, K.A., Goldberg, J., Rogers, B.L., & Tucker, K.L. (2001). Relationship between use of television during meals and children's food consumption patterns. *Pediatrics*, 107(1), e7.

Coon, K.A., & Tucker, K.L. (2002). Television and children's consumption patterns: a review of the literature. *Minerva Pediatrica*, 54(5), 423–436.

Dart, J. (2008). The internet as a source of health information in three disparate communities. *Australian Health Review*, 32(3), 559–569.

Daube, M., & Walker, N. (2008). Advocating for tobacco control in Western Australia, 1971 to the present. In Cancer Council Western Australia, The Progress of Tobacco Control in Western Australia: Achievements, Challenges and Hopes for the Future (pp. 55–70). Perth: Cancer Council Western Australia. Retrieved from http://www.cancerwa.asn.au/resources/2010-07-07-Tobacco-Control-Monograph.pdf

De Fossard, E. (2008). *Using Edu-tainment for Distance Education in Community Work*. Communication for Behavior Change, Vol. 3. New Delhi: Sage.

Donovan, R., & Henley, N. (2010). *Principles and Practice of Social Marketing: An International Perspective*, 2nd edn. Melbourne: IP Communications.

Dugassa, B.F. (2016). Free media as the social determinants of health: the case of Oromia regional state in Ethiopia. *Open Journal of Preventative Medicine*, 6, 65–83.

Giammattei, J., Blix, G., Marshak, H.H., Wollitzer, A.O., & Pettitt, D.J. (2003). Television watching and soft drink consumption: associations with obesity in 11 to 13 year old children. *Archives of Pediatrics and Adolescent Medicine*, 157(9), 882–843.

Goris, J.M., Peterssen, S., Stamatakis, E., & Veerman, J.L. (2010). Television food advertising and the prevalence of childhood overweight and obesity: a multicountry comparison. *Public Health Nutrition*, 13(7), 1003–1012.

Halford, J.C.G., Boyland, E.J., Brown, V., Highes, G.M., Stacey, L., McKean, S., & Dovey, T.M. (2007). Beyond-brand effect of television food advertisements on food choice in children: the effects of weight status. *Public Health Nutrition*, 11(9), 897–904.

HDA (Health and Development Africa) (2007). *Soul City, It's Real: Evaluation Report.* Series 7. Retrieved from https://www.soulcity.org.za/research/evaluations/series/soul-city/soul-city-its-real-evaluation-report-2007

Henson, C., Chapman, S., McLeod, L., Johnson, N., McGeechan, K., & Hickie, I. (2009). More us than them: positive depictions of mental illness on Australian television news. *Australian and New Zealand Journal of Psychiatry*, 43, 554–560.

Internet self-diagnosis increasing (2016). *Australian Pharmacist*, 35(2), 22.

IoM (Institute of Medicine) (2003). *The Future of the Public's Health in the 21st Century*. Washington, DC: National Academies Press.

Johnston, J. (2013). *Media Relations: Issues and Strategies,* 6th edn. Sydney: Allen & Unwin.

Kelly, B., Smith, B., King, L., Flood, V., & Bauman, A. (2007). Television food advertising to children: the extent and nature of exposure. *Public Health Nutrition*, 10(11), 1234–1240.

Kickbusch, I., Pelikan, J.M., Apfel, F., & Tsouros, A.D. (2013). *Health Literacy: The Solid Facts*. Copenhagen: WHO Regional Office for Europe. Retrieved from http://www.euro.who.int/__data/assets/pdf_file/0008/190655/e96854.pdf

King, L., Hebden, L., Grunseit, A., Kelly, B., & Chapman, K. (2012). Building the case for independent monitoring of food advertising on Australian television. *Public Health Nutrition*, 16(12), 2249–2254.

Klin, A., & Lemish, D. (2008). Mental disorders stigma in the media: review of studies on production, content, and influences. *Journal of Communication*, 13(5), 434–449.

Lowry, R., Wechsler, H., Galuska, D.A., Fulton, J.E., & Kann, L. (2002). Television viewing and its associations with overweight, sedentary lifestyle, and insufficient consumption of fruits and vegetables among US high school students: differences by race, ethnicity, and gender. *Journal of School Health*, 72(10), 413–421.

Magarey, A.M., Daniels, M., & Boulton, T.J. (2001). Prevalence of overweight and obesity in Australian children and adolescents; reassessment of 1985 and 1995 data against new standard definitions. *Medical Journal of Australia*, 174, 561–565.

Metcalf, B., Hosking, J., Jeffery, A., Voss, L., Henley, W., & Wilkin, T. (2010). Fatness leads to inactivity, but inactivity does not lead to fatness: a longitudinal study in children. *Archives of Disease in Children*, 95(6), 1–6.

Moodie, C., Bauld, L., Ford, A., & Mackintosh, A.M. (2014). Young women smokers' response to using plain cigarette packaging: qualitative findings from a naturalistic study. *BMC Public Health*, 14, 812.

Morley, B., Chapman, K., Mehta, K., King, L., Swinburn, B., & Wakefield, M. (2008). Parental awareness and attitudes about food advertising to children in Australian television. *Australian and New Zealand Journal of Public Health*, 32(4), 341–347.

NCI (National Cancer Institute) (2002). *Making Health Communication Programs Work*. Bethesda, MD: National Institutes of Health, US Department of Health and Human Services. Retrieved from https://www.cancer.gov/publications/health-communication/pink-book.pdf

Neville, L., Thomas, M., & Bauman, A. (2005). Food advertising on Australian television: the extent of children's exposure. *Health Promotion International*, 20(2), 105–112.

Oritz, P., & Khin, E.K. (2018). Traditional and new media influence on suicidal behaviour and contagion. *Behavioral Sciences and the Law*, 36(2), 245–246.

O'Shaughnessy, M., & Stadler, J.M. (2016). *Media and Society*, 6th edn. Melbourne: Oxford University Press.

Pfefferbaum, B., Doughty, D.E., Reddy, C., Patel, N., Gurwitch, R.H., Nixon, S.J., & Tivis, R.D. (2002). Exposure and peritraumatic response as predictors of posttraumatic stress in children following the 1995 Oklahoma City Bombing. *Journal of Urban Health*, 79(3), 354–363.

PHAI WA (Public Health Advocacy Institute of Western Australia) (2013). *Advocacy in Action: A Toolkit for Public Health Professionals*, 3rd edn. Perth: Curtin University. Retrieved from www.phaiwa.org.au/wp-content/uploads/2015/12/PHAIWA-Advocacy-in-Action-3rd-Edition.pdf

Piotrow, P.T., & De Fossard, E. (2004). Entertainment-education as a public health intervention. In A. Singhal, M.J. Cody, E.M. Rogers & M. Sabido (Eds), *Entertainment-education and Social Change: History, Research, and Practice* (pp. 39–60). Mahwah, NJ: Lawrence Erlbaum Associates.

Pirkis, J.E, Burgess, P.M., Francis, C., Blood, R.W., & Jolley, D.J. (2006). The relationship between media reporting of suicide and actual suicide in Australia. *Social Science and Medicine*, 62, 2874–2886.

Pirkis, J., & Francis, C. (2012). *Mental Illness in the News and the Information Media: A Critical Review*. Canberra: Department of Health and Aged Care.

Pollard, C.M., Miller, M., Daly, A.M., Crouchley, K.E., O'Donoghue, K.J., Lang, A.J., & Binns, C.W. (2008a). Increasing fruit and vegetable consumption: success of the Western Australian Go for 2&5® campaign. *Public Health Nutrition*, 11(3), 314–320.

Pollard, C.M., Lewis, J.M., & Binns, C.W. (2008b). Selecting interventions to promote fruit and vegetable consumption: from policy to action, a planning framework case study in Western Australia. *Australia and New Zealand Health Policy*, 5(27), 7 pages. Retrieved from http://www.anzhealthpolicy.com/content/5/1/27

Pollard, C.M., Miller, M., Woodman, R.J., Meng, R., & Binns, C.W. (2009a). Changes in knowledge, beliefs, and behaviors related to fruit and vegetable consumption among Western Australian adults from 1995 to 2004. *American Journal of Public Health*, 99(2), 355–361.

Pollard, C.M., Daly, A.M., & Binns, C.W. (2009b). Consumer perceptions of fruit and vegetables serving sizes. *Public Health Nutrition,* 12(5), 637–643.

Roberts, M., Pettigrew, S., Chapman, K., Miller, C., & Quester, P. (2012). Compliance with children's television food advertising regulations in Australia. *BMC Public Health,* 12, 846.

Robinson, J., Cox, G., Bailey, E., Hetrick, S., Rodrigues, M., Fisher, S., & Herrman, H. (2016). Social media and suicide prevention: a systematic review. *Early Intervention in Psychiatry*, 10, 103–121.

Salmon, J., Campbell, K., & Crawford, D. (2006). Television viewing habits associated with obesity risk factors; a survey of Melbourne school children. *Medical Journal of Australia,* 184(2), 64–67.

Saylor, C.F., Cowart, B.L., Lipovsky, J.A., Jackson, C., & Finch, A.J. (2003). Media exposure to September 11: elementary school students' experiences and posttraumatic symptoms. *American Behavioral Scientist*, 46(12), 1622–1642.

SCI (Soul City Institute) (2015). *Audience Reception Report.* Soul City Series 12. Retrieved from https://www.soulcity.org.za/research/evaluations/series/soul-city/soul-city-series-12/soul-city-series-12-audience-reception-report/view

Singhal, A., & Rogers, E.M. (2003). *Combating AIDS: Communication Strategies in Action.* New Delhi: Sage.

Singhal, A., & Rogers, E.M. (2004). The status of entertainment-education worldwide. In A. Singhal, M.J. Cody, E.M. Rogers & M. Sabido (Eds), *Entertainment-education and Social Change: History, Research, and Practice* (pp. 3–20). Mahwah, NJ: Lawrence Erlbaum Associates.

Sørensen, K., Van den Broucke, S., Fullam, J., Doyle, G., Pelikan, J., Slonka, Z., & Brand, H. (2012). Health literacy and public health: a systematic review and integration of definitions and models. *BMC Public Health*, 12(80), 13 pages. Retrieved from https://bmcpublichealth.biomedcentral.com/track/pdf/10.1186/1471-2458-12-80

Stack, S. (2003). Media coverage as a risk factor in suicide. *Journal of Epidemiology and Community Health*, 57, 238–240.

Sterin, J.C., & Winston, T. (2018). *Mass Media Revolution*, 3rd edn. New York: Routledge.

Story, M. (2003). Television and food advertising: an international threat to children? *Nutrition & Dietetics*, 60(2), 72–73.

Strasburger, V.C., Wilson, B.J., & Jordan, A.B. (2014). *Children, Adolescents, and the Media*, 3rd edn. Thousand Oaks, CA: Sage.

Sudak, H.S., & Sudak, D.M. (2005). The media and suicide. *Academic Psychiatry*, 29(5), 495–499.

UNAIDS (Joint United Nations Programme on HIV/AIDS) (2005). *Getting the Message Across: The Mass Media and the Response to HIV/AIDS*. UNAIDS Best Practice Collection. UNAIDS Ca. No. UNAIDS/05.29E. Retrieved from http://data.unaids.org/Publications/IRC-pub06/jc1094-mediasa-bp_en.pdf

Usdin, S., Singhal, A., Shongwe, T., Goldstein, S., & Shabalala, A. (2004). No short cuts in entertainment-education: designing Soul City step-by-step. In A. Singhal, M.J. Cody, E.M. Rogers, & M. Sabido (Eds), *Entertainment-education and Social*

Change: History, Research, and Practice (pp. 153–175). Mahwah, NJ: Lawrence Erlbaum Associates.

Van den Broucke, S. (2014). Health literacy: a critical concept for public health. *Archives of Public Health*, 72 (10), 2 pages. Retrieved from https://archpublichealth.biomedcentral.com/articles/10.1186/2049-3258-72-10

Wake, M., Hesketh, K., & Waters, E. (2003). Television, computer use and body mass index in Australian primary school children. *Journal of Paediatrics and Child Health*, 39, 130–134.

Wakefield, M.A., Hayes, L., Durkin, S., & Borland, R. (2013). Introduction effects of the Australian plain packaging policy on adult smokers: a cross-sectional study. *BMJ Open* 3, e003175 (9 pages).

Wardle, J., Carnell, S., Haworth, C., & Plomin, R. (2008). Evidence for a strong genetic influence on childhood adiposity despite the force of the obesogenic environment. *American Journal of Clinical Nutrition*, 87(2), 398–404.

Watson, W.L., Lau, V., Wellard, L., Hughes, C., & Chapman, K. (2017). Advertising to children initiatives have not reduced unhealthy food advertising on Australian television. *Journal of Public Health*, 39(4), 787–792.

WHO (World Health Organization) (2010). *Set of Recommendations on the Marketing of Food and Non-alcoholic Beverages to Children*. Retrieved from http://whqlibdoc.who.int/publications/2010/9789241500210_eng.pdf

WHO (World Health Organization) (2018). *Social Determinants of Health*. Retrieved from http://www.who.int/social_determinants/sdh_definition/en/

Winsten, J.A. (1994). Promoting designated drivers: the Harvard Alcohol Project. *American Journal of Preventative Medicine*, 10(3), S11–S14.

Winsten, J.A., & DeJong, W. (2001). The designated driver campaign. In R.E. Rice & C.K. Atkin (Eds), *Public Communication Campaigns*, 3rd edn (pp. 290–294). Thousand Oaks, CA: Sage.

Woodward, D.R., Cumming, F.J., Ball, P.J., Williams, H.M., Hornsby, H., & Boon, J.A. (1997). Does television affect teenagers' food choices? *Journal of Human Nutrition and Dietetics,* 10, 229–235.

Zuppa, J.A., Morton, H., & Mehta, K. (2003). Television food advertising: counterproductive to children's health? A content analysis using the Australian Guide to Healthy Eating. *Nutrition and Dietetics*, 60(2), 78–84.

Chapter 13

Social Determinants and the Healthcare System

Yvonne Parry and Eileen Willis

Topics covered

This chapter covers the following topics:

- the healthcare system as part of the social determinants of health
- models of healthcare and the social determinants of health
- access to healthcare as a determinant of health
- access to the Australian healthcare system
- policy initiatives for promoting the social determinants of health

Key terms

catastrophic (healthcare) payments
continuity of care
health access
intersectoral collaboration
market-based model
public policy
quintile
role substitution
separation rates
social determinants
universal health coverage
vertical integration
welfare state

Introduction

Many of the chapters in this book have stressed that social factors, rather than biological or genetic ones, determine people's health. In this chapter, we examine and analyse one specific **social determinant** in terms of how it impacts on the health of individuals and population groups. This socio-political factor is the type of healthcare system available to a nation's citizens. We will argue that access to consistent, timely and appropriate health services is necessary to maintain and promote effective health outcomes for individuals and populations, especially disadvantaged groups.

Social determinants
A number of factors, including social, cultural, economic and political, which can impact on the health of individuals.

In order to demonstrate how a nation's healthcare system can be understood as a social determinant of health, we draw on the World Health Organization's Commission on Social Determinants of Health (CSDH) framework (CSDH et al. 2007). In the first section of the chapter, we summarise the CSDH argument that the healthcare system is a determinant of health that impacts on availability and access to health services. Second, we describe the Australian healthcare system, specifically Medicare. We then identify the features of the Australian healthcare system that are positive social determinants of health, and those that contribute to and maintain inequalities in health. In the final section, we provide examples of **public policy** that might contribute to good health outcomes.

Public policy
Policies brought in by governments to administer education, healthcare, water, sanitation, same-sex marriage and so on.

Social determinants of health

The social determinants of health refer to those factors that impact on people's socio-economic position and, as a consequence, their mortality (rates of death) and morbidity (rates of illness). These include an individual's income, occupation and education. Other factors include welfare and taxation policies, or policies that allow equal opportunity for all groups regardless of gender, race, disability or class. These social factors impact on life chances, which in turn impact on the health status of individuals. The evidence is that an individual's socio-economic position, in interaction with the overall socio-political climate of a country, determines health outcomes such as life expectancy, mortality and morbidity rates (Wilkinson & Pickett 2009; see also Chapters 1, 5, 7 & 14 in this volume).

The CSDH (2008) has divided the determinants into two broad categories: the structurally determined or 'upstream' factors, and factors downstream that impact on the availability of and access to services or resources (see also Chapter 1). The CSDH program is all-encompassing, moving from policies that support a healthy start in life (early childhood and education) through to healthy living (housing, urban and rural landscapes, land rights and environmental issues), to employment (safe and decent working conditions, precarious work and fair representation) to health across the life course (disability, income protection, pensions). It also points to the need for policies that support social justice in terms of taxation and monetary policy, the conduct of the

Intersectoral collaboration
Collaborative actions between government agencies and/or all levels of government on 'health or health equity outcomes or on the determinants of health or health equity' (OECD et al. 2008, p. 21).

Universal health coverage
All people and communities can use the promotive, preventative, curative, rehabilitative and palliative health services they need, of sufficient quality to be effective, and the use of these services does not expose the user to financial hardship.

Health access
Access to primary healthcare for all people, independent of income. This means that individuals should have the opportunity or right to receive affordable, timely and appropriate healthcare in a manner that promotes optimum health.

market, financing, trade and commerce, and anti-discrimination legislation (gender, race, culture, religion, sexual orientation). This suggests that governments need to have policies in place across (downstream) a range of portfolios from the environment to education to gender equity in order to achieve health for all or to close the gap in health inequality. This broad policy scope is encapsulated in the 'health in all policies' approach, or **intersectoral collaboration** (CSDH 2008).

The CSDH makes a distinction between health and the healthcare system (CSDH 2008). The focus in this chapter is not on the macro social determinants of health such as income and employment (see Chapter 6 in this volume), but on how access to the healthcare system is organised to optimise health equity. In the past this was referred to as intermediary determinants of health (Solar & Irwin 2007). The approach taken more recently by the CSDH is to identify key features of a healthcare system that support closing the inequality gap and optimising health access. These are universal coverage and a strong primary healthcare system that includes preventative care, accessible primary care and citizen empowerment (CSDH 2008). This chapter focuses on Medicare as an example of a healthcare system and discusses whether it enhances health access, which in turn increases social equity.

Stop and Think

Since the CSDH began its work in 2005, there has been considerable interest in examining inequality within and between nations, and on what motivates governments to legislate for equality, or to close the gap between the rich and poor (CSDH 2008). A major factor in stimulating this interest was the global financial crisis (GFC) of 2008. The GFC highlighted the issue of government failure to regulate capitalism (banks and major corporations) and the impact this had on individual and national debt. The crisis demonstrated the need for governments to be powerful enough and have sufficient control over national debt to be able to bail out local economies. However, in a contradictory turn, some countries were required by either the European Commission, the European Central Bank or the International Monetary Fund to introduce economic policies that restricted access to services such as health, unemployment or social housing either through user-pays or raising the threshold for access to services (van Gool & Pearson 2014). This led to increases in inequality at the same time as the CSDH was working to get governments to begin introducing policies that increase equality through a range of intersectoral approaches (WHO 2011).

Three recent publications have stimulated further discussion about how possible it might be to close the gap between the rich and poor within and between nations. The first was Wilkinson and Pickett's (2009) book *The Spirit Level*. This provides an evidence-based comparison of the richest 23 countries globally (with populations of over 3 million). The authors establish that it is more than income, both individually and nationally, that determines the health and social well-being of a population. The key factor is inequality between people. In Australia, the government took up the term 'closing the gap', and applied it to its policy direction for Aboriginal Australians (see CSDH 2008 report *Closing the Gap* between Aboriginal Australians and the wider population, Australian Govt 2017).

Health and social problems are linked to the degree of inequality within a nation, or the gap between rich and poor. Countries that have smaller gaps between the haves and the have-nots and provide support for their people are more equal, and have fewer health and social problems overall. Conversely, countries with large gaps have many more social and health problems to tackle. For example, the US, one of the world's richest nations, has poorer outcomes across a range of health and social issues than many less wealthy countries.

Two other publications with similar themes are Thomas Piketty's *Capitalism in the 21st Century* (2013) and Walter Scheidle's *The Great Leveller: Violence and the History of Inequality from the Stone Age to the 21st Century* (2015). Both authors argued that the history of inequality is linked to violence and disaster. Scheidle examines the history of human society from the Stone Age to the present time, Piketty restricts his examination of inequality from the Industrial Revolution to the 21st century. For example, they identify the post-war years of the 1950s and 1960s as a period of increased equality that resulted from the Second World War (loss of life/property at devastating levels). Western governments responded to the disaster through a series of welfare policies that lessened (but did not completely close) the gap between rich and poor. Economies were stimulated by major reconstruction programs, which in turn impacted positively on employment, wages, education and health. It is a pessimistic hypothesis to suggest that equality only follows major disasters.

How can this be? All three arguments seem counter-intuitive.

- Surely those countries with the most wealth should have the best health outcomes?
- Surely we don't need disasters to achieve equality?
- What do you think of their views?

Healthcare system as a structural determinant of health

The Rio Declaration acknowledged two important points about access to healthcare: first, that health is dependent on a range of government policies that enhance equity (hence our point above about intersectoral collaboration) and second, that 'good health requires a universal, comprehensive, equitable, effective, responsive and accessible quality health system' (WHO 2011, p. 2). Section 13 of the Rio Declaration pledged to reorient the health sector towards accessible, available, acceptable and affordable quality healthcare and public health services of the highest standards as a fundamental human right (WHO 2011, p. 5). Many interpret these two statements as support for free and universal healthcare, rather than private for-profit care. The WHO position argues that healthcare systems must be financially accessible to the entire population. However, others may see healthcare as an individual responsibility that should be paid for.

Types of healthcare systems and impact on access

One way of determining whether or not a healthcare system provides equitable care that is accessible, available, acceptable and affordable is to examine how the service is financed and whether the system offers universal and relatively free coverage for all citizens. According to Docteur and Oxley (2003), there are three basic models of health delivery and financing. These healthcare systems differ in several ways: whether the funding is public or private, whether the care is provided by private practitioners or publicly paid providers, and who accepts responsibility for the provision and management of public or private healthcare.

Welfare state
Provision by government of social services such as education, healthcare, old-age pensions. Often free, or co-payments or means tested and funded through taxation.

The first is the public-integrated model. In countries that have this model, public hospitals and services are funded by the government as part of the **welfare state**. This makes it a welfare-based model, in which insurance and provision functions are not separated. Doctors and other health professionals can be public employees paid on a salary or, if in private practice, contracting their services to the government. There is universal population coverage, regardless of income, and this coverage is simple to provide. Thus, health access is not dependent on the person's ability to buy health, but on the government's responsibility to provide it as a right for all citizens. Healthcare is paid for through taxation. Those earning more income pay higher taxes and levies towards the healthcare system, and those requiring more care receive it—the healthy and rich subsidise sicker and poorer citizens. Costs and the delivery of the system are directly covered by the government (Docteur & Oxley 2003). This model is used in Australia (in the public hospital sector).

The second approach is the public-contract service delivery model. This model of healthcare uses public funds to contract private companies to provide healthcare (Docteur & Oxley 2003). An example in Australia is the primary healthcare services provided by general practitioners. GPs are private providers paid on a fee-for-service basis by the Commonwealth through Medicare (Willis et al. 2015). The public contract model does provide incentives to prevent ill health and can be very responsive to patient needs. For example, in Australia the federal government provides incentives for GPs to become more efficient, increase their productivity and offer new services. As there is only one funding body, this model is efficient and has low administration costs (Docteur & Oxley 2003), but access may be limited by the facts that a patient may have to make a co-payment or pay a gap fee and that providers are not evenly distributed.

The third and final model, the private insurance model, is an insurance-based system where delivery relies on the private sector, with the insurance and services delivered by private companies. In some countries, such as Switzerland, it is mandatory to take out private health insurance. In others it is voluntary, as in the US (Docteur & Oxley 2003) prior to the introduction of the *Affordable Care Act* during the Obama administration. The Act made insurance compulsory in the US, based on the notion that health is a human right (Rak & Coffin 2013; see Chapter 5).

Private insurance companies can charge what the market will pay, and in some instances access to care depends on the type of cover. Affordability for the consumer is an issue with this model. In the 1990s, in an effort to manage increasing costs, the US introduced managed care plans (Docteur & Oxley 2003). This change allowed insurers to select clients and providers and restrict patient treatments and service access (Docteur & Oxley 2003). Where private health insurance is the major form of health cover, unless the government provides healthcare to some members of society, such as the poor and elderly, large segments of the population may not be covered by any form of health insurance and therefore have limited access to care.

Case Example 13.1

Access to healthcare by different social groups in Australia

Research conducted into the needs of homeless families (Parry et al. 2016) found that parents identified the lack of health services for their children, and accessibility and cost, as issues affecting their lives.

Barry and Jenny (pseudonyms) worked for a large global manufacturing organisation that closed. Due to an economic downturn they could not find employment and thus could not pay their bills. They sold their house at a loss and were left with debts.

> We tried to rent privately but it was so expensive ... we used all our savings ... we spent time with friends, you know on the couches and stuff ... as we have no relatives in this state and couldn't afford to leave. We ended up exhausted with the worry of it all ... no money for any housing and then we all (3 children) got sick. We didn't want to use a GP as we know it's expensive, with all the gap fees and then the cost of drugs. So, we used Emergency Departments (ED). We know you are not supposed to and we feel embarrassed and sometimes we wait for hours but it's the only way we can access health. We even get the kids immunised there.

The inability to access health is inefficient and costly for health systems, governments, the public, community and individuals. The WHO recognises that integrated and interdisciplinary primary healthcare is 10 times more effective than waiting for families to access health services. The use of emergency departments for primary healthcare is not cost-effective (Parry 2012). Changes to affordable primary healthcare can undermine universal health access and the public-integrated model.

Stop and Think

It is acknowledged by governments and professional bodies, such as the Australian Medical Association (AMA), that particular population groups have less access to healthcare, leading to higher rates of morbidity and mortality. However, the solutions to this are complex. The AMA would like more doctors to work in outer suburbs and in rural and remote regions, but doctors in these areas are likely to earn less than their peers in inner-city practices.

- How would you tackle this issue if you were Minister for Health?
- If you were a health professional in private practice, would you go to a rural area?
- One solution would be for the government to bond medical practitioners to rural areas. What do you think of this as a solution? Discuss with your tutor why this could not happen in Australia.

Australian healthcare system

Market-based model
A system where access to education, health and housing must be paid for by the individual, and those who are sick or incapacitated must provide for their own income protection.

As noted above, healthcare systems around the world can be divided into three broad categories, the first two welfare-based models and the third a **market-based model**. A welfare-based model assumes that health is a basic human right and that all citizens should have equal and timely access to healthcare. As a consequence, governments usually take some responsibility for organising and funding the healthcare system. A market model argues that, in a democracy, citizens should be able to choose how much and what kind of healthcare they wish to purchase. Under the market model, citizens pay for healthcare; under the welfare model, the government provides and manages the care through a state-run system or the funding of an insurance scheme. Pure market or pure welfare models do not exist. Most countries, including the US, have a mix of both.

The Australian healthcare system is a mixture of market (private insurance model) and welfare provision (public-integrated and public-contract models). The foundation of the current Australian healthcare system is Medicare. It was established in 1984 by the Hawke federal Labor government at a time when up to 35 per cent of Australians had no health cover (Willis 2015). The first point to note about Medicare is that it is a compulsory (everyone must be in the scheme) and universal (everyone is covered by the scheme, regardless of income) health insurance scheme based on the principle of equal access for all Australians. It is funded through taxation and a progressive levy on all taxpayers. This levy is set at 2 per cent of each person's income. For those on high incomes who do not have private health insurance, the levy increases a further 1–1.5 per cent depending on their income (Australian Govt & ATO 2018). The Medicare levy does not cover the full cost of healthcare, so in reality most Medicare-related health costs are funded through taxation (Willis et al. 2015).

Medicare is divided into two distinct parts: funding for hospitals and funding for primary care and other medical, allied health and nursing services. Funding for hospitals can be viewed under the public integration model. The Commonwealth partly funds the state and territory governments to run the public hospitals. Under the legislation, the states and territories must provide free and timely access to healthcare for all Australians and other eligible persons (Willis et al. 2015). While not a national health service, this component of Medicare effectively provides free hospital care to all Australians and as a healthcare policy is illustrative of accessible, available, affordable and acceptable care that is equitable in reach. For example, if an individual was involved in a motor vehicle accident they would be conveyed by ambulance to a public hospital where they would receive free hospital, medical, nursing and allied healthcare, including free pharmaceuticals during their hospital stay. Follow-up care in rehabilitation or the hospital's outpatient clinics would also be free, although the individual might have to pay a small charge for ongoing pharmaceuticals and wait several weeks or months for an outpatient appointment. Similarly, if an individual required elective surgery such as a hip replacement this could be provided in a public hospital free of charge, but of course with a considerable, but clinically timely, wait.

The second part of Medicare, also funded by the Commonwealth, provides funding to cover primary care from a medical practitioner, and some allied health and nursing services. This aspect of Medicare conforms to the public contract model (Docteur & Oxley 2003). When the Hawke Labor government introduced Medicare in 1984 it hoped these medical services would be free through bulk-billing. The Commonwealth sets the scheduled fee for all medical services and pays doctors 85 per cent of this fee. If a doctor bulk-bills, the patient is not charged the gap fee, so the service is effectively free, but the doctor only receives 85 per cent of the estimated cost of the service. If the doctor charges the scheduled fee, or above the scheduled fee, the patient pays the additional amount. This is called a gap payment. In its original design Medicare provided relatively free access to primary medical care with a low gap fee. Underlying both features of Medicare is an acknowledgment that health and access to affordable care is a basic human right that should be managed and provided by government and paid for through taxation or some form of universal insurance. These aspects of Medicare make it a positive social determinant of health and in theory should ensure health access.

Limits of access to hospital care

The original 1984 Medicare agreements between the state and territory governments and the Commonwealth noted that hospital care must be timely. Timely care is defined as care that is offered within a clinically appropriate period. For example, an individual with a heart attack would receive immediate care. But since not all medical conditions need to be treated straight away, some patients are assigned to elective surgery or outpatient waiting lists. While waiting lists must be made public, and patients must not wait beyond what is considered clinically safe, this is an area where health access becomes problematic. Three problems associated with timely access to hospital care illustrate the complexity of access to healthcare as a social determinant of health even in systems based on the premise that health is a human right. The first problem is the increased numbers requiring care either as an emergency admission or for elective surgery. The increased pressure on public hospitals is partly explained as a result of population growth, the increase in the percentage of people living into their 70s and beyond, thus requiring care for chronic conditions, the increase in education which leads people to demand quality healthcare, the slight drop in the number of people with private health insurance, and the high cost of medical care. As a result, elective surgery in public hospitals may not always be as timely as needed for a patient's comfort or convenience. This can impact on people's general well-being, and on their capacity to earn their living and function in everyday life. The high demand for healthcare services may lead governments with publicly funded hospital systems to use a quota system to restrict the number of procedures as a cost-containment strategy (Curtis et al. 2010).

A second factor is geography. Not all Australians have equal access to public hospitals providing emergency or elective care. Examples include those living in rural and remote areas, particularly Indigenous Australians, and even those living in outer suburbs. Travelling to the city for hospital care brings added expenses, although the Patient Admission Transport Scheme, which reimburses patients from rural and remote areas for travel and accommodation costs while in a city hospital, provides some financial assistance. A major problem is that it is difficult to entice health professionals to work in isolated communities, or the population there may be so low that it is not economically efficient for governments to provide the service. The model of healthcare is a factor in influencing governments to provide the service.

A third factor relates to socio-economic status, including cultural and ethnic disparities in health access. Being poor, and therefore likely to be sicker, is not the only difficulty for low socio-economic populations. Their access to healthcare is also stratified. For example, data from the Australian Institute of Health shows around 28 per cent of all admissions to public hospitals are for people in the lowest **quintile**, while for those in the highest quintile it was 11 per cent. We can assume the latter group has access to private health insurance. The medium waiting time for patients in the lowest quintile was 43 days, while those in the highest waited 32 days. Perhaps more interesting is the relationship between waiting times and source of funding for elective surgery in public hospitals. For patients who entered these hospitals as public patients, 2 per cent waited more than 365 days for their procedure, while only 0.8 per cent of those who entered as a private patient waited more than 365 days (Australian Govt & AIHW 2017). This points to an intriguing problem with the mixed nature of the Australian healthcare system. Those with private health insurance are able to seek timely and usually quicker elective surgery or medical care in a private hospital with the doctor of their choice. Waiting lists are not as long in private hospitals. People without private health insurance must wait until their name comes to the top of a public hospital waiting list. But it also appears that people in higher-income brackets do not have to wait as long for surgery as poorer people, even when both groups are seeking care in a public hospital. The problem is not simply that emergency admissions

Quintile

A quintile represents 20 per cent (a fifth) of the population. The lowest quintile is the poorest group; the highest group is the wealthiest.

Table 13.1 Selected separation statistics by socio-economic status of area of usual residence, public and private hospitals, 2015–16

	Socio-economic status of area of usual residence					
	1 (lowest)	2	3	4	5 (highest)	Total[(a)]
Public hospitals						
Separations	1701604	1428588	1246261	1043098	804402	6272481
Separations per 1000 population[(b)]	329.1	273.5	246.3	213.9	164.7	247.9
Separation rate ratio	1.3	1.1	1.0	0.9	0.7	
Private hospitals						
Separations	601911	722669	865515	954553	1171434	4327287
Separations per 1000 population[(b)]	112.0	134.5	167.3	194.1	235.9	167.8
Separation rate ratio	0.7	0.8	1.0	1.2	1.4	
All hospitals						
Separations	**2303515**	**2151257**	**2111776**	**1997651**	**1975836**	**10599768**
Separations per 1000 population[(b)]	**441.1**	**407.9**	**413.6**	**408.1**	**400.7**	**415.7**
Separation rate ratio	**1.1**	**1.0**	**1.0**	**1.0**	**1.0**	

(a) Total includes separations for which the SES group could not be categorised.

(b) Separation rates are directly age-standardised using populations by SES groups, which do not include persons in areas for which the SES could not be determined. Therefore, the total standardised rates for analyses by SES groups differ from rates calculated by state or territory.

Source: AIHW (2016, p. 63)

Separation rates
The percentage of people who leave hospital before midnight on any one day, whether through being discharged, transferred to another facility, or dying.

take precedence over elective surgery, the lists of people needing surgery are long, and the number of procedures a hospital may perform in any one year may be capped. There is also a problem of selection! Table 13.1 illustrates the issue, with the population divided into five quintiles.

Presumably, access to timely acute care should simply be a matter of increasing resources to the public system. However, the allocation of funds is a political issue that reflects the values of a society and the power of particular interest groups. For example, to encourage people to take out private health insurance, the Howard Federal Coalition government (1996–2007) introduced a 30 per cent rebate for individuals and families with private health insurance, which is now means-tested according to income (Australian Govt & PHIO 2018). This policy decision continues to divert resources from the public health system, providing financial incentive to wealthier people. It increased the percentage of people with private health insurance, which in turn increased profits for private insurers, private hospitals and doctors in private practice (Laris et al. 2008), and may also have increased timely access to care for this population, as shown above in the statistics from public hospitals. Figure 13.1 provides information on the number of people with private health insurance by quintile, illustrating the advantage of being wealthy.

Figure 13.1 Proportion of all persons aged 18 and over with private health insurance, 2011–2012

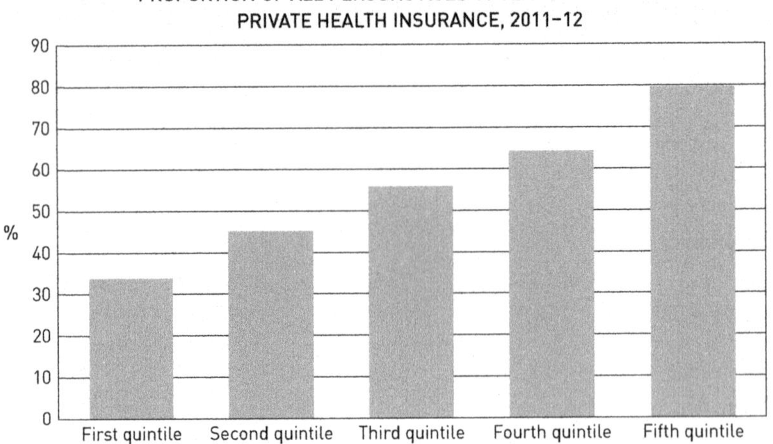

Source: Australian Bureau of Statistics (2018)

Stop and Think

Waiting times for elective surgery are a problem. It is not simply that emergency admissions take precedence over elective surgery, or that the list is just too long, or that the number of procedures a hospital may perform is capped. There appears to be a problem of inequitable selection.

- How can this occur?
- Does this mean that doctors, governments and health managers discriminate against poorer people?
- If you do not think this is the case, how might the statistics in Table 13.1 be explained?

Case Example 13.2

Closing the Gap policy

In Australia, a major equity policy is the Indigenous Closing the Gap policy, which is truly intersectoral with targets across employment, early childhood, health and education. In 2017, the Prime Minister reported on the outcomes and targets. One of the key targets was to halve the mortality rate for children under five by 2018. The 2017 report showed that while there had been some improvement and the gap has narrowed, it has not closed. Between 1998 and 2015, the gap narrowed by 33 per cent, but there is still a 31 per cent mortality gap. Some of this inequality in outcomes is attributed to Indigenous mothers continuing to smoke while pregnant, which may result in low birth rates, and to more robust statistics that may explain what appears to be poor progress for this target, but are really about more accurate reporting. However, there were also positive trends—more mothers were attending antenatal classes. More importantly, a detailed look at the figures show that New South Wales has better outcomes than the Northern Territory. This suggests that differences in outcomes depend on more than being Indigenous.

- What factors in the Northern Territory and Western Australia make it more difficult to close the gap there than in New South Wales? See Table 13.2.

Table 13.2 Infant mortality rates per 1000 live births, by Indigenous status, New South Wales, Queensland, Western Australia, South Australia and the Northern Territory, 2011–15

Jurisdiction	Number of deaths		Rate per 1000 live births		Ratio	Rate difference
	Indigenous	Non-Indigenous	Indigenous	Non-Indigenous		
NSW	118	1581	4.0	3.3	1.2	0.6
Qld	175	1183	6.7	4.1	1.6	2.6
WA	77	327	5.6	2.1	2.7	3.5
SA	31	257	6.5	2.7	2.4	3.8
NT	99	45	13.8	3.4	4.0	10.4
Total of 5 jurisdictions	**500**	**3393**	**6.1**	**3.3**	**1.9**	**2.8**

Source: AIHW (2017)

Limits of access to primary care

The CSDH sees primary care as the cornerstone of health access and encourages governments to prioritise this component of the system. However, just as access to hospitals can be problematic, so too is access to primary medical care. Costs, distance and the problem of supply are major barriers to accessing primary care such as GP services. When Medicare was introduced it was hoped that the majority of doctors would bulk-bill. However, doctors are free to charge any fee they like and some charge above the scheduled fee, leaving patients to pay a gap fee. To assist low-income individuals and families to manage the costs of primary care, various Commonwealth governments have introduced safety nets to help them manage the rising cost of co-payments. The first is the Family Safety Net. In 2018, the threshold was $461.30 for an individual or family, after which Medicare reimburses the individual or family the full scheduled fee. However, since many specialist doctors charge above the scheduled fee (Willis 2015) the patient may still have a high gap fee to pay. To counter this, a second safety measure, called the Extended Medicare Safety Net, was introduced by the Howard government. In early 2018, the cut-off point was $668.10 for disadvantaged individuals and families and $2093.30 for other families and individuals, after which point 80 per cent of their out-of-pocket expenses are reimbursed (Australian Govt & DHS 2018). Another important factor is the cap that was imposed by the federal government on GP Medicare reimbursement between 2013 and 2017. This cap has been removed, and the government is moving to index doctors' fees. Importantly, throughout the freeze on Medicare reimbursements to doctors, many GPs continued to bulk-bill at the very high rate of around 82 per cent (Elkins & Schurer 2017). Despite this, recent reports suggest that Australians have rates of out-of-pocket expenses for healthcare that are second only to those of the US (Russell 2014, 2015), although they are not yet so high as to be defined as **catastrophic payments**. Table 13.3, based on Department of Health statistics, illustrates the slow but steady increase in out-of-pocket expenses in Australia.

Catastrophic (healthcare) payments
The situation where healthcare costs are so high that a family or individual has to go without other basic goods such as food, or go into debt.

The issue of fees for primary medical care is further complicated by the corporatisation of medicine (White 2001). Many small GP clinics have amalgamated to form large multi-purpose clinics controlled by the doctors themselves or by multi-national firms. These clinics provide access to care without an appointment, so attract patients who cannot access a family doctor. While this means that patients can access diagnostic tests on-site and get immediate medical care, the profit motive for owners has led to increased charges linked to **vertical integration** and a lack of **continuity of care**. To counter these trends the Coalition federal government (2015–18) introduced a reform package with three arms: a review of the medical benefits schedule, the Practice Incentive Program (Caruso et al. 2008), and the establishment of the Healthcare Homes Program. Healthcare Homes provides funding to the practices who sign up, independently of Medicare reimbursement. The Healthcare Homes program aims to integrate care for patients with chronic diseases. Its focus is on integrating care for the patient, and offering GPs incentives for quality outcomes. This differs from the current Medicare program that rewards the volume of patients a practice consults, rather than the quality of the outcome (Scott 2017).

Vertical integration
A company provides access to services from other companies within its premises or organisation, for example radiology and pathology services are provided in the same complex as a GP service.

Continuity of care
Access to the same healthcare team over a period of time so that the care plan is coordinated.

Table 13.3 Average patient $ contribution per service for out-of-hospital medical services

	2016–17	2015–16	2014–15	2013–14	2012–13	2011–12	2010–11	2009–10
Aust	60.97	58.49	54.60	51.61	48.12	44.98	41.74	37.06
NSW	66.13	63.44	59.04	56.02	52.27	48.98	45.62	40.60
VIC	60.32	57.72	53.81	50.76	47.24	43.91	40.04	35.48
QLD	58.02	55.78	52.38	49.77	46.55	43.53	40.83	35.69
SA	50.68	48.23	45.36	42.75	40.40	37.68	34.83	31.37
WA	61.95	60.21	56.18	52.33	48.05	44.85	41.99	37.45
TAS	47.84	45.00	41.84	40.03	37.54	35.83	33.96	31.24
NT	73.54	68.93	64.12	59.35	57.12	53.99	49.65	42.58
ACT	63.52	61.09	56.45	53.73	50.57	47.62	44.96	41.25

Source: Australian Govt (2018a)

Distance, supply and access

In addition to costs, distance and the shortages of GPs and medical specialists in rural and outer suburbs in Australia create access problems. The problem manifests in two ways. First, there are fewer health professionals per capita working in rural and remote regions, and second, the structure of the primary care component of Medicare (public contract model) means that health services in rural and remote regions are anti-competitive. For example, in rural and remote areas the number of GPs per capita is considerably less than the higher-income densely populated urban areas of the capital cities. The low populations in rural areas create regional monopolies, as the rural GPs are self-employed practitioners with no or restricted competition. This gives them the significant advantage of charging gap fees strengthened by medical shortages, professional dominance and limited alternatives for services. The result is significant disparity in health access between rural and urban populations. However, data in support of this argument is mixed. Medicare's own data suggests that bulk-billing rates are high at around 85 per cent (Hunt 2017), however, research by Bradbury and colleagues shows that in rural New South Wales the rate of same-day appointments available was as low as 47 per cent, while the bulk-billing availability was 21 per cent across 184 practices (Bradbury et al. 2017).

This inequity in access extends to some urban populations. For example, many outer suburban areas have limited health access. This limits after-hours access and places a strain on other services (Australian Govt 2018c). Areas of socio-economic disadvantage also have higher numbers of patients per GP (Australian Govt 2018c).

Stop and Think

Did you know that ...

In 2009–2011, people living in *Remote* and *Very remote* areas had mortality rates 1.4 times higher than those of people living in *Major cities*. For nearly all causes of death, rates were higher for people living outside *Major cities*, with people in *Remote* and *Very remote* areas faring the worst. Coronary heart disease was the leading cause of death for all areas, and mortality rates were 1.2–1.5 times higher in rural and remote areas than in *Major cities*. In *Remote* and *Very remote* areas, the rate of dying due to a land transport accident was more than four times as high as in *Major cities*. In *Remote* and *Very remote* areas, death rates due to diabetes were between 2.5 and four times as high. For suicide, the rate is 1.8–2.2 times as high as in *Major cities* (AIHW & Australian Govt 2017, p. 248).

Cost, access, distance, undersupply and long waits for an appointment can deter people from accessing primary care, or they may seek inappropriate care such as attending a public hospital emergency department. For example, in 2014, 44 per cent of presentations to public hospital emergency departments were for what is known as semi-urgent and 9 per cent were for non-urgent or GP-type presentations, that is, illnesses that could be dealt with more effectively by the patient's family doctor (AIHW 2014b). What the data indicate is that 40–50 per cent of people who present at a public hospital emergency department for primary care should really have seen a local GP. While it is not clear exactly why these people do not seek primary care from a GP, the research does show that low socio-economic groups the world over cannot afford appropriate primary medical care or do not have access to it. Parry's (2012) research found that parents from the lowest quintile areas were six times more likely to use emergency departments for paediatric primary healthcare, in part due to a lack of GP services. We also know that there are more presentations to emergency departments on weekends (AIHW 2014a).

Health access reform

Most western countries have attempted to deal with the problems of health access over the last 30 years through a series of reforms. In the early 1990s, reforms focused on increasing the productivity and efficiency of existing services by setting targets that attempted to ensure better access. Examples included providing incentive funding to hospitals if patients on elective surgery waiting lists did not have long waits. In Australia, public hospitals have to publish waiting times so that the public can see how efficient they are (Willis 2015). More recent reforms to increase patient access have included increasing the number of health professionals that have been educated and trained, and extending the skills and practice of health professionals other than doctors through a process of **role substitution**. Nurse practitioners are one example of this. Nurse practitioners can prescribe a limited number of drugs and order diagnostic tests, but role substitution has been minimal in Australia with the exception of Assistants in Nursing and Personal Care Workers substituting for registered and enrolled nurses, particularly in aged care (Willis et al. 2016).

Role substitution

The process whereby one profession takes up the role and skills of another.

This discussion on health access has assumed that all sick people need is access to a GP and a hospital. This is not always the case. Comprehensive healthcare also means access to pharmaceuticals, dental care and ongoing services for those with a mental illness or a chronic condition and for the elderly. Where these services are not provided in a free and timely manner, because they are outside the remit of the welfare state, some populations will have reduced life chances. Of course, even where there is excellent health access, if populations do not have access to employment, education or housing their health status will deteriorate.

Case Example 13.3

Access to dental care in Australia

Dental care in Australia is an area of healthcare outside of Medicare. While most states and territories have some form of school-based dental service, and the Commonwealth provides funding under the Child Dental Benefit Schedule, these schemes do not cover all orthodontic work, which is often classified as 'cosmetic'. A major cost issue for many families without private health insurance looms when one of their children requires orthodontic work. Consider the following family situation.

Margaret is a single mother with three boys aged seven to 13. She has been unemployed for some time, and has only just obtained a one-year contract teaching for a private provider. She has no health insurance, and relies on Medicare. Her middle son requires orthodontic work as his teeth are crowded in the front of his mouth. Failure to remedy the issue will probably result in loss of permanent teeth when his is older. He tends not to smile, due to his unsightly teeth, and is being teased at school. Margaret obtained a free quote from a local dentist who estimated the cost of corrective treatment at $6000 over 18 months. Margaret's mother who is in her 70s doesn't consider that the teeth are a 'problem'—her own bottom row of teeth are crooked and she says she got by in life, married and had a good job.

- Do you think the quality of your teeth is marker of your parent's socio-economic status, or just a matter of fashion?
- Do you think orthodontic care to straighten teeth should be funded under a national dental program similar to Medicare?
- Funding would be an issue for a national dental program. How do you think the population would react to an increase in the Medicare levy to fund a dental care program that covered corrective treatment?
- How would you argue against the proposition that corrective treatment to straighten teeth is simply cosmetic?
- What would you say to the boy's grandmother about dental care in the 21st century?

Reflection Exercise

Consider the three issues outlined below, in terms of what federal and/or state and territory governments might have to do to ensure they provide free, universal access to healthcare.

- Governments do not necessarily have to make a profit; however, private companies need to or they will go out of business and in the long run this impacts negatively on the Australian economy. Given this, it is simply good business sense for private medical insurers to limit the cover provided to young people who require mental healthcare overnight and long stays in hospital for treatment.

- The AIHW reports that in 2014, 36 per cent of people in Australia were eligible for free dental care, although COAG noted that in 2015 government funding was only available for around 20 per cent of this group (Australian Govt 2018b, p. 1).
- Australia's rate of births by caesarean section is above the OECD average, and is increasing. The increase is higher in the private sector (42 per cent of births, compared to 28 per cent increase in the public sector). This would appear to suggest that women with private health insurance birthing in private hospitals are at a disadvantage, given that they are more likely to have a caesarean (Australian Govt 2018d).

Good business sense does not necessarily make for good healthcare. People with a mental health issue may require long-term care. Long-term care is expensive. There is a tendency for public hospitals to discharge mental health patients into the care of community services and their families. While this might be seen as best for the patient, asking families to care for a relative with a mental health issue, without having knowledge of the full clinical factors, is problematic. It may not be the best option, yet it appears that both the public and the private sectors find long-term care too expensive.

Dental care in Australia is provided mainly through private providers and is expensive. Services provided to low-income populations by the six states and two territories are not consistent. For example, Victoria provides services for Indigenous people, refugees, asylum seekers, pregnant women and homeless people. In Western Australia, specific groups targeted for state government dental care are residents in aged care homes and those living in remote regions, while in Tasmania it is provided for those living in remote regions and Indigenous people. There are two issues to note here. The services offered by the states are not consistent, making any intervention by the federal government difficult. Second, the service provision suggests that there is a dearth of dentists in rural and remote regions (Australian Govt 2018b).

Untangling the issues behind the high caesarean rate in the private hospital sector is vexed. It may well be that birthing women with private health insurance are older and more at risk, or overweight and at risk. Older women develop more comorbidities during pregnancy than younger women. However, it is worth asking if there are other considerations. Research by Einarsdottir et al. (2012) shows that the increase in caesarean rates correlates with changes to health insurance policy, which imposed penalties on young people who did not take out health insurance once they hit 30 years of age, and the Extended Medicare Gap, which reimbursed women who sought a private obstetrician for the birth of their child.

Summary

The social determinants of health are divided into those that directly relate to an individual's characteristics, such as gender or race, and to policies that are structural and intermediary, or upstream or downstream. Health access is a downstream determinant of health. An examination of health access as a social determinant of health requires understanding what kind of healthcare a particular country has in place. Most countries in the developed world have one of three types of healthcare systems. The first is the public integrated model, which is usually funded through taxation. The second is the public contract service delivery model, which uses public funds to contract private companies to provide healthcare. Both models have the capacity to provide universal and relatively free access to healthcare. The third model is the private fee-for-service approach. This model limits health access to those who can afford the care. The type of healthcare system a nation has is influenced by the values of that society, the kind of government, and its social policies. Health access as a social determinant is also underpinned by an understanding of health as a social right, rather than health as an individual responsibility. In order to examine the health access of a particular system it is necessary to investigate the policies governing the provision of healthcare. In Australia, for example, Medicare both facilitates and limits access to healthcare. Access to GPs is based on the public contract service delivery model whereby GPs are paid to deliver the service as private providers. As a consequence, they may not offer after-hours services or services to people in remote or rural areas. Public hospital care is free and universal. However, there is considerable strain on healthcare systems, and governments worldwide are attempting to reduce costs.

Tutorial exercises

Go to the webpage http://www.abc.net.au/news/2017-12-11/whats-middle-class-depends-on-where-you-live-the-conversation/9241586. Do the test that determines if you are in the middle class or not.

1. Did you agree with your class allocation? What difference do you think this makes to your life chances?
2. Identify those aspects of the social determinants of health that are part of the healthcare system. Identify the factors that are not part of the healthcare system.
3. Discuss what can be done by health professionals to address the social determinants of health. What limitations do health professionals face in tackling social determinants outside of the health system?
4. Examine the Closing the Gap policy for Indigenous people.
5. Identify one intersectoral policy and be prepared to discuss this in your tutorial.
6. What are the strengths of the Australian healthcare system in terms of access, availability and affordability? Back up your claims with evidence from the chapter.
7. Find other students in your tutorial group who come from regional or rural areas and discuss the health services available in their town. Compare this with services available in suburbs in the city, or your regional town.

Further reading

CSDH (Commission on the Social Determinants of Health) et al. (2007) *Challenging Inequality through Health Systems*. Retrieved from http://www.who.int/social_determinants/resources/csdh_media/hskn_final_2007_en.pdf?ua=1_

CSDH (Commission on Social Determinants of Health) (2008). *Closing the Gap in a Generation: Health Equity through Action on the Social Determinants of Health*. Retrieved from http://www.who.int/social_determinants/thecommission/finalreport/en/

Docteur, E., & Oxley, H. (2003). *Health-care Systems: Lessons from the Reform Experience*. Paris: OECD. Retrieved from www.oecd.org/dataoecd/5/53/22364122.pdf

Piketty, T. (2013). *Capital in the 21st Century*. Cambridge, MA: Harvard University Press.

Scheidle, W. (2015). *The Great Leveller: Violence and the History of Inequality from the Stone Age to the 21st Century*. Princeton, NJ: Princeton University Press.

Solar, O., & Irwin, A. (2007). *A Conceptual Framework for Action on the Social Determinants of Health.* Draft Discussion Paper for the Commission on Social Determinants of Health. Retrieved from http://www.google.com.au/url?sa=t&rct=j&q=&esrc=s&source=web&cd=1&ved=0ahUKEwiw6dSog53ZAhUQ5rwKHW8uAhkQFggsMAA&url=http%3A%2F%2Fwww.who.int%2Fsocial_determinants%2Fresources%2Fhealth_equity_isa_2008_en.pdf&usg=AOvVaw31R5LIfRF9q_HAvhsp9hjJ

Websites

http://www.abc.net.au/news/2015-10-28/social-class-survey-where-you-fit-in-australia/6869864

This web page allows you to determine where you sit in terms of social and cultural class.

http://www.commonwealthfund.org/interactives-and-data/maps-and-data

This website from the Commonwealth fund provides a number of interactive maps that explore health equality in the US.

www.equalitytrust.org.uk/why

This website from the Equality Trust provides background to the ideas behind the movement for Closing the Gap.

http://www.who.int/social_determinants/thecommission/finalreport/en/>

This website is the home of the Commission on Social Determinants of Health—you can sign up to the web page and keep up to date.

https://closingthegap.pmc.gov.au/

This web page is the home of the federal government policy initiatives, Closing the Gap for Aboriginal Australians.

www.who.int/social_determinants/thecommission/finalreport/en/index.html

This is the home page of the WHO Commission on Social Determinants of Health.

http://www.health.gov.au/internet/main/publishing.nsf/content/health-care-homes#two

This is the home page for consumers interested in Health Care Homes.

https://www.aihw.gov.au/reports/rural-health/rural-remote-health/contents/access-to-health-services

The home page of the Australian Institute of Health and Welfare provides information on rural health.

References

AIHW (Australian Institute of Health and Welfare) (2014a). *Emergency Departments: At the Front Line.* Retrieved from https://www.aihw.gov.au/getmedia/1bfbff5c-d3db-40c8-8a48-310269825fcd/8_8-emergency-dept.pdf.aspx

AIHW (Australian Institute of Health and Welfare) (2014b). *Australia's Health 2014.* Australia's Health Series No. 14. Cat. No. AUS 178. Canberra: Australian Institute of Health and Welfare.

AIHW (Australian Institute of Health and Welfare) (2017). *Aboriginal and Torres Strait Islander Health Performance Framework 2017 Report.* Retrieved from https://www.pmc.gov.au/sites/default/files/publications/indigenous/hpf-2017/index.html

AIHW (Australian Institute of Health and Welfare) & Australian Govt (2017). *Australia's Health 2016.* Retrieved from https://www.aihw.gov.au/getmedia/9844cefb-7745-4dd8-9ee2-f4d1c3d6a727/19787-AH16.pdf.aspx?inline=true

Australian Govt (2017). Closing the Gap: Prime Minister's Report 2017. Canberra: Department of the Prime Minister and Cabinet. Retrieved from https://closingthegap.pmc.gov.au/sites/default/files/ctg-report-2017.pdf

Australian Govt (2018a). *Annual Medicare Statistics: Financial Year 1984–85 to 2016–2017.* Retrieved from http://www.health.gov.au/internet/main/publishing.nsf/Content/Annual-Medicare-Statistics

Australian Govt (2018b). *A Discussion on Public Dental Waiting Times Information in Australia 2012–14 to 2016–17*. Retrieved from https://www.aihw.gov.au/getmedia/df234a9a-5c47-4483-9cf7-15ce162d3461/aihw-den-230.pdf.aspx?inline=true

Australian Govt (2018c). *General Practice Statisitics: GP Workforce Statistics 2001–2 to 2016–17*. Retrieved from http://www.health.gov.au/internet/main/publishing.nsf/content/general+practice+statistics-1

Australian Govt (2018d). *National Maternity Services Plan: The Current Environment.* Retrieved from http://www.health.gov.au/internet/publications/publishing.nsf/Content/pacd-maternityservicesplan-toc~pacd-maternityservicesplan-chapter2

Australian Govt & AIHW (Australian Institute of Health and Welfare) (2017). *Admitted Patient Care: 2015–2016*. Retrieved from https://www.aihw.gov.au/getmedia/3e1d7d7e-26d9-44fb-8549-aa30ccff100a/20742.pdf.aspx?inline=true

Australian Govt & ATO (Australian Taxation Office) (2018). *Income Thresholds and Rates for Medicare Levy Surcharge.* Retrieved from https://www.ato.gov.au/Individuals/Medicare-levy/Medicare-levy-surcharge/Income-thresholds-and-rates-for-the-Medicare-levy-surcharge/

Australian Govt & DHS (Department of Human Services) (2018). *Medicare Safety Net.* Retrieved from https://www.humanservices.gov.au/individuals/services/medicare/medicare-safety-net

Australian Govt & PHIO (Private Health Insurance Ombudsman) (2018). *Australian Government Private Health Insurance Rebate*. Retrieved from https://www.privatehealth.gov.au/healthinsurance/incentivessurcharges/insurancerebate.htm

Bradbury, J., Nancarrow, S., Avila, C., Pit, S., Potts, R., Doran, F., & Freed, G. (2017). Actual availability of appointments at general practices in regional New South Wales, Australia. *Australian Family Physician*, 46(5), 321–324. https://www.racgp.org.au/afp/2017/may/actual-availability-of-appointments-at-general-practices-in-regional-new-south-wales,-australia/

Caruso, E., Cisar, N., & Pipe, T. (2008). Creating a healing environment: an innovative educational approach for adopting Jean Watson's theory of human caring. *Nursing Administration Quarterly*, 32(2), 126–132.

CSDH (Commission on Social Determinants of Health) (2008). *Closing the Gap in a Generation: Health Equity through Action on the Social Determinants of Health*. Retrieved from http://www.who.int/social_determinants/thecommission/finalreport/en/

CSDH (Commission on Social Determinants of Health), Doherty, J., Loewenson, R., Francis, V., & Members Knowledge Network (2007). *Challenging Inequity through Health Systems: Final Report.* Knowledge Network on Health Systems. Retrieved from http://www.who.int/social_determinants/resources/csdh_media/hskn_final_2007_en.pdf?ua=1

Curtis, A., Russell, C., Stoelwinder, J., & McNeil, J. (2010). Waiting lists and elective surgery: ordering the queue. *Medical Journal of Australia*, 192(4), 217–220.

Docteur, E., & Oxley, H. (2003). *Health-care Systems: Lessons from the Reform Experience*. Paris: OECD. Retrieved from www.oecd.org/dataoecd/5/53/22364122.pdf

Einarsdóttir, K., Kemp, A., Haggar, F., Moorin, R., Gunnell, A., Preen, D. ... & Holman, D. (2012). Increase in caesarean deliveries after the Australian private health insurance incentive policy reforms. *Plus One*, 7(7), 7(7), e41436. https://doi.org/41410.41371/journal.pone.0041436

Elkins, R., & Schurer, S. (2017). *FactCheck: Are Bulk-billing Rates Falling, or at Record Levels?* Retrieved from https://theconversation.com/factcheck-are-bulk-billing-rates-falling-or-at-record-levels-72278

Hunt, G. (2017). *Strongest Bulk Billing Rates since Medicare's Inception.* Retrieved from http://www.health.gov.au/internet/ministers/publishing.nsf/Content/health-mediarel-yr2017-hunt046.htm

Laris, P., Gleeson, S., & Alperstein, G. (2008). *Social Determinants of Health: Areas for Action.* Sydney: Australian Health Promotion Association (NSW Branch).

OECD (Organisation for Economic Cooperation & Development), Public Health Agency of Canada & WHO (2008). *Health Equity through Intersectoral Action: An Analysis of 18 Country Case Studies.* Retrieved from http://www.google.com.au/url?sa=t&rct=j&q=&esrc=s&source=web&cd=1&ved=0ahUKEwiw6dSog53ZAhUQ5rwKHW8uAhkQFggsMAA&url=http%3A%2F%2Fwww.who.int%2Fsocial_determinants%2Fresources%2Fhealth_equity_isa_2008_en.pdf&usg=AOvVaw31R5LIfRF9q_HAvhsp9hjJ

Parry, Y.K. (2012). Understanding the relationship between the social determinants of health (SDH), Paediatric Emergency Department use and the provision of primary care: a mixed methods analysis. PhD thesis. Adelaide: Flinders University, School of Medicine.

Parry, Y.K., Grant, J., & Burke, L. (2016). A scoping study: children, policy and cultural shifts in homelessness services in South Australia: are children still falling through the gaps? *Health and Social Care in the Community*, 24(5), e1–e10.

Piketty, T. (2013). *Capital in the 21st Century.* Cambridge, MA: Harvard University Press.

Rak, S., & Coffin, J. (2013). Affordable Care Act. *Practice Management, March/April.* Retrieved from https://www.researchgate.net/profile/Janis_Coffin/publication/239943452_Affordable_Care_Act/links/589b619a92851c942ddad86a/Affordable-Care-Act.pdf

Russell, L. (2014). *Analysis of the 2014–2015 Health Budget: Unfair and Unhealthy.* Retrieved from https://ses.library.usyd.edu.au/bitstream/2123/11981/1/2014-15healthbudget.pdf

Russell, L. (2015). *Analysis of the Federal Health Budget and Related Provisions 2015–2016.* Retrieved from http://apo.org.au/files/Resource/analysis_of_the_federal_health_budget_and_related_provisions.pdf

Scheidle, W. (2015). *The Great Leveller: Violence and the History of Inequality from the Stone Age to the 21st Century.* Princeton, NJ: Princeton University Press.

Scott, A. (2017). *ANZ Melbourne Institute Health Sector Report: General Practice Trends.* Retrieved from http://mabel.org.au/__data/assets/pdf_file/0005/2334551/ANZ-MI-Health-Sector-Report.pdf

Solar, O., & Irwin, A. (2007). *A Conceptual Framework for Action on the Social Determinants of Health.* Draft Discussion Paper for the Commission on Social Determinants of Health. Retrieved from http://www.google.com.au/

url?sa=t&rct=j&q=&esrc=s&source=web&cd=1&ved=0ahUKEwiw6dSog53ZAhUQ5rwKHW8uAhkQFggsMAA&url=http%3A%2F%2Fwww.who.int%2Fsocial_determinants%2Fresources%2Fhealth_equity_isa_2008_en.pdf&usg=AOvVaw31R5LIfRF9q_HAvhsp9hjJ

van Gool, K., & Pearson, M. (2014). *Health, Austerity and Economic Crisis: Assessing the Short-term Impact in OECD Countries.* Retrieved from http://dx.doi.org/10.1787/5jxx71lt1zg6-en

WHO (World Health Organization) (2011). *Rio Political Declaration on Social Determinants of Health.* Retrieved from http://www.who.int/sdhconference/declaration/en/

WHO (World Health Organization) (2018). *Universal Health Coverage and Health Financing.* Retrieved from http://www.who.int/health_financing/universal_coverage_definition/en/

Wilkinson, R., & Pickett, K. (2009). *The Spirit Level.* London: Allen Lane.

Willis, E., Price, K., Bonner, R., Henderson, J., Gibson, T., Hurley, J. … & Currie, T. (2016). *Meeting Residents' Care Needs: A Study of the Requirements for Nursing and Personal Care Staff.* National Aged Care Staffing and Skills Mix Project Report. Retrieved from http://www.anmf.org.au/documents/reports/National_Aged_Care_Staffing_Skills_Mix_Project_Report_2016.pdf

Willis, E., Reynolds, L., & Kelehere, H. (2015). *Understanding the Australian Healthcare System.* Sydney: Elsevier.

Chapter 14

Social Determinants of Health on a Global Scale

Deborah Gleeson and Susan Chong

Topics covered

This chapter covers the following topics:

- the global distribution of infectious diseases and non-communicable diseases
- inequities in health within and between countries
- global economic, political and health system determinants of health
- action to address the social determinants of health at the global level

Key terms

comprehensive primary healthcare
globalisation
Health in All Policies
inequities in health
infectious diseases
non-communicable diseases
structural determinants of health
Sustainable Development Goals
transnational corporations
universal health coverage

Introduction

In the last few centuries, there have been dramatic improvements in life expectancy and health around the world. These improvements have been largely due to reductions in infectious diseases, improvements in food and water quality, better housing and living conditions, better nutrition, and healthcare technologies such as vaccines and antibiotics (Baum 2016). However, the gains have not been shared equally between countries and population groups, with the world's poorest countries and people continuing to bear the highest burden of disease, injury and premature death.

There are stark differences in life expectancy and infant mortality in different parts of the world. For example, a girl born in Australia in 2015 can expect to live for 84.8 years, whereas a girl born in Sierra Leone in the same year has a life expectancy of only 50.8 years (WHO 2017a). The Australian girl's risk of dying before the age of five is less than 0.04 per cent whereas the girl born in Sierra Leone has more than a 12 per cent chance of dying before her fifth birthday—a risk 300 times greater than that of her Australian counterpart (WHO 2017a).

In 2005, the World Health Organization set up the Commission on the Social Determinants of Health to investigate global inequities in health, make recommendations for how these inequities could be reduced, and catalyse a global effort to address them (CSDH 2008). Three years later, the CSDH released its report, which concluded that **inequities in health** are rooted in the distribution of power, money and resources at both global and local levels (CSDH 2008, p. 2). Therefore, improving health requires an understanding of the social determinants of health at the global level, and action directed to correcting inequities at both the global and local levels (see also Chapters 1, 5, 7, 9 & 13 in this volume).

Inequities in health
Unfair and avoidable differences in health status (between regions, countries or population groups).

The Millennium Development Goals (MDGs), agreed between the 191 member states of the UN in 2000, represented the first large-scale, concerted global effort to reduce poverty, hunger, disease and other problems experienced primarily by low- and middle-income countries. The MDGs involved eight goals which the UN countries committed to address by 2015. This major effort, along with a substantial investment in funding for health programs, including maternal and child health and nutrition, contributed to a substantial decline in maternal and child mortality during that period, although key targets were not met (Boerma et al. 2018).

The MDGs were superseded by the **Sustainable Development Goals** (SDGs) in 2015 (UN n.d.). These are a set of 17 goals and 169 targets, with a greater focus on economic and environmental sustainability than the MDGs.

Sustainable Development Goals
A set of 17 development goals agreed between UN member states in 2015 to address the global challenges of poverty, inequalities and climate change.

SDG3 ('Ensure healthy lives and promote well-being for all at all ages') is explicitly focused on health. It includes a set of 13 targets that aim to reduce maternal and child mortality and prevent premature death, illness and injuries from a range of causes. SDG3 also includes targets related to strengthening health systems by achieving universal health coverage, providing affordable medicines and vaccines, providing adequate numbers of health professionals, and strengthening the capacity to manage global health risks (UN n.d.). Many of the other SDGs are also related to, and in some cases intrinsic to, health, such as SDG2 (zero hunger), 6 (clean water and sanitation), 13 (climate action) and 10 (reduce inequalities).

In this chapter, we explore the global distribution of health and disease and the influence of social determinants of health on these patterns. We examine the global burden of both infectious and non-communicable diseases, focusing on differences between developing and developed countries. We also discuss the role of global economic, political and health system factors in shaping global health inequities, and conclude by examining current action to address the social determinants at the global level.

Infectious diseases on a global scale

Historical records show that infectious or communicable diseases have afflicted humankind for thousands of years. For example, malaria was described in 2700 BCE by Chinese physicians (Cox 2010). During the medieval period, Central Asia and Europe were devastated by the Black Plague, which caused up to 200 million deaths (Benedictow 2004). A century ago, it is estimated that 50–100 million people died during the 1918 influenza pandemic (Johnson & Mueller 2002). In the last two centuries, major advances in medical science and technology for prevention and treatment, such as immunisation and antibiotics, have resulted in steep declines of **infectious diseases**. Yet communicable diseases such as tuberculosis (TB) remain among the top causes of death globally (WHO 2015). They present a major health problem in many parts of the world, and among vulnerable populations in all societies.

Infectious diseases
Infections caused by micro-organisms such as bacteria, viruses, fungi and microparasites. Many infectious diseases are transmissible from person to person either directly or indirectly. Common communicable diseases include influenza, measles, sexually transmitted infections and malaria.

The past few decades have seen certain infectious diseases become an increasing threat to public health at national and global levels. Outbreaks of new infectious diseases such as Ebola and Zika in the Latin American, West African and Middle Eastern regions have spread to other parts of the world (WHO 2014; Musso et al. 2015). The incidence of three major infectious diseases—HIV, TB and malaria—has been declining globally, but parts of the world continue to bear a disproportionate burden of these diseases and associated mortality.

Globally, it is estimated that there were 36.7 million people living with HIV and 1.8 million people infected with HIV in 2016 (UNAIDS 2017). The burden of disease is concentrated in developing regions, especially in low- and middle-income countries (LMICs), particularly those in sub-Saharan Africa. Overall, infection rates decreased between 2010 and 2016 but in some regions infection rates continued to increase, specifically in Eastern Europe and Central Asia among people who inject drugs (UNAIDS 2017). Deaths due to AIDS decreased in that period due to the increased availability and accessibility of anti-retroviral treatment. The rate of decrease varied across regions, with particular regions experiencing a slow or no decline in deaths. Globally, the leading cause of death among women aged 15–49 years in that period was AIDS-related illnesses (UNAIDS 2017; see also Chapter 4).

Developed countries have taken great strides in controlling and treating HIV and AIDS. Australia was one of the first countries to detect the transmission of HIV. The rapid actions in prevention and public health interventions mitigated the spread of the virus; the collaboration and partnerships among government agencies, researchers, clinicians and the community sector has been recognised as a model HIV response internationally. The HIV prevalence rate in Australia, at approximately 0.13 per cent with 19 097 people living with HIV (as of end 2015) is low compared to the rate in other developed countries (Kirby Institute 2016). Most of the HIV cases occur among men who have sex with men, and to lesser extent among people who inject drugs, and sex workers (Kirby Institute 2016). Among Aboriginal and Torres Straits Islanders it was estimated there were 574 people living with HIV in 2016 (Kirby Institute 2017). The breakthrough in biomedical prevention and treatment, including post-exposure prophylaxis and anti-retroviral drugs, has significantly curbed transmission and improved the quality of life for people living with HIV in Australia.

The HIV situation and the response to the epidemic in LMICs is starkly different. Political, social and economic contexts are recognised to influence the spread of the epidemic, as these factors affect people's risk of and vulnerability to HIV, and the treatment and care of people living with HIV (Seeley et al. 2012). The response to the epidemic in LMICs occurs in settings with limited resources (due to poverty) and complex interactions/intersection of structural forces (Auerbach et al. 2011) including cultural norms, gender inequity and power relations (Mbonye et al. 2012), economic livelihoods (MacPherson et al. 2012), and people's behaviour and practices. For example, girls may not have access to educational opportunities due to being care-givers and lacking financial means. This could impede access to HIV prevention awareness and materials, and in many cases pressure them to engage in transactional sex or sex work, thus increasing their risk of HIV infection.

Tuberculosis is a disease caused by the bacterium *Mycobacterium tuberculosis* and its modern strains first appeared about 15 000–20 000 years ago (Sreevatsan et al. 1997). Through medical understanding of the TB pathogen, from the 18th century onwards infections were controlled through public health strategies of improving housing, sanitation and nutrition. A vaccine for TB, the Bacille Calmette-Guerin or BCG vaccine, was developed in the early 20th century and further curbed infections (Luca & Mihaescu 2013). The re-emergence of TB followed the HIV pandemic; TB is a common co-infection for people with HIV and caused 40 per cent of deaths (Gupta et al. 2015). Tuberculosis kills more people than any other infectious disease and is the ninth leading cause of death worldwide (WHO 2017b). There were 10.6 million cases of TB reported in 2016, and 1.7 million deaths, most of which occurred in poor and resource-limited countries (WHO 2017b). India has the highest number of TB infections and, along with Indonesia, China, Philippines, Pakistan, Nigeria and South Africa, account for 64 per cent of total TB cases in the world (WHO 2017b).

Treatment for TB is available (but the accessibility of drugs varies between poor and rich countries) and successful recovery requires the disease to be fully treated. The infected person should be diagnosed and treated quickly to stop the spread of the disease, and adhere to and complete the course of medicine (six to nine months). Otherwise, treatment can be compromised by the spread of multi-drug-resistant TB which requires a longer treatment period, is costlier and produces more adverse effects (Albanna & Menzies 2011).

Malaria cases are concentrated in tropical and subtropical regions. The disease is spread by the female *Anopheles* mosquitoes that transmit parasites (mainly *Plasmodium falciparum* and *Plasmodium vivax*) through bites to humans. Across the world, 91 countries reported a total of 216 million malaria cases in 2016 (WHO 2017c).

African nations bear the greater disease burden, with 90 per cent of cases and 91 per cent of deaths reported in this continent (WHO 2017c). Deaths due to malaria are highest, at 70 per cent, among infected children under five years of age (WHO 2017c). The disease can be treated with antimalarial medications but severe malaria and late treatment can be life-threatening. Malaria prophylaxis can be provided to prevent the disease but is not always feasible for the local population due to its high cost, the side effects of long-term use, and limited availability in poor countries (Fernando et al. 2011).

According to the WHO (2017c), cases of malaria decreased between 2010 and 2015, and the disease burden in affected countries has markedly reduced. However, in 2016 an estimated 216 million cases were reported (compared with 237 million cases in 2010) and prevention, diagnosing and treatment of malaria continues to be a major challenge, particularly as LMICs bear the greater burden of disease.

The countries with a high disease burden of malaria, TB and/or HIV share similar challenges in their attempts to control and prevent the spread of these diseases, and to treat people who are infected. Most are LMICs grappling with poverty, which undermines efforts to address the social determinants of health, producing health inequities along with inequities in employment, gender equity, housing, food security and social support.

Moreover, the health systems in most LMICs are in need of strengthening to build health infrastructure (e.g. hospitals), develop and improve health policy, provide better access to healthcare and protect people against the financial burden of ill health (WHO 2010). As such, there is much reliance on international donors to provide technical assistance and financing to strengthen the health sector and progress development. This is a major concern, as there is some uncertainty in whether official development assistance can be sustained (OECD 2018). Greater investment is crucial to finance the increased healthcare spending needed to close the gap in health inequities within and among countries (Dieleman et al. 2016), particularly as the burden of diseases will be concentrated in developing countries for the foreseeable future.

Furthermore, HIV and TB are highly stigmatised diseases. People living with HIV or infected with TB experience stigma and discrimination in many settings, including the workplace, schools and universities, accommodation, healthcare centres, travel, and in social contexts (Stangl et al. 2013). For example, stigma is a major inhibitor to people living with HIV disclosing their status to family, friends and colleagues, thus reducing their likelihood of seeking social and other support, and exacerbating their social isolation (Smith et al. 2008; see also Chapter 4).

Another key factor known to undermine the HIV response is laws or legislative frameworks that prohibit certain activities and behaviours. In countries that allow for punitive laws and discriminatory law enforcement that prosecute same-sex relations, sex work and drug use, there is an increased risk of HIV transmission, non-disclosure of HIV status and barriers to seeking treatment and care (UNDP HIV & AIDS Group 2012). For example, transgender people face discriminatory laws based on gender identity that intensify marginalisation across every aspect of their life experience from education and employment to health (Baral et al. 2011).

The emergence of drug-resistant infectious diseases is another challenge worldwide, as some medicines which were previously effective in curing a disease have lost their efficacy in killing the targeted bacteria and other micro-organisms. New drugs have to be developed to replace standard therapy; extensively drug-resistant TB has emerged, with limited treatment options and a high mortality rate. For LMICs this means that more resources (which they can ill-afford) have to be directed to community education and awareness, detection of drug resistance, and complex multi-drug therapies that require intensive monitoring and management.

Stop and Think

International passengers (both Australians and non-residents) arriving in Australia have to complete an incoming passenger card that includes declarations relating to customs and quarantine. Specifically, a passenger who is not an Australian citizen has to answer the question: 'Do you have tuberculosis?'

- There are many infectious diseases in the world. Why is the government particularly concerned about TB?
- What would be the health consequences, for the passenger and others, if a passenger had TB?
- What would be the health consequences, for the passenger and others, if a passenger had TB but did not know they were infected?

Case Example 14.1

Malaria in Myanmar

Malaria is a global health priority that affects close to 100 countries. Sub-Saharan Africa bears the heaviest burden of the disease, with approximately 90 per cent of the cases and deaths worldwide (WHO 2017c). The disease also affects regions closer to Australia such as south-east Asia, in which two countries—Indonesia and Myanmar—report the most cases. Myanmar reports more than half the deaths caused by malaria (WHO 2017c). However, Myanmar has made tremendous progress in reducing morbidity and mortality in the last decade.

Between 2012 and 2015 there was a reduction of cases by 82 per cent and of deaths by 93 per cent (WHO 2018a). The incidence of malaria reduced by 49 per cent during the same period. The decrease is due to the wide distribution of insecticide-treated mosquito nets and artemisinin-based combination therapy.

These achievements are remarkable as Myanmar is one of the poorest countries in Asia, but since 2011 the government has made governance, economic and social reforms and its economy is growing steadily. The National Malaria Elimination Plan 2016–2030 sets out the aim to achieve malaria-free status by 2030 (NMCP 2017), which is predicated on SDG3.3 ('By 2030, end the epidemics of AIDS, tuberculosis, malaria and neglected tropical diseases and combat hepatitis, water-borne diseases and other communicable diseases'). The implementation of the Plan will be carried out in several phases. The current phase focuses on three key interventions: case detection and management, disease prevention and entomology surveillance. This will require cross-sectoral collaboration among government bodies such as the health, transport and education ministries, and international agencies such as Médecins sans Frontières working in-country on anti-malaria interventions. Partnering with community and village health workers is integral to the sustainable prevention, detection and treatment of malaria. For example, community health workers can demonstrate the use of mosquito nets and alert health authorities to cases.

Myanmar continues to address challenges that could impede progress towards achieving the goal of eradicating malaria, including a health system that requires strengthening to provide accessible and affordable quality healthcare, and infrastructure and rural development such as schools, transport and energy projects (Global Fund 2014). Human resources in the health sector have to be expanded and expertise in health system components such as the supply chain (including equipment and medicines) and financial management need to be developed. Roads have to be built to reach remote villages where the poorest and most affected people are located, to increase awareness, diagnosis and treatment. Some of these areas are not under government control—the conflict zones add to the difficulties of expanding coverage of health services and education. Further complications are the mobility and migration of the population across borders and the geography and landscape of Myanmar—dense forests, agricultural fields, river basins, urban areas and border towns.

While effective prevention and treatment have lowered the rates of transmission and deaths, the rise in drug and insecticide resistance is a threat to malaria eradication efforts in Myanmar and other affected countries (Mu et al. 2016; Newby et al. 2016). A vaccine is not yet available but a promising candidate is undergoing clinical trials (WHO 2016a). Philanthropic bodies such as the Bill and Melinda Gates Foundation directly fund research into developing a malaria vaccine that could reduce disease and control transmission (Breman & Brandling-Bennett 2011).

As a low-income country, Myanmar has received support from bilateral and multilateral donors to implement its National Malaria Strategic Plans. The Global Fund is the main funder, having invested close to US$140 million by 2017 (Global Fund 2018). The funding stream from international donors is unlikely be sustained over the long term. Myanmar will have to raise domestic funds for its malaria programs—a difficult task due to competing health priorities in a resource-limited setting.

Non-communicable diseases: a growing global problem

Non-communicable diseases
NCDs are cardiovascular diseases (e.g. heart attack and stroke), diabetes, cancers and chronic respiratory diseases such as chronic obstructive pulmonary disease and asthma. These diseases, which are not transmitted from one person to another, account for the majority of deaths globally and share a common set of behavioural risk factors (tobacco consumption, poor nutrition, physical inactivity and harmful use of alcohol).

While infectious diseases are an ongoing challenge in many countries, **non-communicable** (non-infectious) **diseases** (NCDs) are now the leading global cause of death (WHO 2011). In 2008 they accounted for almost two-thirds (over 60 per cent) of the 57 million deaths (WHO 2011, p. 1). Many LMICs experience a double burden of continuing infectious disease epidemics along with rising rates of NCDs.

The burden of NCDs is overwhelmingly experienced by LMICs (WHO 2011). People in low-income countries tend to get sicker earlier in life, and die earlier from NCDs than people in high-income countries. Nearly 30 per cent of deaths from NCDs in LMICs occur under the age of 60 (in comparison with 13 per cent of deaths under the age of 60 in high-income countries) (WHO 2011, p. 10). The burden of NCDs is also increasing more quickly in LMICs than in high-income countries (WHO 2017d).

Risk factors for NCDs have the greatest effects on LMICs (and on the poorest groups in these countries). For example, approximately 80 per cent of the world's smokers reside in LMICs (WHO 2018b). In most countries, rates of taking up smoking are higher and rates of smoking cessation are lower in lower socio-economic groups (Hosseinpoor et al. 2012). A study of smoking rates in 48 LMICs found that, among men, the smoking rate was over 2.5 times higher for poor men than rich men (Hosseinpoor et al. 2012). Since the main risk factors for NCDs can be modified, many of these deaths could be prevented by adequately funded preventive health and treatment interventions (WHO 2011).

Poverty, along with other social determinants such as education, income and employment status, are closely intertwined with NCDs. Poverty makes people more vulnerable to NCDs and contributes to premature death from NCDs, in LMICs as well as in high-income countries (Niessen et al. 2018). NCDs also tend to reduce household income, contributing to poverty at the household level (WHO 2011), and can result in impoverishment through catastrophic healthcare costs (Nugent et al. 2018). At the household level, unhealthy behaviours, poor physical status as a result of NCDS and the high cost of healthcare lead to loss of household income. When those who get sick or die are the income-earners in a family, there is often not enough money to pay for sufficient good-quality food or education. People become trapped in a cycle of poverty and disease—loss of income increases their exposure to risk factors and the risk of disease.

At the level of countries, NCDs put a strain on health system resources, reduce workforce productivity and reduce national income, slowing economic development (WHO 2011). The health systems in LMICs are less equipped to address a high burden of NCDs and their risk factors (WHO 2011).

Case Example 14.2

NCDs in Pacific island countries

When we think of the Pacific islands, the images that often come to mind are the sandy white beaches and swaying palm trees we see in travel brochures, but the reality for the people who live in these countries is very different from this idyll.

The Pacific islands have some of the highest rates of NCDs in the world—including cardiovascular diseases, cancer, chronic respiratory diseases and diabetes (Hou et al. 2016). Diabetes affects over 20 per cent of the adult population in more than half of the Pacific island countries where rates have been measured (Hawley & McGarvey 2015). Diabetes is a particular problem because treatment options are very limited in the Pacific islands, and people who have diabetes tend to have much shorter lives than their counterparts in countries like Australia.

Smoking is a major risk factor for hypertension, diabetes and cancer and is prevalent in all Pacific island countries. More than half of all adult males smoked daily in some countries in 2012, including Kiribati and Papua New Guinea (Ng et al. 2014). The prevalence of overweight and obesity in Pacific island countries, another major NCD risk factor, has been estimated at 32.1–93.5 per cent, and more than half the population is overweight in all countries except Papua New Guinea (Hawley & McGarvey 2015).

The high burden of NCDs in the Pacific islands is the result of a complex mix of social, political and economic factors. Over time, there has been a shift from a subsistence economy (where people grow enough food for themselves and their families, and some to trade for basic necessities) to a cash economy, where people need money to purchase goods (Thow & Snowdon 2010). The increasing movement of people into urban centres, seeking work, has reduced access to farm land and traditional foods, and the need to work outside the home has made traditional cooking methods inconvenient for many people (Thow & Snowdon 2010).

Local food production has declined, and in some cases farming is no longer economically worthwhile. Fishing has become an increasingly important commercial export activity, and Pacific islanders increasingly consume cheaper imported processed fish rather than local fresh fish (Thow & Snowdon 2010). Climate change also presents a major problem: arable land in low-lying coral atolls like Kiribati is becoming inundated as sea levels rise. There are more frequent and extreme weather events like cyclones that cause damage to crops and infrastructure, and changes to fish habitats (Bell et al. 2016).

These changes have resulted in major shifts in dietary patterns. The traditional diet of root crops and fish has been replaced with mostly imported foods which are generally highly processed, high in saturated fat, refined carbohydrates, sugar and salt, and have low nutritional value (fatty meats, instant noodles, white rice, soft drinks) (Hawley & McGarvey 2015). These imported foods are often lower in price than local traditional foods, and widely accessible through supermarkets and fast-food outlets (Thow & Snowdon 2010). People have become more sedentary due to the transition away from subsistence farming (Hawley & McGarvey 2015).

Treating NCDs is a major economic burden for Pacific island countries, which have high health expenditure as a proportion of GDP and as a proportion of government expenditure. For example, Anderson (2012) found that in Vanuatu, the cost of treating someone who was newly diagnosed with diabetes was around five times higher than the per capita expenditure on health for the population, and the cost of providing medication for diabetes was eight to 65 times higher than the amount allocated per person. For both economic and health reasons, a major investment is being made in addressing the causes of NCDs in the Pacific region.

Inequities in health and structural determinants of health

Although there have been overall gains in life expectancy and health, the gap between the health outcomes of rich and poor countries, and between higher and lower socio-economic groups within countries, has been widening (see also Chapters 7 & 13). The CSDH (2008, p. 37) reported that in 1980 the world's richest countries had a gross national income (GNI) per capita 60 times the GNI per capita of the poorest countries. By 2005 the richest countries had 122 times the GNI per capita of the world's poorest countries.

Even wealthy countries experience systematic inequalities in health outcomes according to people's socio-economic position in society (Mackenbach 2012). In the US, for example, a comprehensive review of studies of survival rates showed that rapidly rising income inequality has been reflected in widening gaps in life expectancy and mortality rates between middle- and high-income Americans and their poorer counterparts (Bor et al. 2017). As shown in the seminal work of Adler et al. (1994), these differences exist not only between the wealthiest and poorest parts of society—there is a gradual increase in health status at every step up the socio-economic hierarchy.

In all societies, the population groups who are most disadvantaged are the most vulnerable. For example, people who are most likely to have unhealthy diets (and therefore higher rates of overweight and obesity, and diet-related diseases) are disadvantaged population groups with lower incomes and education levels, and poor working and living conditions (Friel et al. 2015).

When thinking about health at the global level, we need to consider the **structural determinants of health**. These are factors that relate to the organisation of society, the way institutions operate and the economic and political context (Solar & Irwin 2010; Crammond & Carey 2016; see also Chapters 7 & 13).

Structural determinants of health
Factors embedded in the way society operates, including policies and institutions, and economic and political factors, which are beyond the control of individuals.

Key structural factors that shape people's socio-economic position in society include income, education, employment and occupational status (Solar & Irwin 2010). Structural determinants also include the economic and political factors that give rise to and maintain these patterns, including institutions (e.g. government agencies, education and health systems) and social and public policies (e.g. social security and taxation, housing policies, education and health policies) (Solar & Irwin 2010). These structural determinants operate far above the level of the individual and affect very large groups of people simultaneously.

Structural determinants can be thought of as the fundamental or underlying factors that affect health outcomes through a complex and multi-layered set of intermediary factors such as the material circumstances of people's lives (e.g. their ability to afford healthy food and adequate housing), psychosocial factors (e.g. stress and social support) and behavioural risk factors such as consumption of alcohol and tobacco (Solar & Irwin 2010; Crammond and Carey 2016). A core principle of public health is that to improve health outcomes, we need to address the root causes of ill health rather than just ameliorating their effects (Crammond & Carey 2016).

The next two sections explore how some of the structural determinants of health operate at the global level.

Stop and Think

The daily smoking rate among Australian adults declined from 23.8 per cent in 1995 to 14.5 per cent in 2015 (ABS 2015). In Papua New Guinea, the adult smoking rate was estimated at 26.3 per cent in 2016 (WHO 2017e).

- What structural factors might contribute to the difference in smoking rates between Australia and Papua New Guinea?

Global economic and political determinants of health

As discussed earlier in the chapter, the CSDH (2008) described how inequities in health are underpinned by the unequal distribution of power, money and resources at the global level. These imbalances shape daily living conditions around the world. Many determinants of these large-scale inequalities are located in global political and economic arrangements.

Globalisation
The global integration of economic arrangements and the increasingly fluid movement of people, ideas, technology, goods and services across national borders.

A group of forces that are collectively referred to as **globalisation** powerfully shape health inequities at the global level. The increasing integration of economies into a global system means that societies are more exposed to forces that operate beyond national borders (Schrecker et al. 2008).

Globalisation has both positive and negative effects. Integration into a global economy can, under certain conditions, drive economic growth and reduce poverty (Schrecker et al. 2008). But it can also create and worsen inequities between rich and poor countries. For example, foods such as cereals can be produced relatively cheaply in countries like the US, where farmers are subsidised heavily by the government; the surplus is exported to developing countries (Otterson et al. 2014). This has contributed to food insecurity by increasing reliance on imported foods and displacing local food production (Otterson et al. 2014).

One of the factors underpinning the massive global inequities in power and resources that we see today is the legacy of Third World debt. Many poor countries borrowed money in the 1960s and 1970s when interest rates were extremely low; they have never been able to afford to repay those debts. High interest rates and oil prices from the 1980s onwards, combined with falling commodity prices, caused the 'debt trap' (Schrecker et al. 2008). In affected countries, vital resources are diverted to debt repayment with little hope of ever significantly reducing the level of debt, instead of being spent on public services like health and education. The Jubilee Debt Campaign UK estimates that 27 countries are currently experiencing debt crisis. Ghana, for example, spends an estimated 30 per cent of government revenue annually servicing debt repayments (JDC n.d.).

The International Monetary Fund, which plays a leading role in the global economic arena, has been criticised for applying strict conditions to its loans to developing countries. These have forced many countries to privatise services, deregulate markets, reduce taxes and reduce government funding on health, education, housing and other social programs (Stuckler & Basu 2009; Labonte 2015; Baum 2016). Rather than reducing debt, these types of policies increased health inequalities and undermined health systems in many countries, leading to rises in maternal and child mortality rates (Stuckler & Basu 2009; Baum 2016). Many developing countries are still dependent on loans and funds from donors, which often come with restrictions on how they can be spent. These restrictions often fit better with the priorities of the wealthy countries and the donors than with what the recipient countries perceive as their most pressing needs.

Transnational corporations

TNCs are companies that have their headquarters in one country but operate through subsidiaries in one or more other countries, thus crossing national boundaries.

Powerful actors at the global level include wealthy countries such as the US and EU, donors and **transnational corporations** (TNCs). The US is the biggest funder of global health and retains a great deal of influence on how the funding is spent (Fidler 2010). Development assistance for health increased by more than 500 per cent from 1990 to 2005, and by 2007, funding from private donors accounted for nearly a quarter of global health funding (McCoy et al. 2009). The Bill and Melinda Gates Foundation has been particularly dominant—by 2009 it contributed more money to fund global health than any government except the US and UK (McCoy et al. 2009). TNCs also wield enormous power in setting global agendas due to their economic resources (Ottersen et al. 2014). As de Jonge (2017, p. 10) describes:

> Global corporations now have revenues that rival the entire GDP of many countries. Of the 100 largest economies, 50 are global corporations while 49 are countries. The combined sales of the world's top 200 corporations account for over a quarter of world GDP. Sheer economic weight means that TNCs can and do exert a great deal of influence over decision makers and over peoples' lives generally. This influence is compounded by close connections and communities of interest linking TNCs to each other.

Many TNCs have played key roles in exacerbating health inequities and contributing to rising rates of NCDs (Kickbusch et al. 2016). For example, the tobacco, alcohol and processed food industries are increasingly turning their attention to marketing and advertising in developing countries (Moodie et al. 2013). They sometimes undermine public health efforts through a range of strategies, including publishing dubious research, co-opting health experts, lobbying decision-makers and persuading the public to oppose regulation of their activities (Moodie et al. 2013). Due to the enormous influence of global corporations on health, the term 'commercial determinants of health' has been coined to capture the 'strategies and approaches used by the private sector to promote products and choices that are detrimental to health' (Kickbusch et al. 2016, p. e895). Due to their global reach, TNCs are often able to evade the efforts of governments to regulate them by shifting their activities from one country to another.

Case Example 14.3

Global marketing of infant formula

Breastmilk is by far the best food for infants. Exclusive breastfeeding is recommended by the WHO and UNICEF (2003) for at least the first six months of a baby's life, along with continued breastfeeding for at least two years. Breastfeeding has many protective health effects for both babies and mothers (Kaplan & Graff 2008; Victora et al. 2016), and is particularly important in protecting infants' health in disadvantaged settings. It also has economic benefits for households and nations, and reduces health system spending (Baker et al. 2016).

Rates of exclusive breastfeeding, however, remain low. They were estimated at below 50 per cent in most countries and around 35 per cent in LMICs by 2013 (Victora et al. 2016). In LMICs, wealthy mothers are much more likely to breastfeed exclusively than poor mothers (Victora et al. 2016).

Aggressive marketing of breastmilk substitutes (infant formula) has been a primary contributor to low breastfeeding rates (Kaplan & Graff 2008). A global baby food industry has developed, with sales of US$32 billion by 2007 (Smith et al. 2014). The total volume of infant formula sales increased by 40.8 per cent from 2008 to 2013, with the greatest rate of growth in middle-income Asian countries including China, Indonesia, Malaysia, Thailand and Vietnam (Baker et al. 2016).

Promotion of breastfeeding, together with more effective regulation of infant formula marketing in recent years, has led to a flattening of demand for commercial infant formula in many developed countries. However, demand has continued to increase in LMICs (Smith et al. 2014). For example, in China, increasing demand and heavy marketing of formula drove the decline in breastfeeding for infants up to six months of age from 67 per cent in 1998 to 28 per cent by 2012 (Smith et al. 2014). China is now the largest global market for breastmilk substitutes. This contributed to a public health crisis in 2008, when an episode of melamine-contaminated Chinese formula led to the death of six infants and the hospitalisation of more than 50000 (Tang et al. 2015). Fears about contamination led to the importation and panic-buying of large quantities of infant formula from other countries, including Australia, which led to shortages of some products in those countries (Tang et al. 2015).

Baker et al. (2016) estimate that the global expenditure on infant formula marketing exceeded $US4 billion in 2014. Formula is marketed directly to mothers through a range of different strategies, including traditional forms of marketing (e.g. print advertisements and billboards) and television and online advertising, along with distribution of samples and discounted products (Piwoz & Huffman 2015). Baby food manufacturers also use health professionals and health services to market their products; for example, through baby care information and product packages given to mothers in hospitals and at maternal and child health services (Kaplan & Graff 2008; Baker et al. 2016).

The International Code of Marketing of Breast-milk Substitutes was adopted by the World Health Assembly in 1981 as part of a global effort to reduce unethical marketing, but by 2016 only 39 of 194 countries had fully implemented it in their laws (WHO et al. 2016). Marketing remains common even in countries that have implemented the provisions (Piwoz & Huffman 2015). Australia banned direct advertising of infant formula to consumers in 1983, but companies have continued to promote their brands to the public by advertising baby food and toddler formula (Smith & Blake 2013).

Inequities in health are to some extent produced and maintained through international trade and investment agreements intended to liberalise trade (remove barriers to trade between countries). These barriers can be tariffs (import taxes) or non-tariff barriers such as government regulations for food safety, product labelling and the provision of services, where such regulations disadvantage foreign companies or make trade between countries more costly or difficult.

Trade agreements, along with globalisation and economic integration more generally, have driven large-scale changes in the availability, composition, accessibility and prices of foods, and ultimately changes in diet and its consequences—overweight, obesity and NCDs (Friel et al. 2013). Trade agreements have also reduced the range of policies, laws and regulations that governments can use to promote and protect health (Gleeson & Friel 2013; Labonte 2015).

For example, Samoa banned imports of turkey tails from the US (a fatty meat product popular in the Pacific islands) in 2007 in an attempt to reduce overweight and obesity, but had to remove the ban in 2011 in order to join the World Trade Organization (WTO) (Thow et al. 2010).

Some trade and investment agreements provide avenues for corporations to sue governments for compensation in international tribunals, claiming that the investor protections afforded by the agreement have been breached. A well-known example is the challenge to Australia's tobacco plain packaging laws brought by the tobacco company Philip Morris Asia (Gleeson & Friel 2013). The claim was unsuccessful, but the case took six years and was very costly to defend (Hutchens & Knaus 2018). The threat of such legal cases can deter governments from implementing public health policies or delay their introduction. In New Zealand, plans to introduce plain packaging of tobacco products were put on hold while the case was underway in Australia (Crosbie et al. 2018).

Health system determinants: global dimensions

In many countries, large numbers of people still lack access to affordable healthcare. Health systems in LMICs often lack basic infrastructure and are ill-equipped to meet the needs of their populations and provide financial protection against the costs of ill health (Mills 2014). This can be a result of donor funding directed to specific diseases and programs, and/or lack of government investment in healthcare facilities and personnel. India, for example, spent only 4.1 per cent of GDP on health in 2014 (Bhatia 2016), in comparison with Australia which spent 9.8 per cent of GDP per capita on health in the same year (Glover 2016). Only 26.7 per cent of India's health expenditure was funded by governments, with the remainder funded through private sources. Out-of-pocket health costs in India are high and only around half of the population is covered by health insurance (Bhatia 2016).

Stop and Think

- How do you think underfunding of the healthcare system affects health outcomes in India, for both infectious diseases and NCDs?

There are stark variations in access to medications, vaccines and treatments in different parts of the world. In 2004, almost one-third of the world's population lacked access to essential medicines (WHO 2004). While much has been done to correct this imbalance, some 400 million people still lacked access to basic healthcare by 2015, including access to medicines and vaccines (WHO & World Bank 2015). Most pharmaceutical research and development is conducted in western countries, and funding is overwhelmingly weighted towards diseases that mainly affect people in developed countries. Only around 1 per cent of research and development funding is directed toward the 'neglected tropical diseases' that affect approximately 1.7 billion people in LMICs (Rottingen et al. 2013; UN 2016).

High medicine prices present another major barrier to access for people in developing countries. High prices result primarily from intellectual property protections such as patents for new medicines, which prevent anyone else from making or selling the drug for a period of time—at least 20 years, for most countries that are members of the WTO. Patents and other types of intellectual property protection delay the availability of cheaper generic medicines. A large number of bilateral and regional trade agreements have extended and expanded intellectual property protections further than those required by the WTO, making it increasingly difficult for countries to provide affordable access to medicines (Lopert & Gleeson 2013).

Global shortages of health workers present another pressing problem for health systems. In 2006, there was a global shortage of 4.3 million health professionals, according to the WHO (2006). Shortages are particularly dire in the poorest countries and regions with the greatest unmet health needs. For example, sub-Saharan Africa experiences 24 per cent of the world's burden of disease but has a very small proportion (3 per cent) of the world's health workforce (Taylor et al. 2011).

At the global level, shortages of health workers have resulted in large-scale migration of health workers from poor countries to wealthy countries. This is commonly referred to as the 'brain drain'. Brain drain is partly the result of active recruitment of health workers by wealthy countries, and partly the result of health workers seeking to migrate to countries where they will have better pay and working conditions and access to a better life-style (Taylor et al. 2011). This brain drain exacerbates existing health workforce shortages in LMICs, weakens their health systems and makes it more difficult to provide essential services and to reduce health inequities (Mackey & Liang 2012).

Action to address global health inequities

Since the release of the CSDH report, there has been a concerted global effort to address the inequities of social determinants of health. The CSDH recommended three approaches to addressing inequities in health: improving people's daily living conditions; working towards a fairer distribution of power, money and resources; and developing capacity to monitor the problem and evaluate actions to address it (CSDH 2008, p. 2).

The most important action is to correct systemic inequalities in socio-economic status within and between countries (Niessen et al. 2018). Within countries, national governments have an important role in redistributing resources, for example through taxation, and in providing welfare programs and other essential services such as health and education, which ameliorate the effects of income inequality (Blas et al. 2008).

An approach that has been shown to be effective in addressing the structural determinants of health is known as **Health in All Policies** (HiAP). It is based on the fact that many of the conditions which are important for improving health require action that goes beyond the health sector; other sectors need to be engaged (Donkin et al. 2018).

Health in All Policies
HiAP is a cross-sectoral approach to addressing the social determinants of health.

HiAP is based on the idea of 'intersectoral action for health', one of the key concepts in the WHO's 1978 Alma-Ata Declaration, and the concept of healthy public policy which is central to the 1986 Ottawa Charter for Health Promotion (Kickbusch 2010). It uses a systematic approach to 'examine determinants of health, which can be influenced to improve health but are mainly controlled by policies of sectors other than health' (Shito et al. 2006). At the global level, a HiAP approach suggests that the health effects of international economic policies and trade agreements need to be taken into account and balanced against economic interests. There is an important role for health workers and their professional associations in advocating for health to be higher on the agenda in both national and international policies.

Within the health sector, **universal health coverage** is very important in providing essential healthcare services and affordable medicines and vaccines, as well as protecting people against the potentially catastrophic effects of ill health (WHO & World Bank 2017; see also Chapter 13).

Universal health coverage
The provision of access to health services for the whole population, without financial hardship.

Comprehensive primary healthcare is an important approach that aims to meet the immediate needs of individuals and communities while addressing the political, economic and social structures that create health inequity (Legge et al. 2007).

Comprehensive primary healthcare
A multi-disciplinary model of healthcare that includes community involvement, multi-sectoral collaboration, prevention and action on the social determinants of health.

Addressing imbalances in global health requires a concerted global effort, with developing countries included as partners rather than simply as recipients of funding. Change requires empowerment, participation and mobilisation of the communities most affected. Civil society, including community groups, non-government organisations and social movements, has a very important role to play in driving change at the global level (Blas et al. 2008). An example is the People's Health Movement (PHM n.d.), a global network of health activists and organisations, mainly from LMICs, which was founded in Bangladesh in 2000. PHM provides a critique of the global economic system, advocates for comprehensive primary healthcare and a fair distribution of resources, and monitors the activities of the WHO and other players in global health.

Case Example 14.4

Global initiatives to address infectious diseases

Since the early 2000s, there has been unprecedented global action in supporting poor and developing countries to manage HIV, TB and malaria.

The Global Fund to Fight AIDS, TB and Malaria (Global Fund) was established as a funding institution to raise funds (about US$4 billion annually) and provide resources for countries in need of programs. Fundamental to its work is its partnerships with governments, civil society, the private sector and people affected by the diseases to ensure a holistic and comprehensive approach to achieve a 'world free of HIV, TB and malaria'. The partnership and unparalleled investment resulted in more than 22 million lives saved, from 2000 to 2016.

The WHO 'End TB' strategy (WHO 2015) set goals to reduce incidence of TB by 90 per cent between 2015 and 2035, and is aligned to SDG3.3 that focuses on HIV, TB and malaria. To achieve the targets, the strategy proposed three essential pillars: integrated patient-centred care and prevention; bold policies and supportive systems; and intensified research and innovation. Importantly, both national governments and international donors had to increase their financing to implement the three components and advance research for better diagnostics, vaccines and treatment.

The SDG3.3 agenda is to end the epidemics of AIDS, TB, malaria and neglected tropical diseases by 2030. To align with this goal, and to control and eliminate malaria within the time-frame, WHO produced the Global Technical Strategy for Malaria 2016–2030. Its intention is to reduce malaria mortality rates and incidence rates, eliminate malaria in endemic countries, and prevent re-establishment of malaria in malaria-free countries (WHO 2016a, b). The framework for achieving these goals involves three main strategies: providing access to prevention, diagnosis and treatment for all those who need it; working towards eliminating malaria; and transforming surveillance into core prevention.

Concurrently, the global Roll Back Malaria partnership, comprising malaria endemic countries, donors, public and private sectors, and research institutions, launched the RBM Action and Investment to Defeat Malaria 2016–2030 (AIM) (RBM 2015). The focus is to advocate for increased investment to achieve the targets set for SDG3.3 and a malaria-free world. This advocacy document outlines actions for global collaboration among stakeholders including governments, civil society and affected communities, and non-health sectors working on development and human security.

The increasing influence of globalisation on health calls for strong global health governance. The WHO has an important leadership role in co-ordinating action on global health, and providing guidance and technical assistance to member countries. Influential WHO initiatives include the Framework Convention for Tobacco Control and the Global Strategy for Women's, Children's and Adolescents' Health. However, the WHO has no power to enforce its guidelines and resolutions. It is also chronically underfunded by member states and is reliant on donors, who largely tie their funding to particular disease prevention programs (Legge 2012).

Despite examples of good practice from around the world, progress remains patchy (Donkin et al. 2018) and there are significant challenges to systematically addressing health inequities through action on the social determinants of health (Baker et al. 2017). Much work remains to be done if the SDGs are to be achieved by 2030.

Reflection Exercise

Jessica, a diabetes educator, takes up a position in a diabetes clinic in a public hospital in Nuku'alofa, the capital of Tonga. On her first day, a 48-year-old woman named Loa,* who was diagnosed with Type 2 diabetes two years previously, comes in for an appointment.

Jessica has read about the high rates of Type 2 diabetes in the Pacific islands. From her training, she knows it is very important for Loa to have a good diet, to be physically active and to maintain a healthy weight.

Loa's chart shows that she received counselling about physical activity and nutrition when her diabetes was diagnosed, but her weight has continued to increase. Jessica looks around the consultation room and notes the posters encouraging people to be more active and eat less fat and salt. She gently enquires about Loa's nutritional intake, level of physical activity and understanding of the advice she has received. Loa clearly understands the health information, but finds it difficult to maintain changes to her diet and to be more active.

Jessica asks Loa more about her life. She discovers that Loa and her family came to Nuku'alofa 10 years ago from one of the smaller islands, like many other families, to look for work. Well-paid jobs are scarce. To make ends meet, Loa has had to take on two casual jobs, while caring for her three children.

Loa's family lives in a makeshift settlement in a low-lying marsh area on the outskirts of Nuku'alofa. Loa has tried to grow taro and other root vegetables the family used to eat, but the water in the marsh is too salty. While neighbours sometimes share their fruit and vegetables, fresh food is often too expensive for her to buy, so the family mainly eats white rice and instant noodles with tinned corned meat and fish canned in oil. When she shops for food, she is surrounded by advertising for soft drinks and packaged snack foods. Loa is often too tired from work and caring for her children to prepare and cook nutritious meals, and it is often both cheaper and easier to buy fast food that fills them up. It is difficult to walk around the settlement due to the marshy ground and she doesn't feel safe walking alone—this makes it difficult for her to get enough exercise.

- What does this case example suggest about the structural factors that have contributed to Loa's diabetes?
- What would need to change in Loa's life to enable her to change her life-style?
- How could Jessica help Loa and others like her?

This chapter shows that simply providing health information and encouraging people to live healthier lives does not ensure that everyone has an equal chance to be healthy. Improving people's daily living conditions is central to addressing inequities in health (CSDH 2008). In Loa's case, this might include strategies such the Tonga Health Promotion Foundation's community gardening program, which provides soil, seedlings and gardening equipment to communities to enable them to grow food. Other strategies might include providing better housing and vocational training. An example of tackling the underlying structural factors would be working with different sectors of government to support and subsidise locally grown food, and limit marketing of unhealthy foods.

* This scenario has been fictionalised and any resemblance to any person is unintended.

Summary

Gains in health and life expectancy over the last few centuries have not been equally shared. Stark, and widening, differences remain in health outcomes in different parts of the world. At the global level, there have been steep declines in infectious diseases due to advances in treatment and prevention, but infectious diseases still present a major problem in LMICs and in vulnerable groups in all societies. LMICs also experience a disproportionate burden of NCDs and their risk factors.

To understand the causes of these health inequities, we need to understand how the structural determinants of health operate at the global level. Global economic and political determinants of health include globalisation and the increasing integration of the global economy, manifested in issues like Third World debt, the health-damaging effects of various TNCs and the constraints that international trade agreements place on government efforts to protect health. Structural determinants include health system factors such as underresourcing of health systems, lack of access to medicines, vaccines and treatments, and shortages and migration of health workers.

The WHO (CSDH 2008) recommends three approaches to addressing inequities in health: improving people's daily living conditions; working towards a fairer distribution of power, money and resources; and developing capacity to monitor the problem and evaluate actions to address it. Some effective national strategies include redistributive policies (e.g. taxation), provision of welfare services, universal health coverage and comprehensive primary healthcare, and Health in All Policies approaches. At the global level, reducing health inequities requires participation by developing countries and affected communities, along with concerted global strategies and strong global health leadership.

Tutorial exercises

1. Read the executive summary of the 2016 Report of the UN Secretary-General's High-Level Panel on Access to Medicines, or the fact sheet available at http://www.unsgaccessmeds.org/final-report/. What recommendations did the High-Level Panel make, and how will they address the problems of access to medicines in developing countries?
2. In small groups, choose one of the specific targets under SDG3, 'Ensure healthy lives and promote well-being for all at all ages' (https://sustainabledevelopment.un.org/sdg3). What structural determinants of health would need to be addressed, to meet the target you have chosen? What action should be taken to address these structural determinants?
3. Discuss what you think will happen to infectious diseases in the future. Are they likely to be successfully contained or controlled? What is happening now that could cause re-emergence of infectious diseases? What global factors could slow down progress?

Acknowledgments

We would like to acknowledge the contributions of Dr Rebecca Fanany, who wrote an earlier version of the lecture material on which this chapter is based, and Dr Tarryn Phillips, who kindly provided advice on the Reflection Exercise.

Further reading

CSDH (Commission on Social Determinants of Health) (2008). *Closing the Gap in a Generation: Health Equity through Action on the Social Determinants of Health.* Final Report of the Commission on Social Determinants of Health. Retrieved from http://www.who.int/social_determinants/thecommission/finalreport/en/

Donkin, A., Goldblatt, P., Allen, J., Nathanson, V., & Marmot, M. (2017). Global action on the social determinants of health. *BMJ Global Health*, 3, e000603. doi:10.1136/bmjgh-2017-000603

Jones, K.E., Patel, N.G., Levy, M.A., Storeygard, A., Balk, D., Gittleman, J.L., & Daszak, P. (2008). Global trends in emerging infectious diseases. *Nature*, 451(7181), 990.

Niessen, L.W., Mohan, D., Akuoku, J.K., Mirelman, A.J., Ahmed, S., Koehlmoos, T.P., Trujillo, A., Khan, J., & Peters, D.H. (2018). Tackling socioeconomic inequalities and non-communicable diseases in low-income and middle-income countries under the Sustainable Development Agenda. *Lancet*, 391(10134), 2036–2046. doi:10.1016/S0140-6736(18)30482-3

Otterson, O.P., Dasgupta, J., Blouin, C., Buss, P., Chongsuvivatwong, V., Frenk, J. et al. (2014). The Lancet-University of Oslo Commission on Global Governance for Health: the political origins of health inequity—prospects for change. *Lancet*, 383, 630–667.

Solar, O., & Irwin, A. (2010). *A Conceptual Framework for Action on the Social Determinants of Health. Social Determinants of Health Discussion Paper 2 (Policy and Practice).* Geneva: World Health Organization.

UN (2016). *Report of the United Nations Secretary-General's High Level Panel on Access to Medicines: Promoting Innovation and Access to Health Technologies.* Retrieved from http://www.unsgaccessmeds.org/final-report/

UNAIDS (Joint United Nations Programme on HIV/AIDS) (2017). *Ending AIDS: Progress Towards the 90-90-90 Targets Global AIDS Update.* Geneva.

UNDP HIV & AIDS Group (2012). *Global Commission on HIV and the Law: Risk, Rights and Health.* New York: UN Development Programme.

WHO (World Health Organization) (2011). *Global Status Report on Noncommunicable Diseases 2010.* Geneva: World Health Organization.

Websites

http://www.un.org/sustainabledevelopment/sustainable-development-goals/

This website is maintained by the UN. It is the primary source of information about the 2030 Agenda for Sustainable Development and the 17 Sustainable Development Goals and associated targets.

http://www.who.int/social_determinants/thecommission/en/

This page on the World Health Organization's website contains links to the final report of the Commission on Social Determinants of Health and related publications.

http://www.euro.who.int/en/publications/policy-documents/declaration-of-alma-ata,-1978

This page links to the WHO Declaration of Alma-Ata, which outlines a global vision for comprehensive primary healthcare.

https://www.theglobalfund.org/en/

This website contains information on the Global Fund's efforts to fight AIDS, TB and malaria. It documents grants made to countries and the results from those investments.

https://rollbackmalaria.com/

This website details the coordinated action against malaria involving over 500 members worldwide of the Roll Back Malaria Partnership.

http://www.stoptb.org/

This website is about the global effort to accelerate progress on access to TB diagnosis and treatment; research and development for new TB diagnostics, drugs and vaccines; and tackling drug-resistant and HIV-associated TB.

https://www.gnpplus.net/

The Global Network of People Living with HIV describes its work in improving the quality of life of its communities through global advocacy, community strengthening and knowledge management.

https://www.gavi.org/

The Global Alliance for Vaccines and Immunization is a public–private global health partnership committed to increasing access to immunisation in poor countries.

https://hivlawcommission.org/

The Global Commission on HIV and the Law interrogated the relationship between legal responses, human rights and HIV.

References

ABS (Australian Bureau of Statistics) (2015). *National Health Survey: First Results, 2014–15*. Retrieved from http://www.abs.gov.au/ausstats/abs@.nsf/Lookup/by%20 Subject/4364.0.55.001~2014-15~Main%20Features~Smoking~24

Adler, N.E., Boyce, T., Chesney, M.A., Sheldon, C., Folkman, S., Kahn, R.L., & Syme, S.L. (1994). Socioeconomic status and health: the challenge of the gradient. *American Psychologist*, 49(1),15–24.

Albanna, A.S., & Menzies, D. (2011). Drug-resistant tuberculosis. *Drugs*, 71(7), 815–825. doi:10.2165/11585440-000000000-00000

Anderson, I. (2012). *The Economic Costs of Noncommunicable Diseases in the Pacific Islands*. Final Report, November 2012. Retrieved from http://www.worldbank.org/content/dam/Worldbank/document/the-economic-costs-of-noncommunicable-diseases-in-the-pacific-islands.pdf

Auerbach, J.D., Parkhurst, J.O., & Cáceres, C.F. (2011). Addressing social drivers of HIV/AIDS for the long-term response: conceptual and methodological considerations. *Global Public Health*, 6(Suppl.3), S293-S309. doi:10.1080/17441692.2011.594451

Baker, P., Friel, S., Kay, A., Baum, F., Strazdins, L., & Mackean, T. (2017). What enables and constrains the inclusion of the social determinants of health inequities in government policy agendas? A narrative review. *International Journal of Health Policy and Management*, 7(2), 101–111.

Baker, P., Smith, J., Salmon, L., Friel, S., Kent, G., Iellamo, A., Dadhich, J.P., & Renfrew, M.J. (2016). Global trends and patterns of commercial milk-based formula sales: is an unprecedented infant and young child feeding transition underway? *Public Health Nutrition*, 19(14), 2540–2550.

Baral, S., Beyrer, C., & Poteat, T. (2011). *Human Rights, the Law, and HIV among Transgender People*. Working Paper prepared for the Third Meeting of the Technical Advisory Group of the Global Commission on HIV and the Law, 7–9 July 2011.

Baum, F. (2016). *The New Public Health*. 4th edn. Melbourne: Oxford University Press.

Baum, F., Freeman, T., Lawless, A., Labonte, R., & Sanders, D. (2017). What is the difference between comprehensive and selective primary health care? Evidence from a five-year longitudinal realist case study in South Australia. *BMJ Open*, 7, e015271. doi:10.1136/bmjopen-2016-015271

Bell, J., Taylor, M., Amos, M., & Andrew, N. (2016). *Climate Change and Pacific Island Food Systems*. Copenhagen and Wageningen: CCAFS and CTA.

Benedictow, O.J. (2004). *The Black Death, 1346–1353: The Complete History*. Woodbridge, UK: Boydell & Brewer.

Bhatia, M. (2016). The Indian health care system, 2015. In E. Mossialos, M. Wenzl, R. Osborn & D. Sarnak (Eds), *2015 International Profiles of Health Systems* (pp. 77–85). Washington, DC: The Comonwealth Fund.

Blas, E., Gilson, L., Kelly, M.P., Labonte, R., Lapitan, J., Muntaner, C., et al. (2008). Addressing social determinants of health inequities: what can the state and civil society do? *Lancet*, 372, 1684–1689.

Boerma, T.J., Requejo, J., Victora, C.G., Amouzou, A., George, A., Barroso, C., et al. (2018). Countdown to 2030: tracking progress towards universal health coverage for reproductive, maternal, newborn, and child health. *Lancet*, 391(10129),1538–1548. doi:10.1016/S0140-6736(18)30104-1

Bor, J., Cohen, G.H., & Galea, S. (2017). Population health in an era of rising income inequality: USA, 1980–2015. *Lancet*, 389, 1475–1490.

Breman, J.G., & Brandling-Bennett, A.D. (2011). The challenge of malaria eradication in the twenty-first century: research linked to operations is the key. *Vaccine*, 29, D97–D103. doi:10.1016/j.vaccine.2011.12.003

Bygbjerg, I.C. (2012). Double burden of noncommunicable and infectious diseases in developing countries. *Science*, 337(6101), 1499–1501.

Cox, F.E.G. (2010). History of the discovery of the malaria parasites and their vectors. *Parasites and Vectors*, 3(1), 5.

Crammond, B.R., & Carey, G. (2016). What do we mean by 'structure' when we talk about structural influences on the social determinants of health inequalities? *Social Theory and Health*, 15(1), 84–98.

Crosbie, E., & Thompson, G. (2018). Regulatory chills: tobacco industry legal threats and the politics of tobacco standardised packaging in New Zealand. *New Zealand Medical Journal*, 131(1473), 25–41.

CSDH (Commission on Social Determinants of Health) (2008). *Closing the Gap in a Generation: Health Equity through Action on the Social Determinants of Health.* Final Report of the Commission on Social Determinants of Health. Geneva, World Health Organization.

de Jonge, A. (2017). The evolving nature of the transnational corporation in the 21st century. In A. de Jonge & R. Tomasic (Eds), *Research Handbook on Transnational Corporations* (pp. 9–38). Cheltenham, UK: Edward Elgar.

Dieleman, J.L., Templin, T., Sadat, N., Reidy, P., Chapin, A., Foreman, K. … & Kurowski, C. (2016). National spending on health by source for 184 countries between 2013 and 2040. *Lancet*, 387(10037), 2521–2535. doi:10.1016/S0140-6736(16)30167-2

Donkin, A., Goldblatt, P., Allen, J., Nathanson, V., & Marmot, M. (2018). Global action on the social determinants of health. *BMJ Global Health*, 3, e000603. doi:10.1136/bmjgh-2017-000603

Fernando, S.D., Rodrigo, C., & Rajapakse, S. (2011). Chemoprophylaxis in malaria: drugs, evidence of efficacy and costs. *Asian Pacific Journal of Tropical Medicine*, 4(4), 330–336.

Fidler, D.P. (2010). *The Challenges of Global Health Governance*. New York: Council on Foreign Relations.

Friel, S., Hattersley, L., Ford, L., & O'Rourke, K. (2015). Addressing inequities in healthy eating. *Health Promotion International*, 30(S2), ii77–1188.

Friel, S., Hattersley, L., Snowdon, W., Thow, A.-M., Lobstein, T., Sanders, D., et al. (2013). Monitoring the impacts of trade agreements on food environments. *Obesity Reviews*, 14(Suppl.1), 120–134.

Gleeson, D., & Friel, S. (2013). Emerging threats to public health from regional trade agreements. *Lancet*, 381(9876), 1507–1509.

Global Fund (Global Fund to Fight AIDS, Tuberculosis and Malaria) (2014). *Audit of Global Fund Grants to Myanmar*. Geneva: Global Fund to Fight AIDS, Tuberculosis and Malaria.

Global Fund (Global Fund to Fight AIDS, Tuberculosis and Malaria) (2018). *Myanmar—Country Overview: Grants*. Retrieved from https://www.theglobalfund.org/en/portfolio/country/?loc=MMR&k=b3d59122-9d71-4df9-ae0e-9e4b1b315de8

Glover, L. (2016). The Australian health care system, 2015. In E. Mossialos, M. Wenzl, R. Osborn & D. Sarnak (Eds), *2015 International Profiles of Health Systems* (pp. 11–19). Washington, DC: The Commonwealth Fund.

Gupta, R.K., Lucas, S.B., Fielding, K.L., & Lawn, S.D. (2015). Prevalence of tuberculosis in post-mortem studies of HIV-infected adults and children in resource-limited settings: a systematic review and meta-analysis. *AIDS (London, England)*, 29(15), 1987.

Hawley, N.L., & McGarvey, S.T. (2015). Obesity and diabetes in Pacific Islanders: the current burden and the need for urgent action. *Current Diabetes Reports*, 15, 29. doi:10.1007/s11892-015-0594-5

Hosseinpoor, A.R., Bergen, N., Mendis, S., Harper, S., Verdes, E., Kunsty, A., et al. (2012). Socioeconomic inequality in the prevalence of noncommunicable diseases in low- and middle-income countries: results from the World Health Survey. *BMC Public Health*, 12, 474.

Hou, X., Anderson, I., & Burton-McKenzie, E.-J. (2016). *Pacific Possible: Health and Non-Communicable Diseases.* Background Paper. Washington, DC: World Bank.

Hutchens, G., & Knaus, C. (2018). Revealed: $39m cost of defending Australia's tobacco plain packaging laws. *The Guardian*, 1 July 2018. Retrieved from https://www.theguardian.com/business/2018/jul/02/revealed-39m-cost-of-defending-australias-tobacco-plain-packaging-laws

JDC (Jubilee Debt Campaign UK) (n.d.). *Jubilee Debt Campaign*. Retrieved from https://jubileedebt.org.uk/

Johnson, N.P.A.S., & Mueller, J. (2002). Updating the accounts: global mortality of the 1918–1920 'Spanish' influenza pandemic. *Bulletin of the History of Medicine*, 76(1), 105–115.

Kaplan, D.L., & Graff, K.M. (2008). Marketing breastfeeding: reversing corporate influence on infant feeding practices. *Journal of Urban Health: Bulletin of the New York Academy of Medicine*, 85(4), 486–504.

Kickbusch, I. (2010). Health in All Policies: the evolution of the concept of horizontal health governance. In I. Kickbusch & K. Bucket (Eds), *Implementing Health in All Policies: Adelaide 2010* (pp. 11–23). Adelaide: Department of Health, South Australia.

Kickbusch, I., Allen, K., & Franz, C. (2016). The commercial determinants of health. *Lancet*, 4(12), e895–896.

Kirby Institute (2016). *HIV, Viral Hepatitis and Sexually Transmissible Infections in Australia: Annual Surveillance Report 2016*. Sydney: Kirby Institute, University of New South Wales.

Kirby Institute (2017). *Bloodborne Viral and Sexually Transmissible Infections in Aboriginal and Torres Strait Islander People: Annual Surveillance Report 2017*. Sydney: Kirby Institute, University of New South Wales.

Labonte, R. (2015). Globalization and health. In N. Smelser & P. Baltes (Eds), *International Encyclopedia of the Social and Behavioural Sciences,* 2nd edn, Vol. 10 (pp. 198–205). New York: Elsevier.

Legge, D. (2012). Future of WHO hangs in the balance. *British Medical Journal* 345, e6877. doi:10.1136/bmj.e6877

Legge, D., Gleeson, D., Wilson, G., Wright, M., McBride, T., Butler, P., & Stagoll, O. (2007). Micro–macro integration: reframing primary healthcare practice and community development in health. *Critical Public Health*, 17(2), 171–182.

Lopert, R., & Gleeson, D. (2013). The high price of 'free' trade: US trade agreements and access to medicines. *Journal of Law, Medicine and Ethics*, 41(1), 199–223. doi:10.1111/jlme.12014

Luca, S., & Mihaescu, T. (2013). History of BCG vaccine. *Maedica (Buchar)*, 8(1), 53–58.

Mackenbach, J.P. (2012). The persistence of health inequalities in modern welfare states: the explanation of a paradox. *Social Science and Medicine*, 75, 761–769.

Mackey, T.K., & Liang, B.A. (2012). Rebalancing brain drain: exploring resource allocation to address health worker migration and promote global health. *Health Policy*, 107, 66–73.

MacPherson, E.E., Sadalaki, J., Njoloma, M., Nyongopa, V., Nkhwazi, L., Mwapasa, V. … & Theobald, S. (2012). Transactional sex and HIV: understanding the gendered structural drivers of HIV in fishing communities in southern Malawi. *Journal of the International AIDS Society*, 15(Suppl.1), 1–9.

Mbonye, M., Nalukenge, W., Nakamanya, S., Nalusiba, B., King, R., Vandepitte, J., & Seeley, J. (2012). Gender inequity in the lives of women involved in sex work in Kampala, Uganda. *Journal of the International AIDS Society*, 15(Suppl.1). doi:10.7448/IAS.15.3.17365

Mills, A. (2014). Health care systems in low- and middle-income countries. *New England Journal of Medicine*, 370, 552–557. doi:10.1056/NEJMra1110897

Moodie, R., Stuckler, D., Monteiro, C., Sheron, N., Neal, B., Thamarangsi, T., et al. (2013). Profits and pandemics: prevention of harmful effects of tobacco, alcohol, and ultra-processed food and drink industries. *Lancet*, 381, 670–679.

Mu, T.T., Sein, A.A., Kyi, T.T., Min, M., Aung, N.M., Anstey, N.M. … & Hanson, J. (2016). Malaria incidence in Myanmar 2005–2014: steady but fragile progress towards elimination. *Malaria Journal*, 15, 503. doi:10.1186/s12936-016-1567-0

Musso, D., Roche, C., Robin, E., Nhan, T., Teissier, A., & Cao-Lormeau, V.-M. (2015). Potential sexual transmission of Zika virus. *Emerging Infectious Diseases*, 21(2), 359.

Newby, G., Bennett, A., Larson, E., Cotter, C., Shretta, R., Phillips, A.A., & Feachem, R.G.A. (2016). The path to eradication: a progress report on the malaria-eliminating countries. *Lancet*, 387(10029), 1775–1784. doi:10.1016/S0140-6736(16)00230-0

Ng, M., Freeman, M.K., Fleming, T.D., Robinson, M., Dwyer-Lindgren, L., Thomson, B. et al. (2014). Smoking prevalence and cigarette consumption in 187 countries,

1980–2012. *Journal of the American Medical Association*, 311(2), 183–192. doi:10.1001/jama.2013.284692

Niessen, L.W., Mohan, D., Akuoku, J.K., Mirelman, A.J., Ahmed, S., Koehlmoos, T.P., Trujillo, A., Khan, J., & Peters, D.H. (2018). Tackling socioeconomic inequalities and non-communicable diseases in low-income and middle-income countries under the Sustainable Development Agenda. *Lancet*, 391(10134), 2036–2046. doi:10.1016/S0140-6736(18)30482-3

NMCP (National Malaria Control Programme) (2017). *National Plan for Malaria Elimination in Myanmar 2016–2030*. Yangon, Myanmar: Ministry of Health and Sports Myanmar.

Nugent, R., Bertram, M.Y., Jan, S., Niessen, L.W., Sassi, F., Jamison, D.T., Pier, E.G., & Beaglehole, R. (2018). Investing in non-communicable disease prevention and management to advance the Sustainable Development Goals. *Lancet*, 391(10134), 2029–2035. doi:10.1016/S0140-6736(18)30482-3

OECD (Organisation for Economic Co-operation and Development) (2018). *Development Aid Stable in 2017 with more sent to Poorest Countries.* Retrieved from http://www.oecd.org/development/development-aid-stable-in-2017-with-more-sent-to-poorest-countries.htm

Otterson, O.P., Dasgupta, J., Blouin, C., Buss, P., Chongsuvivatwong, V., Frenk, J. et al. (2014). The Lancet-University of Oslo Commission on Global Governance for Health: the political origins of health inequity: prospects for change. *Lancet*, 383, 630–667.

PHM (People's Health Movement) (n.d.). *People's Health Movement.* Retrieved from http://www.phmovement.org/en

Piwoz, E.G., & Huffman, S.L. (2015). The impact of marketing of breast-milk substitutes on WHO-recommended breastfeeding practices. *Food and Nutrition Bulletin*, 36(4) 373–386.

RBM (Roll Back Malaria) (2015). *RBM Action and Investment to Defeat Malaria 2016–2030*. Retrieved from https://rollbackmalaria.com/

Rottingen, J.-A., Regmi, S., Eide, M., Young, A.J., Viergever, R.F., Ardal, C., et al. (2013). Mapping of available health research and development data: what's there, what's missing, and what role is there for a global observatory? *Lancet*, 382(9900), 1286–1307.

Schrecker, T., Labonte, R., & De Vogli, R. (2008). Globalisation and health: the need for a global vision. *Lancet*, 372, 1670–1676.

Seeley, J., Watts, C.H., Kippax, S., Russell, S., Heise, L., & Whiteside, A. (2012). Addressing the structural drivers of HIV: a luxury or necessity for programmes? *Journal of the International AIDS Society*, 15(Suppl.1), 17397. doi:10.7448/IAS.15.3.17397

Shito, M., Ollila, E., & Koivusalo, M. (2006). Principles and challenges of Health in All Policies. In T. Stahl, M. Wismar, E. Ollila, E. Lahtinen & K. Leppo (Eds), *Health in All Policies: Prospects and Potentials* (pp. 3–20). Helsinki: Ministry of Social Affairs and Health & European Observatory on Health Systems and Policies.

Smith, J., & Blake, M. (2013). Infant food marketing strategies undermine effective regulation of breast-milk substitutes: trends in print advertising in Australia, 1950–2010. *Australian and New Zealand Journal of Public Health*, 37, 337–344. doi:10.1111/1753-6405.12081

Smith, J., Galtry, J., & Salmon, L. (2014). Confronting the formula feeding epidemic in a new era of trade and investment liberalisation. *Journal of Australian Political Economy*, 73, 132–171.

Smith, R., Rossetto, K., & Peterson, B.L. (2008). A meta-analysis of disclosure of one's HIV-positive status, stigma and social support. *AIDS Care*, 20(10), 1266–1275. doi:10.1080/09540120801926977

Solar, O., & Irwin, A. (2010). *A Conceptual Framework for Action on the Social Determinants of Health.* Social Determinants of Health Discussion Paper 2 (Policy and Practice). Geneva: World Health Organization.

Sreevatsan, S., Pan, X.I., Stockbauer, K.E., Connell, N.D., Kreiswirth, B.N., Whittam, T.S., & Musser, J.M. (1997). Restricted structural gene polymorphism in the Mycobacterium tuberculosis complex indicates evolutionarily recent global dissemination. *Proceedings of the National Academy of Sciences*, 94(18), 9869–9874.

Stangl, A.L., Lloyd, J.K., Brady, L.M., Holland, C.E., & Baral, S. (2013). A systematic review of interventions to reduce HIV-related stigma and discrimination from 2002 to 2013: how far have we come? *Journal of the International AIDS Society*, 16(3Suppl.2).

Stuckler, D., & Basu, S. (2009). The International Monetary Fund's effects on global health: before and after the 2008 financial crisis. *International Journal of Health Services*, 39(4), 771–781.

Tang, L., Binns, C.W., & Lee, A.H. (2015). Infant formula crisis in China: a cohort study in Sichuan province. *Journal of Health, Population and Nutrition*, 33(1), 117–122.

Taylor, A.L., Hwenda, L., Larsen, B., & Daulaire, N. (2011). Stemming the brain drain: a WHO global code of practice on international recruitment of health personnel. *New England Journal of Medicine*, 365(25), 2348–2351.

Thow, A.M., Swinburn, B., Colagiuri, S., Diligolevu, M., Quested, C., Vivili, P. et al. (2010). Trade and food policy: case studies from three Pacific Island countries. *Food Policy*, 35, 556–564.

Thow, A.-M., & Snowdon, W. (2010). The effect of trade and trade policy on diet and health in the Pacific Islands. In C. Hawkes, C. Blouin, S. Henson, N. Drager & L. Dube (Eds), *Trade, Food, Diet, and Health: Perspectives and Policy Options* (pp. 147–168). Chichester, UK: Blackwell.

UN (2016). *Report of the United Nations Secretary-General's High Level Panel on Access to Medicines: Promoting Innovation and Access to Health Technologies.* Retrieved from http://www.unsgaccessmeds.org/final-report/

UN (n.d.). *Sustainable Development Goals.* Retrieved from http://www.un.org/sustainabledevelopment/sustainable-development-goals/

UNAIDS (Joint United Nations Programme on HIV/AIDS) (2017). *Ending AIDS: Progress towards the 90-90-90 Targets Global AIDS Update.* Geneva.

UNDP HIV & AIDS Group (2012). *Global Commission on HIV and the Law: Risk, Rights and Health.* New York: UNDP.

Victora, C.G., Bahl, R., Barros, A.J., Franca, G.V.A, Horton, S., Krasevec, J., Much, S., Sankar, M.J., Walker, N., & Rollins N.C. (2016). Breastfeeding in the 21st century: epidemiology, mechanisms, and lifelong effect. *Lancet*, 387, 475–490.

WHO (World Health Organization) (2004). *WHO Medicines Strategy: Countries at the Core 2004–2007*. Geneva: World Health Organization.

WHO (World Health Organization) (2006). *The World Health Report 2006: Working Together for Health.* Geneva: World Health Organization.

WHO (World Health Organization) (2010). *Health Systems Financing: The Path to Universal Coverage. World Health Report 2010.* Geneva: World Health Organization.

WHO (World Health Organization) (2011). *Global Status Report on Noncommunicable Diseases 2010*. Geneva: World Health Organization.

WHO (World Health Organization) (2014). *WHO: Ebola Response Roadmap Situation Report, 24 December 2014*. Geneva: World Health Organization.

WHO (World Health Organization) (2015). *Global Tuberculosis Report 2015*, 20th ed. Geneva: World Health Organization. Retrieved from http://www.who.int/iris/handle/10665/191102

WHO (World Health Organization) (2016a). Malaria vaccine. WHO position paper, January 2016. *WHO Weekly Epidemiological Record*, 4, 33–52.

WHO (World Health Organization) (2016b). *Global Technical Strategy for Malaria 2016–2030*. Geneva: World Health Organization.

WHO (World Health Organization) (2017a). *World Health Statistics 2017: Monitoring HEALTH for the SDGs*. Geneva: World Health Organization.

WHO (World Health Organization) (2017b). *Global Tuberculosis Report 2017*. Geneva: World Health Organization.

WHO (World Health Organization) (2017c). *World Malaria Report 2017*. Geneva: World Health Organization.

WHO (World Health Organization) (2017d). *Noncommunicable Diseases Progress Monitor 2015*. Geneva: World Health Organization.

WHO (World Health Organization) (2017e). *WHO Report on the Global Tobacco Epidemic, 2017: Country Profile—Papua New Guinea*. Retrieved from http://www.who.int/tobacco/surveillance/policy/country_profile/png.pdf?ua=1

WHO (World Health Organization) (2018a). *Help Prevent Malaria*. WHO Myanmar Newsletter Special. Yangon: World Health Organization.

WHO (World Health Organization) (2018b). *Tobacco.* Fact Sheet. Retrieved from http://www.who.int/mediacentre/factsheets/fs339/en/

WHO (World Health Organization) & UNICEF (2003). *Global Strategy for Infant and Young Child Feeding.* Geneva: World Health Organization.

WHO (World Health Organization), UNICEF & IBFAN (2016). *Marketing of Breastmilk Substitutes: National Implementation of the International Code.* Status Report 2016. Geneva: World Health Organization.

WHO (World Health Organization) & World Bank (2015). *Tracking Universal Health Coverage: First Global Monitoring Report.* Retrieved from http://www.who.int/healthinfo/universal_health_coverage/report/2015/en/

WHO (World Health Organization) & World Bank (2017). *Tracking Universal Health Coverage: 2017 Global Monitoring Report*. Retrieved from http://www.who.int/healthinfo/universal_health_coverage/report/2017/en/

Glossary

Agency
The capacity and power of individuals to influence their own lives and shape their society.

Anthropocene
The current geological age during which the combined influence of one species—*Homo sapiens*—has acted with sufficient power and scale to change the Earth system, now viewed as the dominant influence on climate and the environment.

Australia's First Peoples
The preferred term for referring to Aboriginal peoples. It is the collective term for the sovereign peoples of mainland Australia and Tasmania, as well as Torres Strait Islander peoples, the sovereign peoples of the islands between Cape York and Papua New Guinea.

Behavioural determinants
Personal attributes or behaviours that influences an individual's risk of experiencing poor health.

Biological determinants
The inner physiological aspect of health and disease. Genes play a crucial role in underlying biological differences between individuals.

Biological model
The traditional western mode of medicine, which understands disease and illness to be caused by external pathogens or disorders of organs and body systems.

Biological sex
The biologic character or quality that distinguishes male and female from one another as expressed by the person's gonadal, morphologic (internal and external), chromosomal and hormonal characteristics.

Biopsychosocial model
A model which posits that ill health and disease are created through interactions between a person's biological, psychological and social factors.

Catastrophic (healthcare) payments
The situation where healthcare costs are so high that a family or individual has to go without other basic goods such as food, or go into debt.

Climate change
A change in the state of the climate, identified via statistical tests as changes in the mean and/or the variability of its properties that persist for an extended period, typically decades or longer.

Cohort
A group who share the same experiences, in the same time, in the same sequence.

Community engagement
The sustained process of creating meaningful relationships and developing empowering strategies with community members to participate in decision-making, developmental actions and services that affect their lives, in order to create positive change. It includes the monitoring and evaluation of outcomes.

Comprehensive primary healthcare
A multi-disciplinary model of healthcare that includes community involvement, multi-sectoral collaboration, prevention and action on the social determinants of health.

Continuity of care
Access to the same healthcare team over a period of time so that the care plan is coordinated.

Critical reflection
The practice and process of developing awareness about oneself, examining experiences, ideologies, identity, social location, biases, motivations, contradictions and assumptions that might overtly or unconsciously influence behaviours, actions and ways of relating to and engaging with others.

Cultural awareness
An awareness of the impacts of cultural differences on people's actions and healthcare-seeking. It involves awareness of one's own cultural values and the influences of those values on one's conduct.

Cultural competence
Cultural competence involves the ability of healthcare providers and organisations to recognise and respond competently to the cultural and linguistic needs of patients. It requires cultural knowledge and self-awareness.

Cultural idiom of distress
A means for individuals to express their distress within the socio-cultural setting. It is often used as a culturally sanctioned way for an individual to express dissatisfaction with their position or role at a particular time.

Cultural relativism
Understanding other people's behaviour in relation to their culture and the rationale or meaningful context in which that behaviour occurs.

Cultural sensitivity
A capability to build relationships with individuals from different cultures through culturally appropriate conduct and care. It involves recognition of cultural differences and the ability to accommodate them appropriately.

Culture
A system of shared ideas, attitudes and practices that defines the social system of its members. It is a way of life that is shared by group members.

Culture-bound syndrome
A set of symptoms specific to a particular culture and generally not recognised by biomedicine.

Demand
Relationship between the price of a good or service and the amount of that good or service people are willing to buy at that price.

Determinants of health
A range of individual, social, economic, environmental and cultural conditions that have the potential to contribute to or detract from the health of individuals, communities or whole populations.

Deviance
Behaviour which transgresses social expectations and is likely to attract sanctions from other members of a society.

Difference
When an individual possesses characteristics which are dissimilar to, or behaves differently from, the majority of people within a society.

Discrimination
The idea that someone is of less value and should be excluded from social networks and the benefits of society.

Disease
A condition adversely affecting health that has measurable (clinical) symptoms.

Ecological model
A model which understands health and well-being (not merely the absence of disease) to be shaped by human biology, personal behaviour, and psychosocial and physical environments. More recent updates (i.e. socio-ecological models) have added political and economic factors.

Economic welfare
The capacity to make choices due to economic stability at both an individual and societal level—the better your economic welfare, the more choices available to you.

Economics
The study of the choices made in relation to the production, consumption and distribution of goods and services in a scenario of scarcity.

Ecosystem services
The benefits provided by ecosystems that contribute to making human life both possible and worth living. Examples include products such as food and clean water, regulation of the carbon cycle, floods, soil erosion or disease outbreaks, and non-material benefits such as psychological, spiritual and recreational benefits.

Emic
An insider perspective of individuals within a culture.

Entertainment-education
A mass media vehicle which is designed to entertain a wide general audience while changing societal attitudes and norms. It models and normalises behaviour change that promotes health and social development.

Environmental determinants of health
All external factors and conditions that affect people's lives and health. From a health perspective, the definition adopts a more restricted meaning of the chemical, biological and physical agents that impinge on health. Examples include pollution of the air, water or land, exposure to hazards such as noise, vibrations, heat or chemicals, as well as global hazards such as stratospheric ozone depletion and climate change.

Ethnicity
A shared cultural background which is a characteristic of a group within a society.

Ethnocentrism
A profound sense of cultural superiority, which leads to a lack of appreciation of cultural differences and damages relationships with other individuals/groups.

Ethnomedicine
Healing practices commonly observed by members of a culture.

Evaluation
The structured process of assessing the success of a project in meeting its goals, and reflecting on lessons learned.

Explanatory model of illness
The perspective on the nature of illness concerns of an individual and healthcare providers, including its causes and the appropriate health-seeking strategy.

Folk healing
Cultural healing practices and practitioners prevalent in most traditional cultures, generally not part of the professional medical system.

Gender
Socially and culturally constructed categories reflecting what it means to be 'masculine' and 'feminine', and associated expectations of roles and behaviours of men and women.

Gender-based health inequality
The difference in health outcomes between genders.

Globalisation
The global integration of economic arrangements and the increasingly fluid movement of people, ideas, technology, goods and services across national borders.

Health access
Access to primary healthcare for all people, independent of income. This means that individuals should have the opportunity or right to receive affordable, timely and appropriate healthcare in a manner that promotes optimum health.

Health equity
Providing everyone with the resources they individually need to enjoy full and healthy lives. It differs from equality, which provides the same resources to everyone regardless of need.

Health in All Policies
HiAP is a cross-sectoral approach to addressing the social determinants of health.

Health inequality
'Health differences' which are closely connected with social disadvantage and advantage.

Health insurance
A publicly or privately organised risk management scheme that provides protection from financial loss associated with purchasing healthcare.

Health literacy
An individual's ability to successfully seek, identify, interpret and act on health information so as to protect and improve their health.

Health promotion
The process of enabling people to increase control over and to improve their health.

Health
There is no definite meaning of health. Its meaning can be different depending on individuals, social groups and cultures, and can differ at different times. The WHO defines health as 'a state of complete physical, mental and social well-being and not merely the absence of disease or infirmity'.

HIV/AIDS
HIV (Human Immunodeficiency Virus)/AIDS (Acquired Immunodeficiency Syndrome) is a blood-borne virus which emerged in the 1980s in North America and has since spread globally. It is a particularly prominent issue in sub-Saharan Africa. HIV causes the development of AIDS, which marks a certain point of depletion in the immune system and is fatal if left untreated.

Human agency
Our ability to negotiate the social structures and a way to account for individual differences in the life course.

Human rights
An internationally agreed set of principles and standards by which to assess and redress inequality, and to advocate for, and even enforce, a fairer distribution of resources in the world.

Human rights-based approaches
Frameworks for action that are based on international human rights standards and are operationally focused on promoting and protecting human rights through principles of participation, accountability, non-discrimination, empowerment and legality.

Illness
A condition adversely affecting health as perceived by the individual in question.

Individual determinants
The individual characteristics and behaviours of a person. These play an important role in influencing the health outcomes of individuals..

Inequities in health
Unfair and avoidable differences in health status (between regions, countries or population groups).

Infectious diseases
Infections caused by micro-organisms such as bacteria, viruses, fungi and microparasites. Many infectious diseases are transmissible from person to person either directly or indirectly. Common communicable diseases include influenza, measles, sexually transmitted infections and malaria.

Intersectoral collaboration
Collaborative actions between government agencies and/or all levels of government on 'health or health equity outcomes or on the determinants of health or health equity' (OECD et al. 2008, p. 21).

Labelling theory
The process of labelling a person with stigma. Through the process of social interaction, this eventually leads the person to change their self-perception and lose social opportunity.

LGBTIQ
An abbreviation for those who identify as lesbian, gay, bisexual, transgender, intersex and/or queer.

Life and historical times
A way of accounting for cohort effects and how they affect the individual now and in the future.

Life course perspective
The cumulative effects of events from earlier life on later life.

Life event
Abrupt and sudden change in life resulting in significant change in trajectory and stress.

Linked lives
The interdependence with others in our social networks and relationships and how these affect our life course.

Logic model
A graphical or narrative representation of the health promotion process and how it is supposed to work by identifying strategies and desired outcomes.

Market-based model
A system where access to education, health and housing must be paid for by the individual, and those who are sick or incapacitated must provide for their own income protection.

Marketing

The strategies used by commercial or non-profit enterprises—including the use of persuasive media communications such as advertising—that aim to change attitudes so that the consumer feels positive towards, and decides to buy or use, the advertised product or service.

Mass media

The means by which messages are communicated throughout a society, transmitting the same message to large numbers of people over a large geographical area at the same time, for example via television, cinema, radio, the internet, social media, newspapers and magazines.

Media advocacy

Using mass media to stimulate public support and obtain the attention and sympathy of policy-makers and legislators, in order to gain changes in law and policy which have a positive impact on public health.

Mediating factors

Factors which explain the relationship between two other factors or variables (events).

Moral career

A process when a stigmatised individual initially makes sense of the social position of him/herself within the society and later acquires a set idea of what it would be like to hold a specific characteristic.

Multi-level empowerment

Empowerment is commonly understood as an enhanced sense of 'control of destiny' with respect to forces that affect an individual's daily life. Multi-level empowerment is the potential for and process of positive change at individual, family, community, services, system and environmental levels. Changes occur at these separate levels, and are interconnected and interactive.

Needs analysis

A process to assess the health status and needs of individuals, populations and communities.

Non-communicable diseases

NCDs are cardiovascular diseases (e.g. heart attack and stroke), diabetes, cancers and chronic respiratory diseases such as chronic obstructive pulmonary disease and asthma. These diseases, which are not transmitted from one person to another, account for the majority of deaths globally and share a common set of behavioural risk factors (tobacco consumption, poor nutrition, physical inactivity and harmful use of alcohol).

Planetary Boundary Framework

Considers planetary resources and defines a safe operating space for humanity, to map how far humanity has progressed towards irreparably damaging key aspects of Earth's biophysical processes and ecosystems.

Planetary health
The achievement of the highest attainable standard of health, well-being and equity worldwide through judicious attention to the human systems—political, economic and social—that shape the future of humanity and the Earth's natural systems that define the safe environmental limits within which humanity can flourish.

Precautionary Principle
The principle originated as a tool to bridge uncertain scientific information and a political responsibility to act to prevent damage to human health and to ecosystems.

Primary healthcare
Essential healthcare that is accessible to all.

Public health communication
A variety of carefully developed communication strategies aimed at improving or maintaining the health of a population.

Public policy
Policies brought in by governments to administer education, healthcare, water, sanitation, same-sex marriage and so on.

Quintile
A quintile represents 20 per cent (a fifth) of the population. The lowest quintile is the poorest group; the highest group is the wealthiest.

Religion
An organised system of beliefs, practices and rituals that have gradually developed within established traditions. It connects to health and well-being at myriad levels.

Role substitution
The process whereby one profession takes up the role and skills of another.

Scarcity
Limited availability of good and services.

Self-determination
Self-determination became a legal right for all peoples in 1960. Decades later the collective rights of Indigenous peoples to self-determination were articulated in Article 3 of the UN Declaration on the Rights of Indigenous Peoples, which stated 'Indigenous peoples have the right to self-determination. By virtue of that right they freely determine their political status and freely pursue their economic, social and cultural development'.

Semiotics
The study of the meaning of signs and symbols (e.g. images and colours) within a particular culture, how they communicate specific information and influence the interpretation of messages.

Separation rates
The percentage of people who leave hospital before midnight on any one day, whether through being discharged, transferred to another facility, or dying.

Sex
A biological construct based on biological characteristics that enable sexual reproduction.

Sexual diversity
All the diversities of sex characteristics, sexual orientations and gender identities, without the need to specify each of the identities, behaviours or characteristics that form this plurality.

Sexual inequality
Unequal treatment or perceptions of individuals wholly or partly due to their gender or sexuality. It arises from perceived differences in societally prescribed gender roles and sexual norms. Socio-cultural gender and sexuality systems are often dichotomous, hierarchical and detrimental to the functioning of men, women and gender-diverse individuals.

Sexuality
The means by which people experience and express themselves as sexual beings. Human sexuality is characterised by the interaction between biological, physical, psychological, societal and cultural aspects, to name a few key factors.

Sickness
The term is often used interchangeably with disease and illness; sometimes it refers to both. Sickness embodies a sociological meaning and is related to the concept of the 'sick role' theorised by Talcott Parsons.

Social class
The position of a person in a system of structured inequality; it is grounded in unequal distribution of income, wealth, status and power.

Social determinants of health
A range of individual, social, economic, environmental and cultural conditions that have the potential to contribute to or detract from the health of individuals, communities or whole populations.

Social exclusion
The exclusion of individuals from social networks and resources because of their different and stigmatised statuses.

Social gradient in health
Differences in social status that lead to different health outcomes. Individuals who are lower in the social hierarchy tend to have worse health outcomes than those located at higher social levels.

Social justice
Systemic and structural social arrangements that improve equality. They include the fair distribution of resources, equal access to opportunities and rights, and protection of the marginalised and vulnerable.

Social marketing
The application of commercial marketing techniques (including media communications) to the promotion of health and other socially desirable outcomes.

Social mobility
The movement of individuals or groups (e.g. families, social groups) within or between the social strata; or a relative change in an individual's or group's social status.

Social model of health
A model which focuses on the social forces which influence health and well-being.

Social norms
Rules or standards which guide or constrain individuals' actions or behaviour.

Social protection
Factors which protect an individual or group from further disadvantage. It can include government policies aimed to reduce poverty.

Social support
Social support is widely acknowledged as a determinant of health, and as having direct health-giving effects. It is an individual's sense that their needs may be met with assistance and reinforcement from others, whether in practical, instrumental or emotional ways.

Socio-ecological model
A model that conceptualises influences on health in nested layers expanding out from the individual. These layers are seen to influence each other, and in turn shape an individual's health.

Stigma
An attribute or characteristic that separates people from one another. It is used by individuals to interpret specific attributes of others as 'discreditable' or 'unworthy', which results in the stigmatised person becoming devalued.

Stigmatisation
The process of stigmatising a person.

Strengths-based approach
A commitment to actively identifying strengths of an individual, family, community and/or service, as well as assets and available resources, to build and invest in these, respecting and taking into account but choosing not to focus on or reinforce deficits, gaps, negatives or needs.

Structural determinants of health
Factors embedded in the way society operates, including policies and institutions, and economic and political factors, which are beyond the control of individuals.

Structural disadvantage
The disadvantage experienced by some individuals, families, groups or communities because of the way society functions. These disadvantages are systematically rooted in the normal operations of dominant social institutions such

as markets, militaries, employment systems, social networks, health and education and taxation systems. They impact how resources are distributed, how people relate to each other, who has power, who makes decisions and how institutions are organised.

Structure–agency debate
The debate on how much people's decisions are shaped by social institutions and culture compared to their individual will (agency).

Supply
The relationship between price of a good or service and the quantity the suppliers are willing to supply.

Sustainability
The process of living within the limits of available physical, natural and social resources in ways that allow the living systems to thrive in perpetuity.

Sustainable Development Goals
A set of 17 development goals agreed between UN member states in 2015 to address the global challenges of poverty, inequalities and climate change.

Symbolic healing
A healing method that involves the use of religious beliefs to arouse the healing response of an individual.

Timing of lives
Accounts for the age-graded perspective of social markers, roles and events.

Trajectory
A stable path towards a life destination.

Transition
Moving from one life stage to another, or from one life event to another.

Transnational corporations
TNCs are companies that have their headquarters in one country but operate through subsidiaries in one or more other countries, thus crossing national boundaries.

Turning point
A crucial point in time that leads to significant change of direction.

Universal health coverage
All people and communities can use the promotive, preventative, curative, rehabilitative and palliative health services they need, of sufficient quality to be effective, and the use of these services does not expose the user to financial hardship.

Vertical integration
A company provides access to services from other companies within its premises or organisation, for example radiology and pathology services are provided in the same complex as a GP service.

Vulnerable and marginalised people
Distanced from economic, political and social power and resources, because they are perceived as undesirable or without function. This distancing works to exclude marginalised people from systems of protection and integration, increasing their susceptibility to adverse circumstances and harm.

Welfare state
Provision by government of social services such as education, healthcare, old-age pensions. Often free, or co-payments or means tested and funded through taxation.

Well-being
A positive conceptualisation of health: feeling healthy, happy or doing well in life. It can be completely separated from the objectively measured health or disease status of an individual.

Index